Atlas of
GYNECOLOGIC
SURGERY

*Dr. Raymond A. Lee (left) conferring with
Mr. John Hagen (right), the medical illustrator,
about one of the many drawings in this book.*

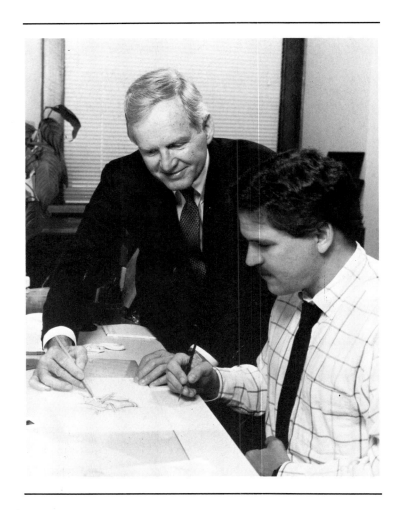

Atlas of
GYNECOLOGIC SURGERY

Raymond A. Lee, M.D.
Chair, Division of Gynecologic Surgery, and
Consultant, Departments of Obstetrics and
  Gynecology and of Surgery
Mayo Clinic and Mayo Foundation
Professor of Obstetrics and Gynecology
Mayo Medical School
Rochester, Minnesota

Illustrated by
John V. Hagen, M.S., A.M.I.

W. B. SAUNDERS COMPANY
Harcourt Brace Jovanovich, Inc.
Philadelphia   London   Toronto   Montreal   Sydney   Tokyo

W. B. SAUNDERS COMPANY
Harcourt Brace Jovanovich, Inc.

The Curtis Center
Independence Square West
Philadelphia, Pennsylvania 19106

Library of Congress Cataloging-in-Publication Data

Lee, Raymond A.

Atlas of gynecologic surgery / Raymond A. Lee; illustrated by
John V. Hagen.

     p.   cm.

ISBN 0–7216–3358–7

   1. Generative organs, Female—Surgery—Atlases.   I. Title.
[DNLM: 1. Genitalia, Female—surgery—atlases.   WP 17 L479a]
RG104.L42   1992

618.1'059—dc20

DNLM/DLC   91–35157

Editor: W. B. Saunders Staff

Designer: Karen O'Keefe

Cover Designer: Joanne Carroll-Suarez

Production Manager: Ken Neimeister

Manuscript Editor: Arlene Friday

Illustration Specialist: Brett MacNaughton

Page Layout Artist: Dorothy Chattin

Indexer: Kathy Garcia

ATLAS OF GYNECOLOGIC SURGERY   ISBN 0–7216–3358–7

Printed in the United States of America.

Last digit is the print number: 9   8   7   6   5   4   3   2   1

*This atlas is dedicated to the patients
for whom it is our privilege to care.*

Preface

Dr. William Worrall Mayo was a general practitioner, as were all physicians in the 1800s, but the sense of accomplishment he received from a successful surgical procedure was especially rewarding. Because of the dangers of infection, surgical practice at that time consisted mainly of repairs of injury to the body surface or extremities. Because of the relative lack of understanding of disorders that affected women and the practice of crude midwifery, diseases in women made up a large share of every physician's practice.

In 1800, it is recorded that Dr. W. W. Mayo was asked to see a young woman with an ovarian tumor that was causing abdominal swelling sufficient to interfere with her ability to eat. Facing certain death, she gave her consent for operation. The patient's husband was a blacksmith and, following specific instructions given by Dr. Mayo, forged some instruments (clamps fitted with hooks made from the teeth of an old mowing machine) necessary for the operation. With the patient under chloroform anesthesia, Dr. Mayo proceeded with the operation, assisted by Mrs. Mayo, the city veterinarian, and another local physician. Young William James and Charles Horace Mayo, his sons, were there too, "peeking through the door" (Will, aged 19, would enter medical school later that year). Dr. Mayo plunged a trocar into the tumor and drained its contents into a tub. He applied the homemade clamps, which had been heating in a charcoal furnace such as solderers used, and proceeded to deliver the tumor, bit by bit, through the incision. The entire tumor weighed some 20 pounds. The operation took nearly an hour, but the patient rallied and was a favorite topic of conversation for some weeks.

Accustomed to helping their father in any way they could, Will and Charlie naturally grew into assisting him at operations. On an earlier occasion, while Dr. W. W. Mayo was doing an operation, the physician giving the anesthetic fainted. Rapidly, Dr. W. W. Mayo moved a cracker box over to the end of the table and instructed young Charlie (possibly 10 or 11 years of age) up onto the stand, and Charlie proceeded to administer the anesthetic. Will Mayo later recounted that "he did it well, with perfect composure." Charlie added a few details: "When she stopped wiggling, Father would tell me to stop; and when she started again, I would drop some more."

There was never any question about the choice of career for the Mayo brothers. Will said, "It never occurred to us that we could be anything but doctors." After graduation from the University of Michigan School of Medicine (Alpha Omega Alpha honor society), Will Mayo (aged 22) returned to Rochester in June 1883, in his words, "to become the greatest surgeon in the world." In August 1883, a tornado struck Rochester, resulting in death and destruction throughout the small community. During the recovery, Mother Alfred Moes, Mother Superior of the Sisters of Saint Francis, a Catholic charitable order, initiated a plan to build a hospital, which was opened in October 1889.

With the advent of anesthesia and aseptic techniques, the science of medicine made tremendous advances. Surgery became accepted as a safe form of treatment, and the Mayo brothers particularly benefited. Like all doctors, the Mayos were initially "physicians and surgeons" and handled their share of the community's childbirths, kidney troubles, typhoid fever, and dreaded diphtheria. But it was surgery that they preferred; as their name and reputation grew, their surgical practice increased. In 1886, W. J. Mayo, with his father, reported several "interesting" cases in the *Minnesota State Medical Society Journal.* They reviewed their experience with catgut suture, drainage tubes, strangulated hernia, colostomy, and compound skull fracture. Drs. Will and Charlie shared their work equally, but gradually they developed their own particular interests and skills.

Dr. Will found that more and more of his time was occupied with pelvic and abdominal operations, whereas Dr. Charlie took over the work on the eye, ear, nose, throat, bones, joints, brain, nerves, and neck. Dr. Will always maintained that this division of labor was the result of Charlie's superiority as a surgeon. "I was driven to cover by a better surgeon," he said; "Charlie drove me down and down until I reached the belly." The surgical practice continued, and the number of abdominal operations at St. Marys Hospital steadily increased from 612 in 1900 to 4000 in 1905. By this time, the Mayos had chosen partners and assistants who helped them concentrate on the surgical side of their practice. Drs. Augustus Stinchfield and Christopher Graham were general diagnosticians who helped screen patients so that the Mayos kept the surgical practice entirely in their own hands.

Dr. Henry S. Plummer originated the idea, and the Mayos agreed with it, that there were specific advantages to specialization in medicine that could be accomplished and dangers avoided only if the group of specialists functioned as a single unit in relation to the patient. The first additions to the surgical staff were trained directly by the brothers, who insisted that surgeons would do all types of surgical procedures, although they could have "special areas of interest."

Dr. James C. Masson was offered the position of Head of a Section of General Surgery in 1915 and quickly became recognized as a very versatile general surgeon with a major interest in urology and gynecology. He later was to develop the Masson fascial stripper and a self-retaining retractor. He went on to describe the techniques of repair of genitourinary fistula. In the 1920s, he described the use of skin grafts and the sigmoid colon for treatment of agenesis of the vagina. He later reviewed the techniques of operative correction of posthysterectomy vaginal vault prolapse, emphasizing that there was "no routine repair, but each needed to be repaired on an individual basis."

Dr. Virgil S. Counseller, a general surgeon, became Head of a Section of General Surgery in 1928; his major interest was in urologic and gynecologic surgery. He developed an international reputation as a skilled, decisive, innovative surgeon. He had wide areas of interest, addressing topics such as stress incontinence, radical hysterectomy for carcinoma of the cervix, and surgical repair of agenesis of the vagina and uterine prolapse.

Dr. Joseph H. Pratt became Head of a Section of General Surgery in 1945. He was an extremely talented and versatile surgeon with remarkable enthusiasm and stamina. His long daily surgical list of gynecologic operations would overwhelm a lesser surgeon. He was particularly known for his ability to operate with equal facility in reconstructive procedures for congenital anomalies and radical operations for malignancy. He was at his best when the surgical condition was the most difficult. In 1958, he was designated the first Chairman of the Division of Gynecologic Surgery in the Department of General Surgery.

Dr. Richard E. Symmonds was the first Mayo Clinic surgeon to do gynecologic procedures who actually initiated his training in obstetrics and gynecology. He completed additional training in general surgery and became Head of a Section of General Surgery in 1956, doing the broad spectrum of general surgical procedures with a special interest in gynecologic surgery. This naturally gifted surgeon (a talent possibly enhanced by his father who, as a general practitioner, taught him how to skin squirrels and rabbits) was known for his practical, sound judgment, his extensive experience, and, most of all, his superb surgical ability. His resolve in his desire to be "the best at what he did" resulted in many successful operations that others thought were impossible and in long-term survival or cures in many patients with malignancy who were thought by some to have unresectable lesions. The author had the privilege of being Dr. Symmonds' colleague (but always as a collegian) for 18 years until his retirement in 1983. Most of the ideas and material in this book are the result of our years of discussion of particular patients or surgical dilemmas that we encountered in individual practice at the Mayo Clinic.

The gynecologic surgical procedures reviewed in this atlas are performed by six surgeons in the Section of Gynecologic Surgery; all have additional and specific training in general surgery. We have joint appointments in the Departments of Surgery and of Obstetrics and Gynecology. Thus, the operative procedures described are the "distillation" of several generations of Mayo surgeons; each is a well-planned procedure that may be modified extemporaneously because of specific disease conditions but avoids wasted motion that prevents the operation from being accomplished safely in a minimum of time. Minor modifications continue to be made; yet, the emphasis remains the same—adequate exposure, accurate and precise dissection of contiguous tissues, perfect hemostasis, approximation of tissue free of tension, and persistent attention to detail.

RAYMOND A. LEE

Acknowledgments

This surgical atlas represents the combined efforts of several individuals within the extended Mayo family. John Hagen, an accomplished and recognized medical illustrator, created every illustration. The separate phases of problem solving, carefully analyzing "working" drawings for accuracy and presentation "as the surgeon would see it," and final rendering were a team effort of surgeon and illustrator. I am sincerely grateful to John Hagen for his commitment to detail and his insistence on excellence.

Most of the illustrations are based on photographs taken during operative procedures. However, in some instances, other illustrations were used as a guide for the new illustrations. The previous work of former Mayo illustrators, Jack Desley, Floyd Hosmer, and William Westwood, was valuable in this process.

From the Section of Publications, which provided complete manuscript preparation services, I wish to thank LeAnn Stee, Assistant Head of the Section, for her expertise and diligent editorial review of the text; my heartfelt thanks to Roberta Schwartz, Supervisor, for her skills of organization and insistence on a schedule that resulted in the atlas being completed on time; and my sincere appreciation for the efforts of Margery Lovejoy, Rose Ann Ptacek-Vitse, and Patricia Calvert, whose expertise and attention to detail produced an accurate manuscript. I am also grateful for the review and insights offered by Clark Nelson of the Mayo Historical Unit.

I especially appreciated the thoughtful suggestions and encouragement I received from Dr. Maurice Webb, good friend and highly esteemed colleague, as he reviewed the entire atlas. I thank Joan Madoll, my secretary, for typing the manuscript.

I also wish to thank Martin Wonsiewicz and his staff at W. B. Saunders Company for their encouragement and confidence in undertaking the publication of this atlas. Finally, I wish to thank the governing board of Mayo Clinic and Mayo Foundation for providing me with an excellent supporting staff and the encouragement to complete this endeavor.

Contents

Vulva

Bartholin's Duct Cyst

Marsupialization

For an acute abscess of a Bartholin duct cyst or a large chronic cyst (clear mucoid material), we prefer incision, drainage, and marsupialization. The incision should be in the mucosa of the labium minus, just outside the carunculae myrtiformes, over the full length of the abscessed wall (Fig. 1). The abscess is permitted to drain, and the interior of the cystic cavity is inspected to ensure that there is no unrecognized loculus or tumefaction.

The lining of the cystic cavity is approximated loosely to the skin edge with fine (4-0) interrupted absorbable sutures (Fig. 2). Care must be taken to obtain perfect hemostasis. Narrow (¼-inch) gauze may be packed into the cavity but is removed in 24 hours.

Excision

An elliptic incision is made in the labium minus just outside the hymenal ring. The fine adhesions to the overlying skin are incised by sharp dissection adjacent to the wall of the cyst (Fig. 3).

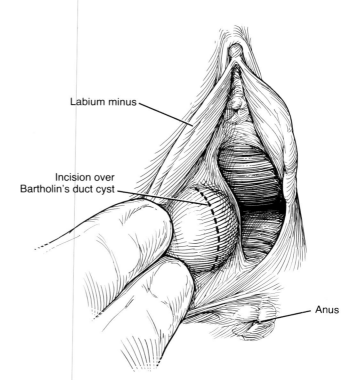

Figure 1

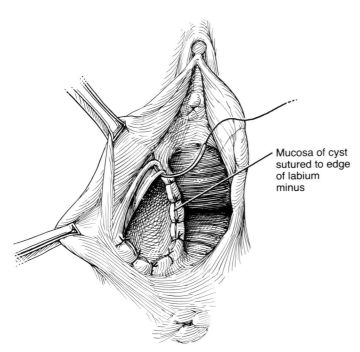

Mucosa of cyst sutured to edge of labium minus

Figure 2

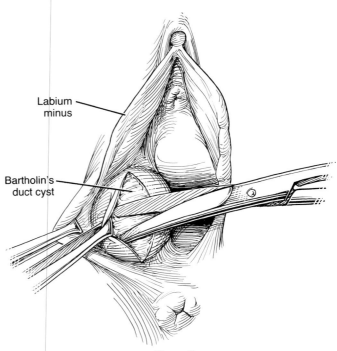

Figure 3

With careful hemostasis, proper traction on the cyst wall, and countertraction on the skin of the labium minus, the proper plane of dissection is visualized and the cystic mass usually can be excised intact (Fig. 4).

If the cyst is entered accidentally, the usually thick mucoid material is evacuated and the surgeon's index finger is inserted into the cystic cavity to aid in applying traction and to ensure complete removal of the cyst (Fig. 5).

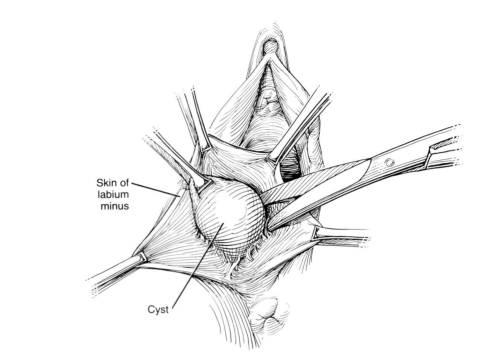

Skin of labium minus

Cyst

Figure 4

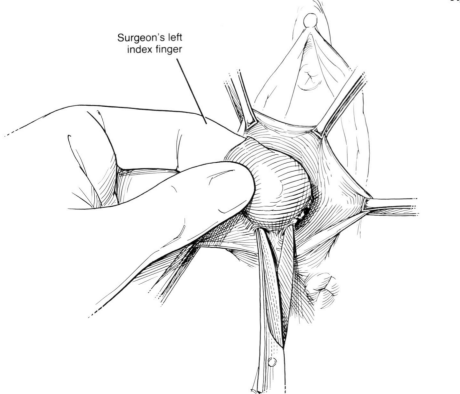

Surgeon's left index finger

Figure 5

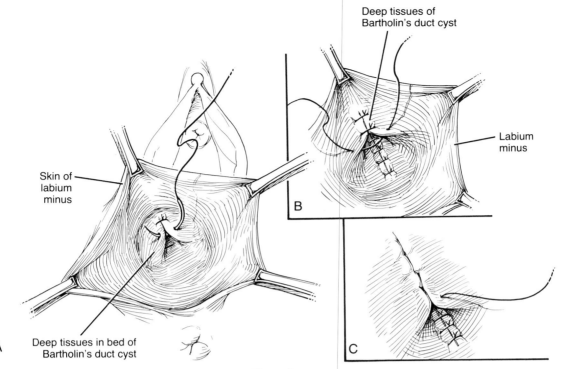

Deep tissues of Bartholin's duct cyst

Labium minus

Skin of labium minus

Deep tissues in bed of Bartholin's duct cyst

A

B

C

Figure 6

Once the cystic mass is excised, thorough hemostasis is obtained by using cauterization and fine sutures. To prevent hematoma formation, the resulting cavity is obliterated with accurate but loose approximation of the surrounding tissue with fine interrupted absorbable suture (Fig. 6A). Each layer of approximated tissue is attached to the underlying layer to eliminate potential dead space (Fig. 6B and C).

The edge of the incision is closed with 4-0 absorbable suture in a subcuticular fashion (Fig. 7). Accurate approximation of tissue without tension and with careful hemostasis minimizes postoperative discomfort and encourages primary healing of the operative site. We prefer not to use a drain.

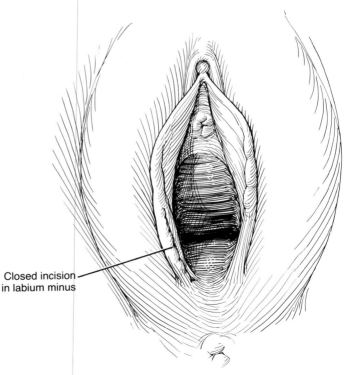

Closed incision in labium minus

Figure 7

Total Simple Vulvectomy

The traditional total vulvectomy consists of resection of the clitoris, mons veneris, and bulbocavernosus fat pad (Fig. 8). An elliptic incision is made through the skin; an adequate margin is obtained to permit frozen-section study, which is done to ensure complete removal of the primary lesion. The incision is continued down through the subcutaneous fat to the level of the deep fascia. A second, inner incision is made in the area of the carunculae myrtiformes. The dissection should begin anterior to the anal orifice in a manner such that the anal sphincter is not damaged.

Traction (up and lateral) applied to the inferior corners of the specimen permits accurate resection of the specimen and facilitates dissection in the proper plane (Fig. 9A). Any bleeding may be controlled with appropriate cautery or fine clamps to direct the blood away from the surgical field. The bulbocavernous and ischiocavernous muscles are removed in addition to the clitoris (Fig. 9B).

If a conservative simple vulvectomy is appropriate, a similar skin incision is accomplished. The dissection extends into the underlying fatty tissue but not to the deep fascia; this procedure thus preserves the clitoris and the muscles of the urogenital diaphragm. The free margins may need to be undermined in preparation for closure.

Closure of the operative site is accomplished with an initial layer of 3-0 absorbable suture to approximate the subcutaneous tissues and to permit a tension-free closure of the skin edges. The skin edges are carefully approximated with 4-0 absorbable suture placed in an interrupted or a subcuticular fashion (Fig. 10). Accurate placement of sutures about the urethra prevents misdirection of the stream of urine. Equal concern for the placement of sutures about the introitus minimizes the potential for dyspareunia.

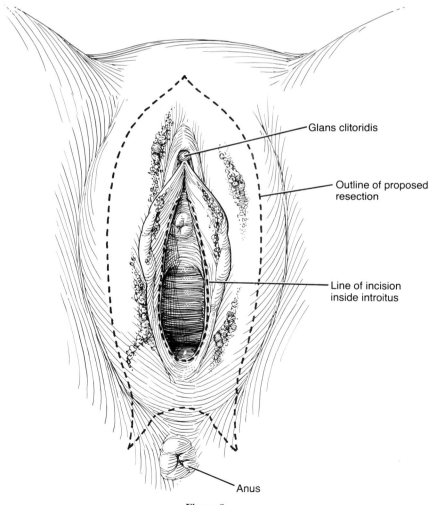

Glans clitoridis

Outline of proposed resection

Line of incision inside introitus

Anus

Figure 8

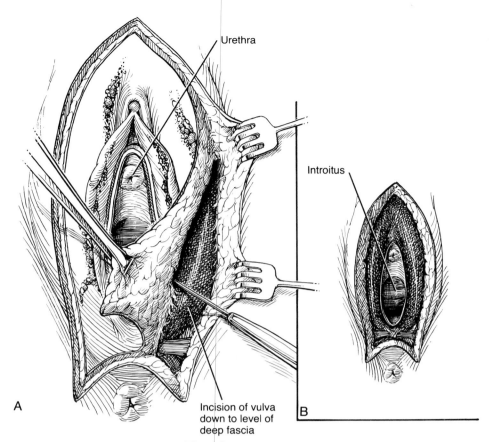

Urethra

Introitus

Incision of vulva
down to level of
deep fascia

A

B

Figure 9

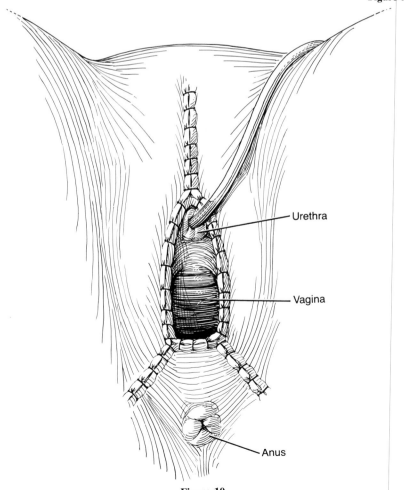

Urethra

Vagina

Anus

Figure 10

Skinning Vulvectomy

A skinning vulvectomy may be the primary treatment for selected conditions. Especially in the young patient, a skinning vulvectomy and immediate skin graft result in a more normal functional and cosmetic result. In this circumstance, the skin is excised to the depth of a layer of loose fibroelastic tissue immediately below the cutis (Fig. 11).

If mobilization of the surrounding tissue with simple skinning vulvectomy does not permit a tension-free closure, a skin graft harvested from the buttocks will suffice as an alternative to primary closure. This has the added advantage of the potential for a more functional and cosmetically acceptable result. A drum of skin (generally, 15 × 10 cm at a thickness of 0.017 inch) is sutured in place with 4-0 absorbable suture (Fig. 12). Overlying fluffs of dressing are held in place with selected ties to the previously placed suture in order to fix the graft in place. The patient is confined to bed for 48 hours, after which she is permitted to ambulate.

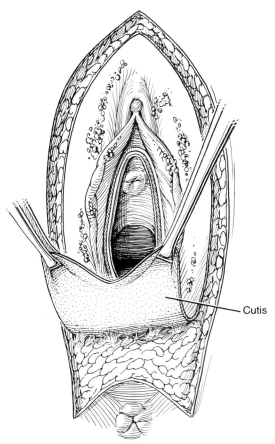

Cutis

Figure 11

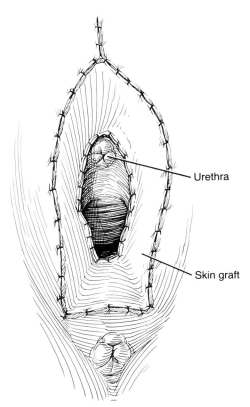

Urethra

Skin graft

Figure 12

Wide Local Excision

In an increasing number of circumstances, modified vulvectomy (wide local excision) and skinning vulvectomy have replaced total vulvectomy with deep removal of the vulvar tissues for the usual in situ lesion of the vulva. A partial vulvectomy is excision of less than 50% of the vulva. With less extensive disease, both laser vaporization and local excision with colposcopic guidance have proved to be effective. Local excision consists of removal of diseased foci with a 0.5-cm margin of microscopically normal tissue (Fig. 13). Accurate loose approximation of the cut edges decreases postoperative discomfort (Fig. 14).

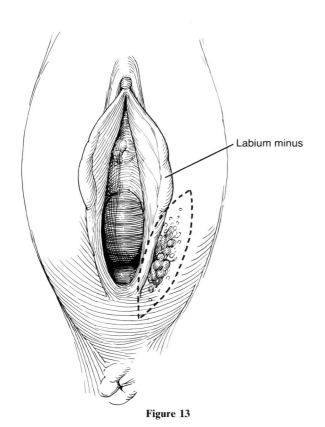

Labium minus

Figure 13

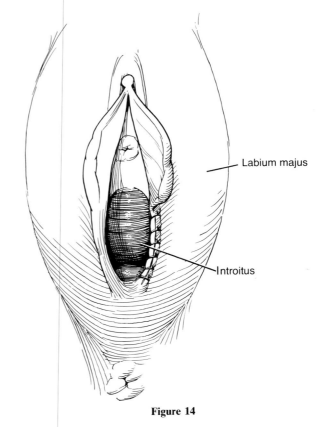

Labium majus

Introitus

Figure 14

Rectangular Flap Closure

Wide local excision of a primary or recurrent lesion in the posterior fourchette may create a difficult area to close. Lack of mobility results in tension on the suture lines and, depending on the location, may create dyspareunia. The initial skin incision is made in a circular fashion about the anus such that there is at least a 1- to 2-cm clearance of the primary lesion (Fig. 15A). This initial incision is continued down to the appropriate depth (usually to expose the capsule of the external anal sphincter) to ensure a margin deep to the lesion (Fig. 15B). The two superior arms of the incision (D and D') are continued in a vertical direction, again with adequate margins lateral to the incision and extended superiorly such that they may be connected (C), usually just inside the introitus. The specimen is then excised with an adequate deep margin, taking the fascia of the deep transverse perineal muscles or, if necessary, resecting the deep perineal muscles to ensure adequate clearance. Once the specimen is excised, complete hemostasis is obtained prior to development of the rectangular flaps.

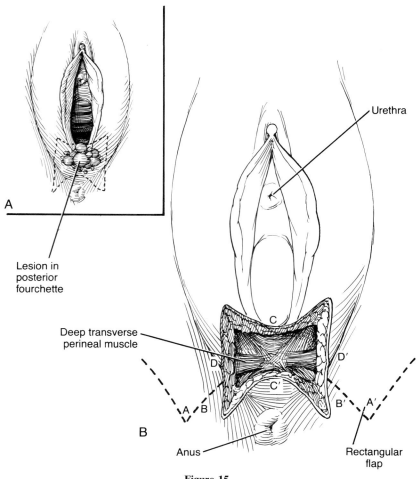

Figure 15

After the frozen-section diagnosis of tissue-free margins is obtained, the flaps are developed (along the stippled lines down to the corners, A and A'). The inner arms of the flap (B and B') should be as long as the defect measured from top to bottom (C to C') (Fig. 15B). The lateral arm should be half the length of the width of the defect (D to D'). The incisions are carried down deeply into the subcutaneous tissue and undermined to facilitate a tension-free approximation in the midline.

The subcutaneous tissues are approximated with 3-0 delayed absorbable suture to thus facilitate the later approximation of the skin edges in a tension-free fashion (Fig. 16). After placement of the rectangular flaps across the introitus (A to A'), the tips (B and B') may be appropriately placed to facilitate a symmetric and cosmetic closure of the perineal incision (Fig. 17). A subcutaneous suction catheter may be placed beneath the flaps.

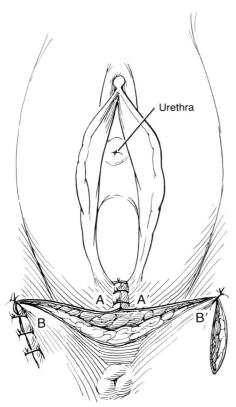

Figure 16
Approximation of rectangular flap in introitus.

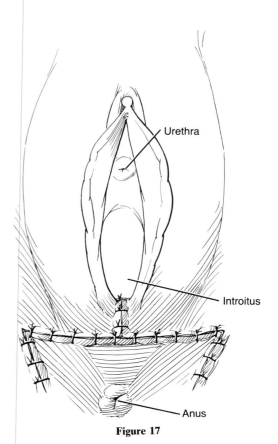

Figure 17

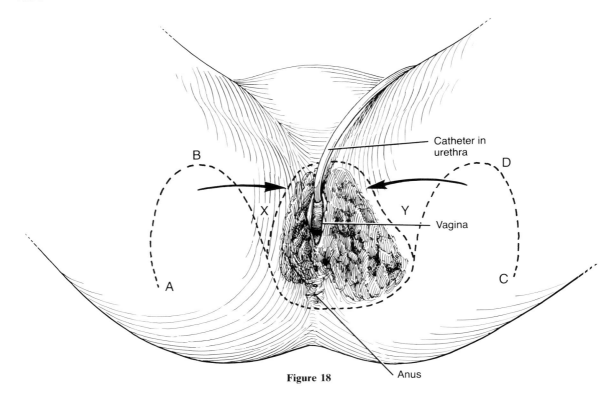

Figure 18

Circular Flap Closure

With lesions that encircle the urethra, vagina, and rectum, several different types of perineal flaps permit effective closure. In the situation shown in Figure 18 (recurrent squamous cell carcinoma), large circular flaps are used; the size of each side is determined by the corresponding defect. To ensure adequate coverage, careful measurements in the superior to inferior direction (*A–B, C–D*) and of the width of the

perineal flap are obtained. The flaps are developed with sufficient subcutaneous tissue and then turned down. The V-shaped wedges (*X* and *Y*) are undermined and moved laterally to cover the harvest site of the circular flap.

Perfect hemostasis must be obtained. Then the flap is sutured in place with 3-0 delayed absorbable sutures (Fig. 19).

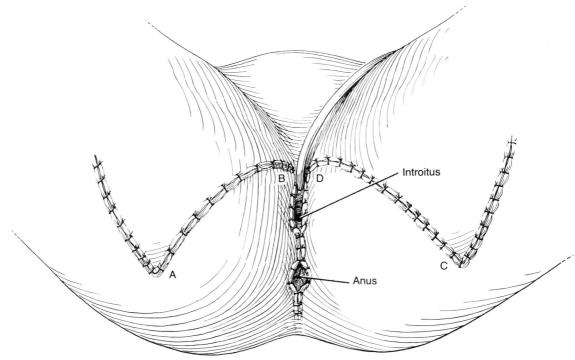

Figure 19

Wide Vulvar Excision and Skin Graft Closure

With diffuse multifocal Paget's disease, a wide local excision with frozen-section examination of the cut edges of the specimens is the best (but not the perfect) means of preventing recurrence (Fig. 20).

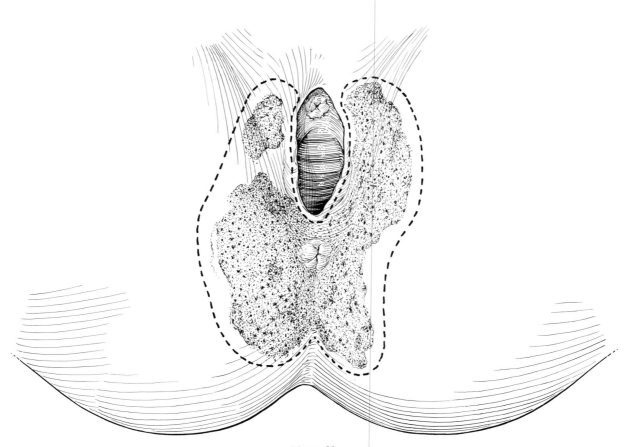

Figure 20

With appropriate traction and countertraction, the involved skin and some underlying subcutaneous tissue are removed. Working from an inferior to a superior direction avoids the chance of bleeding obscuring the line of dissection (Fig. 21).

After the specimen is removed and hemostasis is accomplished with cautery or fine absorbable ties, the area is measured for the proper skin graft. The preserved subcutaneous tissue provides a bed for the graft and optimizes the cosmetic and functional results by preserving the soft, pliable vulva (Fig. 22).

Beginning at the superior margin, the graft is sutured to the edge of the preserved skin with interrupted

4-0 polyglycolic acid suture. The graft shown in Figure 23A was "pie crusted," resulting in a greater accommodation to cover the operative site and also permitting the passage of tissue and lymphatic fluid from the operative area. Proper tension is imperative. If the graft is too tight, fluid may accumulate in the bed. If it is too loose, wrinkling will not permit proper establishment. A soft dressing of gauze fluff is applied to the graft site and fixed in place by tying selected long strands of suture from the outer edge to matching sutures on the inner edge of the introitus (Fig. 23B).

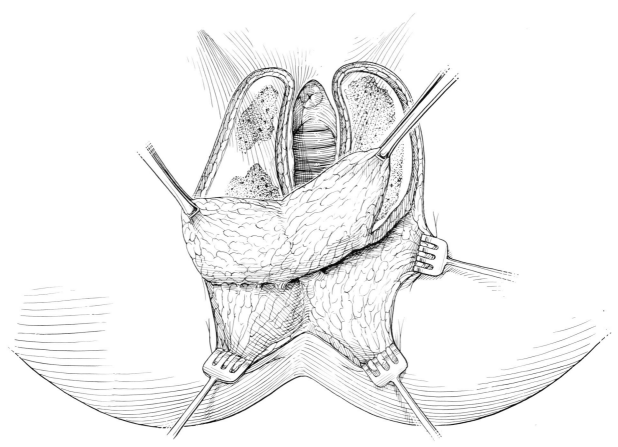

Figure 21

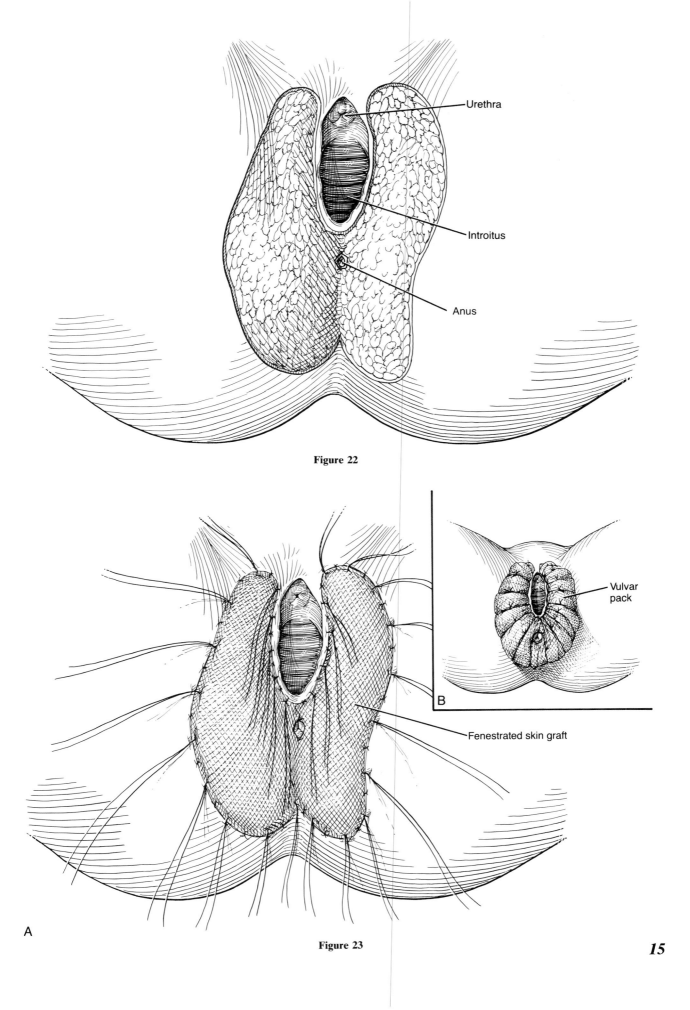

Figure 22

Urethra

Introitus

Anus

Vulvar pack

Fenestrated skin graft

A

B

Figure 23

15

Radical Vulvectomy with En Bloc Bilateral Dissection of the Groin

Because of the predilection of vulvar cancer to invade locally and to metastasize to local lymphatic and regional lymph nodes, the standard treatment for appropriate patients with operable vulvar cancer has been en bloc radical vulvectomy and bilateral groin dissection. If the disease involves the anus, the recto-vaginal septum, or the proximal urethra, wide excision to provide local control may require a modified pelvic exenteration combined with the vulvectomy. In Figure 24*A*, the broken line marks the location of the superior skin incision, which begins at each anterior superior iliac spine and passes to 2 cm above the symphysis pubis and the inguinal ligament. Each corner is fashioned with a V-like incision such that,

with closure, there will not be a dog-ear projection over the spine (Fig. 24*B*).

This incision is continued into the subcutaneous tissue for approximately 7 mm, and undermining (as shown by the fine stippling in the figure) is continued toward the umbilicus (Fig. 24*A*). A thin layer of adipose tissue is left on the preserved skin. The flap thus developed extends down to the symphysis pubis in a tension-free fashion at the time of closure. The superficial fascia is removed down to the aponeurosis of the external oblique muscle, down both sides to the level of the inguinal ligaments, and to the plane of the rectus sheath and the periosteum of the symphysis pubis. This ensures that the contents of the mons pubis (adjacent skin, subcutaneous tissues, and lymphatic channels) are removed completely.

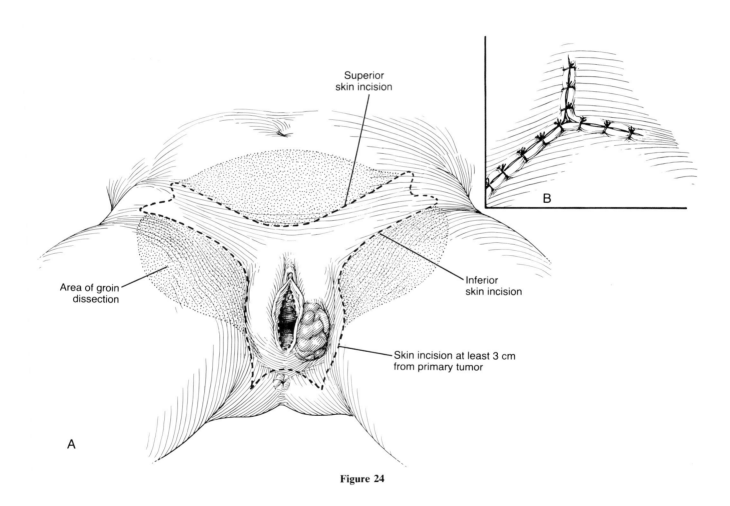

Superior skin incision

Inferior skin incision

Area of groin dissection

Skin incision at least 3 cm from primary tumor

A

B

Figure 24

The inferior skin incision is made 2 cm below and runs parallel to the inguinal ligament and the superior incision. This incision is extended through the skin and subcutaneous tissue, leaving (as with an upper flap) approximately 7 mm of fat beneath the tissue; undermining is again done in an inferior fashion for a distance of about 10 cm down the thigh.

Rakes are placed on the superior edge of the skin overlying the thigh, with countertraction on the skin and subcutaneous tissue of the groin (specimen exposed), to facilitate the dissection of the stippled area down to the fascia lata of the thigh (Fig. 25). With appropriate countertraction on the specimen of skin and the subcutaneous tissue between the superior and the inferior incisions and countertraction with the rake overlying the skin and the subcutaneous tissue of the thigh, the fascia lata is exposed and opened just lateral to the lateral border of the sartorius muscle. The block of skin and subcutaneous tissue (a portion from above and another portion from below the inguinal ligament) contains the lymphatic and areolar tissue down to the aponeurosis of the external oblique and the rectus abdominis muscles and tissue from the anterior thigh inferior to the inguinal ligament. With traction on this specimen medially, the incision in the fascia lata of the thigh is continued laterally and medially to expose, in order, the branches of the femoral nerve and the femoral artery at a level approximately 8 cm below the inguinal ligament.

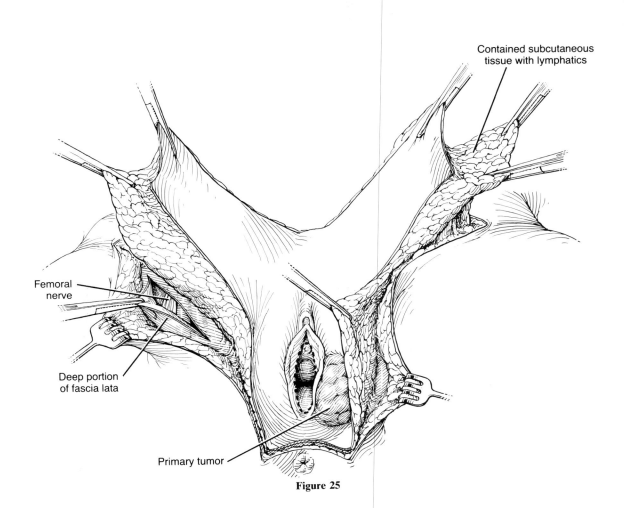

Contained subcutaneous tissue with lymphatics

Femoral nerve

Deep portion of fascia lata

Primary tumor

Figure 25

With appropriate traction on the fascia, which is now pulled superiorly, and scissor dissection immediately adjacent to the wall of the femoral artery, the dissection proceeds toward the inguinal ligament (cephalad direction) (Fig. 26). The external pudendal artery will be encountered, which is clamped, cut, and tied at its origin. This identifies the junction of the saphenous vein with the femoral vein. The proximal end of the saphenous vein is doubly clamped and tied so that a short distance is left from the tie to the junction of this vein with the femoral vein. The overlying skin, subcutaneous tissue, and pedicle of femoral vein are retracted medially, freeing the vein over an area approximately 10 cm below the inguinal ligament.

The specimen continues to be mobilized in a lateral to medial direction, where the distal end of the saphenous vein is clamped, cut, and tied. The contents of the inguinal canal, including the round ligament, are lifted from the underlying soft tissues, clamped, cut, and tied; the proximal cut end of the round ligament is permitted to retract into the canal. The deep inguinal nodes just medial to the femoral vein are removed en bloc with the specimen. This dissection is carried medially to complete the en bloc dissection of the groin as the specimen is sharply dissected off the pectineal muscle and periosteum of the os pubis. Repair of the femoral canal can be accomplished with interrupted 2-0 delayed absorbable sutures placed through the conjoined tendon to the periosteum of the pubic ramus; care is taken that the most lateral suture does not compress or compromise the femoral vein.

A similar dissection is carried out on the left side (Fig. 27). The specimen is then wrapped in a sterile towel and placed between the patient's legs, which are in a lithotomy position. In some patients, the sartorius muscle is incised through its tendinous attachment to the anterior superior iliac spine. A single tie is placed at the site of attachment. The proximal end of the sartorius muscle is freed, mobilized medially, and sutured to the inferior border of the inguinal ligament with interrupted 2-0 delayed absorbable sutures (Fig. 28). The medial border of the sartorius muscle is sutured to the pectineal fascia to ensure coverage of the femoral vein.

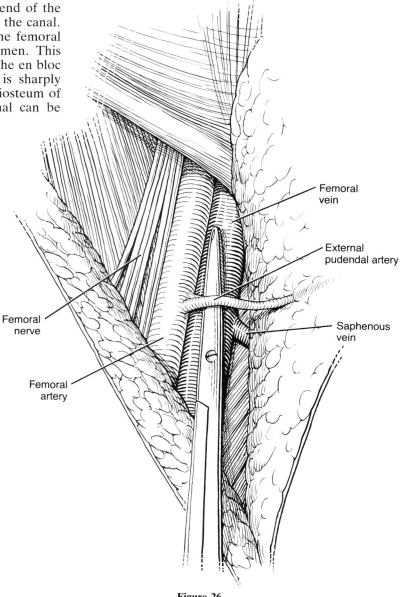

Femoral vein

External pudendal artery

Saphenous vein

Femoral nerve

Femoral artery

Figure 26

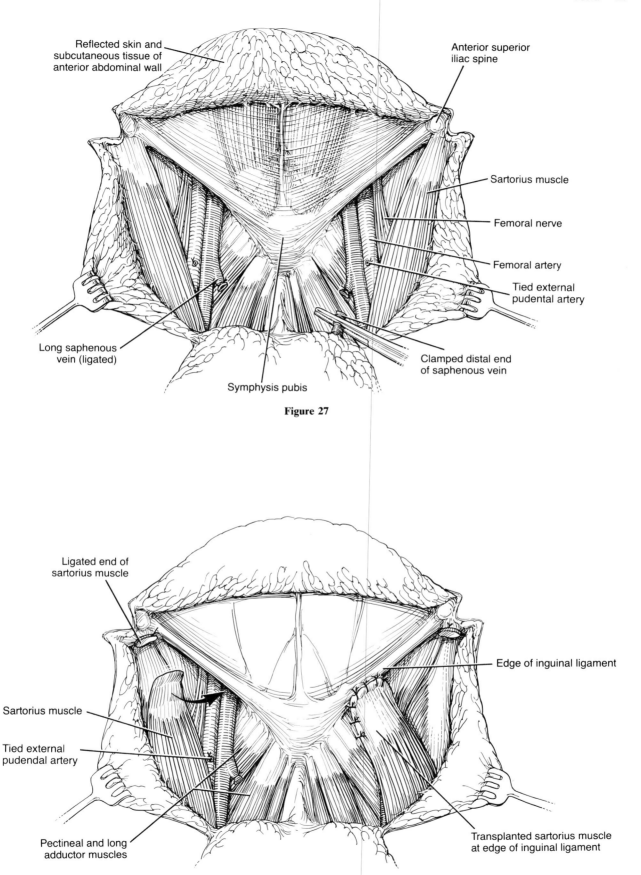

Reflected skin and
subcutaneous tissue of
anterior abdominal wall

Anterior superior
iliac spine

Sartorius muscle

Femoral nerve

Femoral artery

Tied external
pudental artery

Long saphenous
vein (ligated)

Clamped distal end
of saphenous vein

Symphysis pubis

Figure 27

Ligated end of
sartorius muscle

Edge of inguinal ligament

Sartorius muscle

Tied external
pudendal artery

Pectineal and long
adductor muscles

Transplanted sartorius muscle
at edge of inguinal ligament

Figure 28

The vulvar incision is continued along the labial crural folds, extending through the perineal skin and subcutaneous tissue and meeting anterior to the rectum. A margin of at least 3 cm from the primary tumor must be maintained regardless of the location of the tumor. With appropriate traction and countertraction, dissection is continued along the periosteum of the symphysis pubis, the level of the fascia of the deep musculature of the urogenital diaphragm.

Attention is now directed to the inferior aspects of the vulva. Traction is placed on the corners of the vulvar specimen with countertraction to either side of the anal canal, and the incision is continued down to the fascia of the perineum. With sharp dissection, the incision is continued anteriorly, separating the vagina from the anal canal and entering the vagina inside the hymen (Fig. 29). The vaginal walls are incised circumferentially inside the level of the hymen. The amount of the vagina to be excised depends on the site and size of the primary lesion. Countertraction is placed on the specimen as the dissection continues superiorly and flush with the fascia of the perineum, where the internal pudendal vessels are clamped, cut, and tied.

The vulva is now ready for excision. Sharp dissection, working from below in an upward direction, is used; appropriate tissues are clamped at the depth of the perineal fascia and the bulb of the vestibule. The incision is continued in a superior fashion, first on one side and then on the other. It always must be kept in mind that wide clearance of the primary lesion must be accomplished. The specimen has been freed from the ischiopubic rami and contains the bulbocavernous, ischiocavernous, and superficial transverse perineal muscles.

If the location of the primary lesion permits, a small portion of the tissue about the urethra is preserved to facilitate accurate and tension-free closure of the vulvar skin about the urethra. If the primary lesion is adjacent to the urethra, appropriate resection of the urethra should be accomplished; in this case, the patient may require an appropriate operative repair to reestablish urinary continence. The dissection is continued flush with the symphysis pubis, where the clitoris, including the crura, is excised to the depth of the periosteum. The specimen is removed, and complete hemostasis is accomplished before the closure is begun.

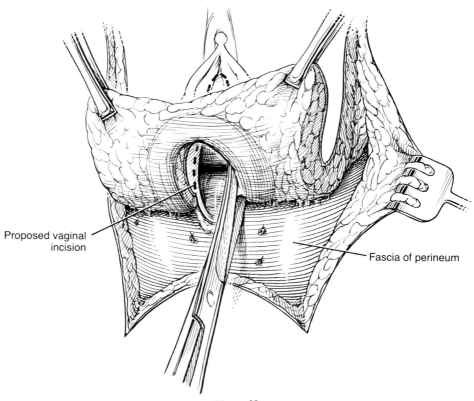

Proposed vaginal incision

Fascia of perineum

Figure 29

A small stab wound is placed through each side of the superior flap, and large suction drains are placed through the flap over the inguinal ligament to end in the femoral canal. It may be necessary to undermine the vagina and adjacent skin of the perineum to permit a tension-free closure of the perineum. The perineal closure is begun at the most inferior aspects in front of the anal canal and extended superiorly in a symmetric fashion (Fig. 30). The subcutaneous tissues are approximated free of tension with fine 3-0 delayed absorbable suture with either subcuticular

or interrupted sutures in the skin. Two or three sutures are placed through the periosteum of the symphysis pubis to incorporate the dorsal fascia of the urethra; this approach ensures a midline location. Closure of the perineum is begun anterior to the rectum, approximating the subcutaneous tissues with 3-0 delayed absorbable suture; this permits a tension-free closure of the skin edges. The suprapubic anterior abdominal wall flap is brought down and sutured to the symphysis pubis with interrupted 3-0 absorbable sutures. This initial step permits lateral approxi-

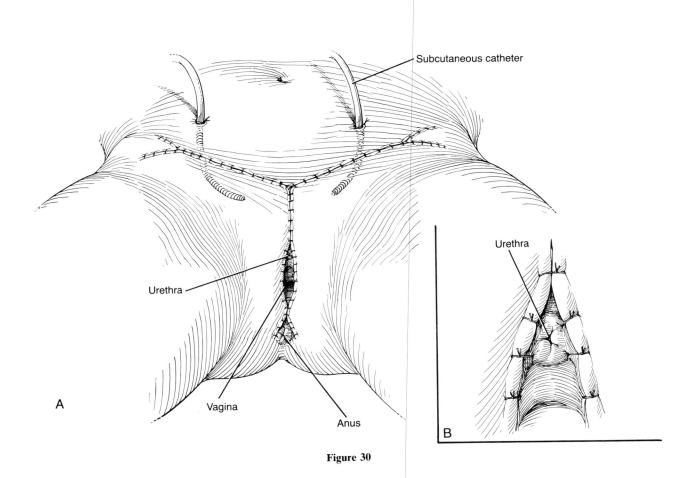

Figure 30

mation of the lateral groin incisions in a symmetric fashion.

The perineum is reconstituted by suturing subcutaneous tissue of the thigh to that of the perivaginal tissues to permit a tension-free closure of the skin of the thigh to the edge of the vaginal wall.

The surgical specimen includes the skin of the groins and underlying subcutaneous tissues and lymph nodes, and it also contains the vulva and its underlying fat, perineal muscles, and lymph nodes (Fig. 31).

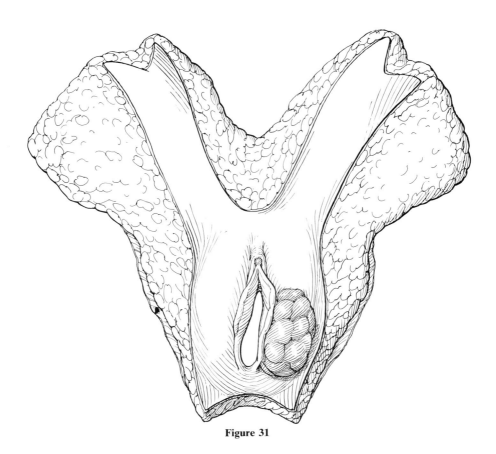

Figure 31

Vagina

Imperforate Hymen

The imperforate hymen is distended because of the hematocolpos. The lines of incision are directed from the 2-o'clock to the 8-o'clock position and from the 10-o'clock to the 4-o'clock position in the wall of the intact hymen (Fig. 32). No suprapubic pressure is applied to hasten evacuation of the dark tar-like accumulated menstrual debris. The vagina is not irrigated. The cervix may be completely effaced and appear simply as a small circular hole at the top of the vagina leading to the uterus. Intrauterine manip-ulation is not attempted. Prophylactic antibiotics are usually given just before the surgical procedure is begun. We prefer not to excise any tissue; when the incision is made, care should be taken that it is not too close to the vaginal edge, because scarring and dyspareunia could result. The suture line is closed in a transverse fashion (opposite the direction of the incision) with interrupted 4–0 delayed absorbable suture (Fig. 33). Reexamination is performed 2 weeks after the operation to ensure complete regression of the uterus and to verify that a hematometra is not present.

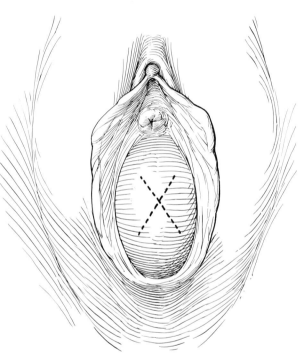

Figure 32
Bulging, intact, imperforate hymen with proposed line of incision.

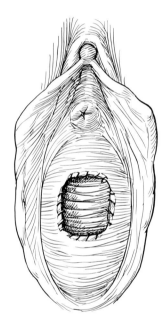

Figure 33
Evacuated hematocolpos with four separate suture lines.

Agenesis of the Vagina

Congenital absence of the vagina continues to challenge gynecologic surgeons who perform reconstructive procedures of the pelvis. We favor a modified McIndoe procedure, which provides excellent results. Increased operative difficulty may be encountered in certain patients. Decreased room for the graft and difficult dissections are typically encountered in patients with short stature; a narrow pubic arch; strong levator muscles; a short or rigid male-type perineum; a pelvic kidney; or a congenitally deep pelvic cul-de-sac. These problems also occur in patients who have had perineal exploration or hymenectomy. In particular, previous operations can make the rectovesical space difficult to dissect and hemostasis difficult to secure—factors that increase the possibility of poor take of the skin graft. Surgical results, as measured by patient satisfaction, are excellent in most patients (95%).

The skin graft harvested from the buttocks is 10 to 12 cm wide and 18 to 20 cm long and has a thickness of 0.017 inch (Fig. 34A). The graft is placed over a condom-covered sponge-rubber mold. The sutures approximating the edges of the skin graft are placed only through the graft and not into the underlying condom or sponge-rubber mold. This technique avoids potential disruption of the skin graft when the sponge-rubber mold is removed 8 to 10 days later. The skin is placed over the mold such that the outer stratified squamous side is adjacent to the condom and the moist layer is on the outside (Fig. 34B).

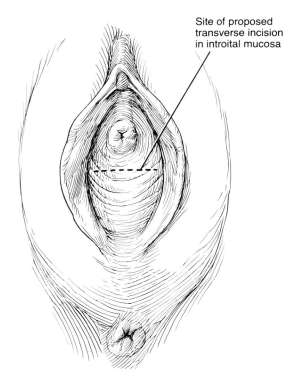

Figure 35

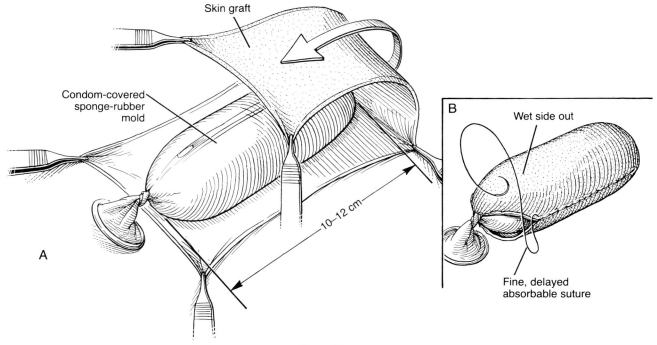

Figure 34

The rectum should be empty, and a no. 16 Foley catheter should be placed through the urethra into the bladder. A transverse or cruciate incision is made approximately 1 cm inferior to the external urethral meatus (Figs. 35 and 36).

The initial dissection of 3 to 4 cm is accomplished with sharp dissection (with Mayo scissors) (Fig. 37), after which an essentially bloodless plane is entered and the rest of the dissection can be accomplished with fingers, sponges, and retractors.

As the fingers are inserted into the vaginal canal, lateral traction is applied to increase its lateral diameter (Fig. 38).

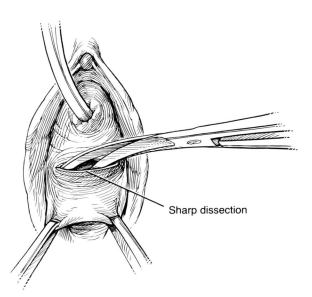

Sharp dissection

Figure 36

Length of transverse incision, 3 cm

Figure 37

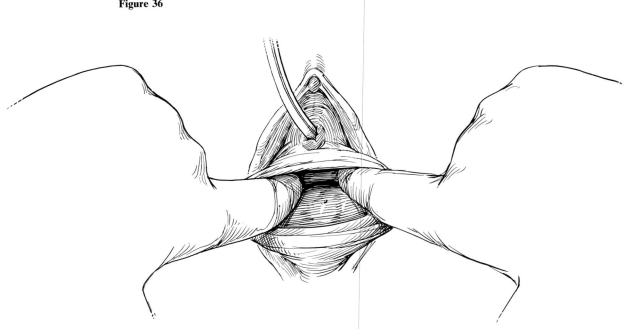

Figure 38

The dissection is carried superiorly such that, with a Deaver retractor elevating the bladder anteriorly and with another holding the rectum posteriorly, one can identify the peritoneum at the apex of the canal (Fig. 39). We generally develop a clear area in the apex of the vagina (peritoneum), freeing the peritoneum for a circumference of about 2 to 3 cm. Theoretically, too wide a dissection at the apex could encourage development of an enterocele. Any bleeding points along the recently developed vaginal space are cauterized; frequently, however, arterial bleeders along the medial edge of the levator muscle in the midvaginal area (3- and 9-o'clock positions) require suture ligature. The skin-covered sponge-rubber mold is inspected in preparation for its insertion in the dissected space (Fig. 40).

The mold is then inserted into the previously developed space, and 0 delayed absorbable sutures are placed through the labia and underlying muscles to hold the mold in place against the potential coughing or straining of the patient (Fig. 41). We generally remove the catheter on the third postoperative day and leave the mold in place for 8 to 10 days. A transparent dressing (Op-Site) is placed on the donor site. If fluid accumulates, it can be removed with a butterfly needle, or the complete dressing can be removed and a new one applied. The dressing is removed at 10 days, at which time the site is epithelialized. The patient is allowed out of bed on the day after operation and is placed on a regular diet.

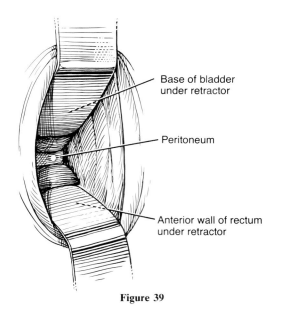

Base of bladder under retractor

Peritoneum

Anterior wall of rectum under retractor

Figure 39

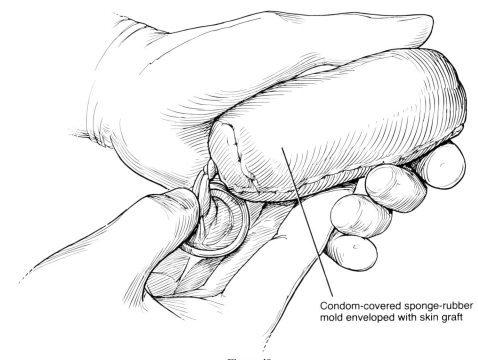

Condom-covered sponge-rubber mold enveloped with skin graft

Figure 40

At 8 to 10 days postoperatively, the patient is returned to the operating room. The labial sutures and the condom-covered sponge-rubber mold are removed. The vaginal canal is irrigated gently with saline. The graft site is inspected to determine its take, which is customarily 100%. Fine sutures (4–0) are used to fix the junction of the skin graft to the edge of the skin of the introitus. After the edges of the skin graft have been sutured to the introitus of the vagina, a polyethylene mold covered with a fine layer of antibiotic cream is inserted into the vagina (Fig. 42).

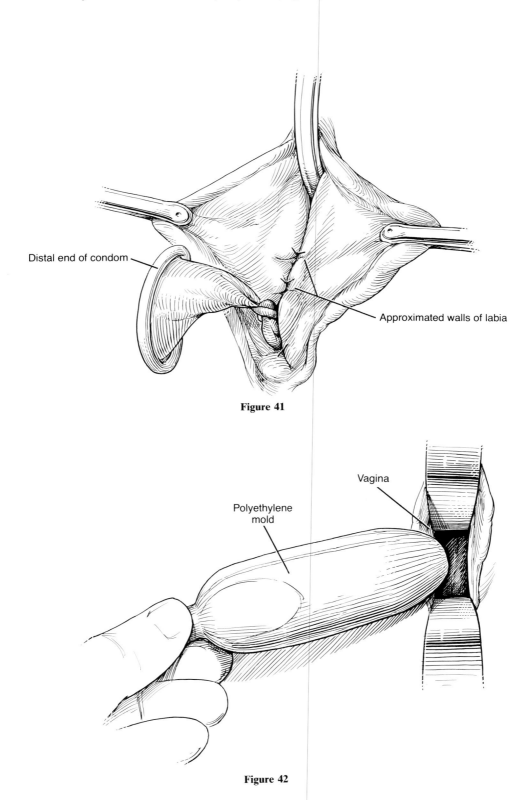

Distal end of condom

Approximated walls of labia

Figure 41

Polyethylene mold

Vagina

Figure 42

Proper development of the vaginal space permits the entire mold to be inserted into the vagina. Because the small nipple protrudes, removal is easy (Fig. 43). We recommend that the patient remove the mold daily, at which time it is washed with soap and water, coated with antibiotic cream, and reinserted. Occasionally, it is necessary for the patient to place pressure posteriorly (toward the rectum) on the nipple end of the mold to facilitate urination. Coitus is usually initiated 2 to 3 months after operation. The mold is worn until the patient is sexually active.

Attention to details in operative technique, including obtaining a generous, viable graft of appropriate dimensions, ensuring sufficient vaginal space (laterally and all the way to the peritoneal reflection), achieving meticulous hemostasis, and using a soft sponge-rubber stent, yields the best results. Appropriate timing of the operation and patient preparation and instruction collectively enhance compliance, which is critical to success. Postoperatively, the patient must avoid potentially injurious activities with the stent in place and must continue to use the stent at all other times until sexual relations occur at regular intervals.

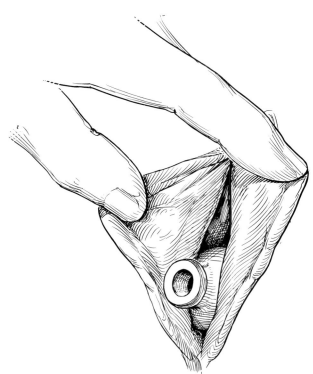

Figure 43
Vaginal canal accepting full length and diameter of polyethylene mold.

Didelphic Uterus and Longitudinal Vaginal Septum Obstructing One Vagina

A large amount of old blood and debris accumulates in the distended, obstructed vagina while the patient continues to have a cyclic menstruation from the opposite side. Given sufficient time, the bloody debris forms a large hematocolpos, which protrudes into the vagina. If it is permitted to develop sufficiently, the expanding mass will partially obstruct and protrude out of the vaginal introitus. Not infrequently, there is an ipsilateral renal agenesis. The patient's symptoms can be corrected with excision of the obstructing vaginal septum (Fig. 44A). An incision is initially made in the center of the bulging mass. (In Figure 44A, the mass is easily identified as it protrudes from the introitus. It is shown in a transverse view in Figure 44B.)

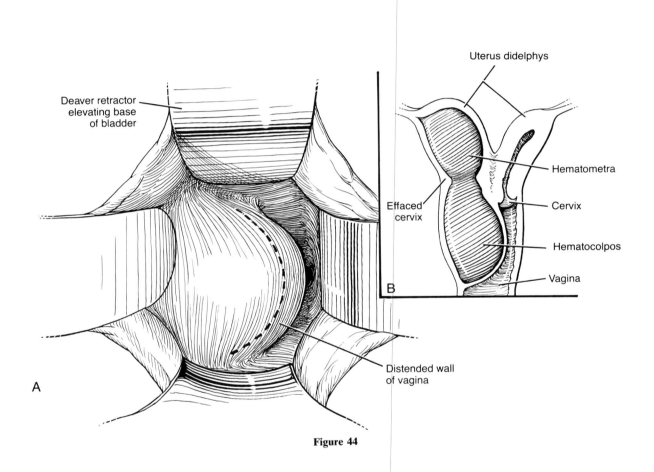

Figure 44

Once the debris is evacuated, palpation demonstrates the thickness and dimensions of the vaginal septum, which then can be completely excised, the cut edges being flush with the adjacent vagina (Fig. 45). The walls of the vagina then are approximated, and he-mostasis is accomplished with interrupted 4–0 delayed absorbable sutures. Total excision of the septum promptly corrects the symptoms and, given sufficient time, results in a remarkably normal vagina. This anomaly has numerous variations and modifications.

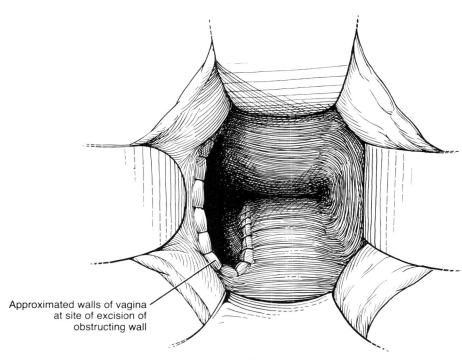

Approximated walls of vagina
at site of excision of
obstructing wall

Figure 45

Vaginal Septum

Longitudinal

Failure of fusion of the lower müllerian ducts that form the vagina results in a vagina with a longitudinal septum (Fig. 46). Usually, a didelphic uterus is also present. The patient generally becomes aware of the septum because of difficulty inserting a vaginal tampon or because of dyspareunia and difficulty with intercourse. Because of these problems, the vaginal septum may need to be removed.

Initially, a straight Kocher clamp is applied 2 to 3 mm from the posterior vaginal wall across the base of the transverse septum, and the septum is incised (Fig. 47A). Placement of 4–0 horizontal mattress suture to approximate the edges of the vaginal wall results in excellent hemostasis. A similar clamp is placed across the vaginal septum approximately 2 to 3 mm from the anterior vaginal wall (floor of urethra and bladder neck). This procedure is continued alternately posteriorly and anteriorly until the apex of the vagina is reached and the septum has been removed (Fig. 47B).

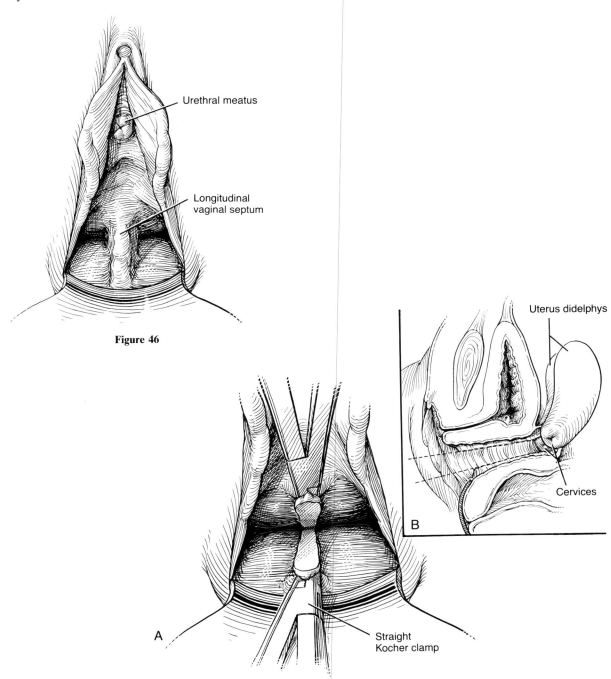

Figure 46

Figure 47

The edges of the vaginal wall are accurately approximated to reduce potential granulation, and a normal, single-barreled vagina results (Fig. 48). Usually, the patient has a double cervix, for which no treatment is necessary.

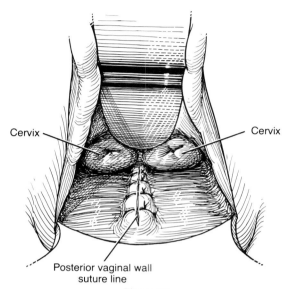

Figure 48

Transverse

Transverse vaginal septum of the vagina may be complete or incomplete and is relatively uncommon (Fig. 49). It occurs most frequently at the junction of the middle third and upper third of the vagina. Generally, the higher the location of the septum in the vagina, the thicker its base and the more difficult it is to correct. The incomplete variety has a small perforation, generally in the center or just off center, but it may be small and difficult to identify. Pregnancy is possible even if the perforation is 1 mm in diameter. Magnetic resonance imaging aids in outlining the thickness of the septum.

Various methods of treatment have been suggested, the easiest being simple dilation; however, we have found that operative resection provides the best results. Patients with a thick, fibrotic septal base sometimes in excess of 1 to 2 cm present several difficult challenges. Of major importance is that the septum be completely removed and that its thick base be excised sufficiently in a peripheral fashion to avoid formation of a constricting ring during healing, which results in dyspareunia. Also, as the base thickens, the space widens, and it is more difficult to bridge the area with normal vaginal epithelium; a split-thickness skin graft may be effective for bridging the defect.

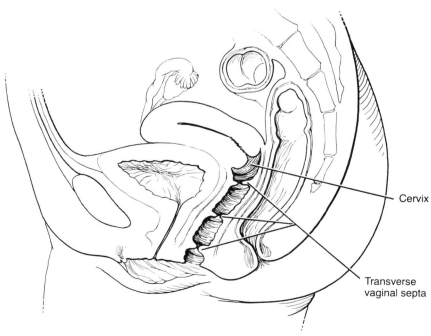

Figure 49

The initial incision in the skin of the septum is made several millimeters inside the lateral extent of the septum (Fig. 50A). Preservation of this skin permits a tension-free approximation once the septum has been removed. After the septum has been incised sufficiently, the index finger is inserted through the newly created defect to palpate the cervix superiorly. The inner aspect of the septum can also be palpated to determine its thickness. Once this is established, the connective tissue portion of the septum is excised, and a small remnant is left adjacent to the anterior, posterior, and lateral walls of the vagina (Fig. 50B). Once the center portion of the septum has been removed, resection of the rest of the septum can then be appropriately tailored to ensure its complete removal and yet allow safe resection by avoiding injury to the bladder or rectum and excessive resection laterally. The thickened wall needs to be removed completely and the vaginal lining needs to be approximated without tension to avoid a postoperative stricture. The vaginal wall may have to be undermined inferiorly and superiorly in sufficient fashion to aid in tension-free approximation (Fig. 50C). The vaginal walls are approximated by incorporating a small portion of the underlying connective tissue with 4–0 or 5–0 delayed absorbable sutures. A sponge-rubber mold covered with a condom is inserted into the vagina for the first 10 days postoperatively, after which it is replaced with a permanent polyethylene mold. If the patient is sexually active, the mold is not required.

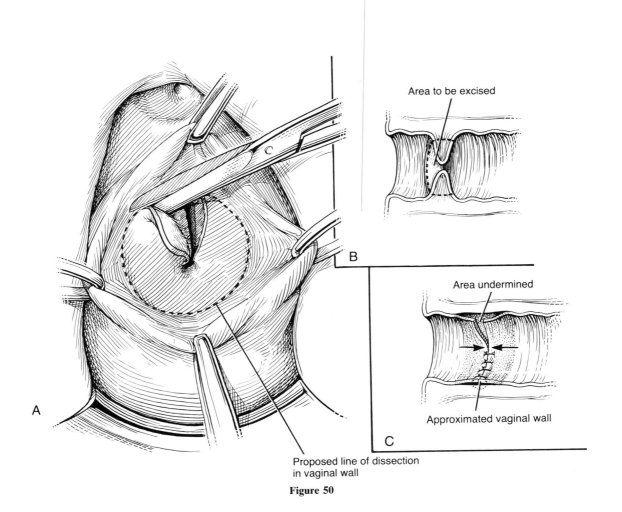

Area to be excised

Area undermined

Approximated vaginal wall

Proposed line of dissection
in vaginal wall

Figure 50

Congenitally High Perineal Body

Occasionally, a patient has a congenitally high perineal body. This is frequently associated with exstrophy of the bladder, but it sometimes occurs without other associated abnormalities. The high perineal body is remarkably consistent in its presentation and is easily misdiagnosed as a congenital anomaly of the vagina when in fact the only abnormality is at the introitus.

Initially, an elliptic incision is made from the 9-, 12-, and 3-o'clock positions through the perineal skin (Fig. 51). This tongue of skin and subcutaneous tissue is then reflected posteriorly. A vertical incision is made into the underlying subcutaneous tissue, extending into the vagina (Fig. 52). The previously developed flap, which is hinged posteriorly, is then swung into the vagina to meet the cut edge of the vaginal walls. This junction is closed in a single layer with 4–0 delayed absorbable sutures (Fig. 53).

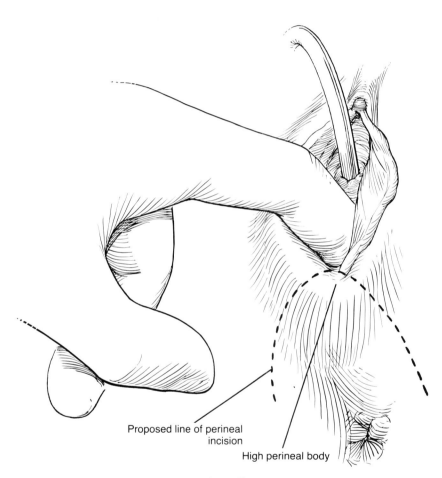

Proposed line of perineal
incision

High perineal body

Figure 51

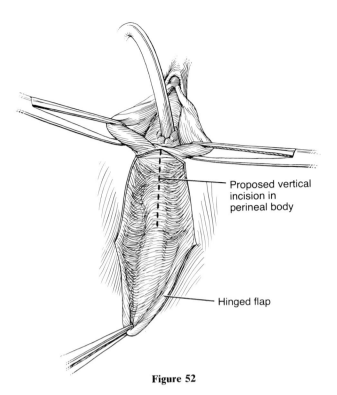

Proposed vertical incision in perineal body

Hinged flap

Figure 52

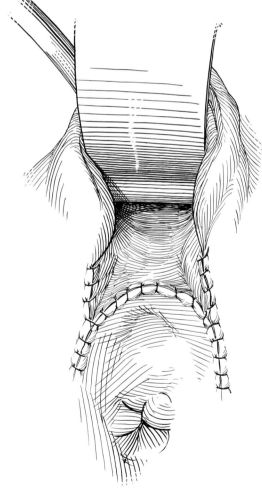

Figure 53

Stricture of the Vagina

Introitus

Narrowing of the introitus may result from overzealous repair of an episiotomy or from a posterior colpoperineorrhaphy. Depending on the depth of the contracture and the involvement of the underlying muscles, various approaches may be required.

Single Incision

The simplest approach is a midline incision of the contracting scar, after which the vaginal skin is mobilized from the underlying, scarred perineal tissues (Fig. 54).

Occasionally, fibrous scar tissue in the subcutaneous area is excessive and requires removal in order to add diameter to the introitus. Once this is accomplished, the vaginal lining is undermined, excellent hemostasis is established, and a tension-free transverse closure is performed (Fig. 55).

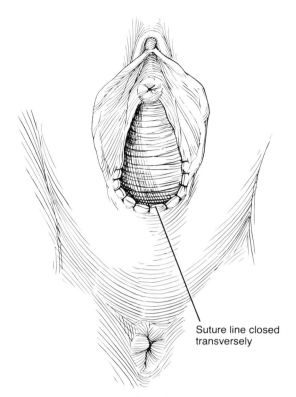

Suture line closed transversely

Figure 55

Multiple Incisions

Occasionally, a single midline incision with conversion to a transverse closure is insufficient. In these circumstances, we have found that three separate vertical incisions (Fig. 56), each converted to a trans-

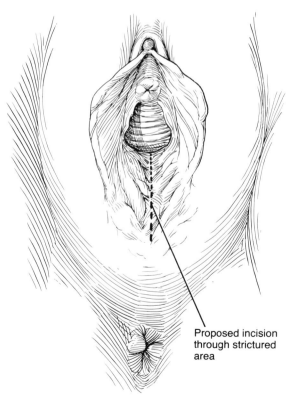

Proposed incision through strictured area

Figure 54

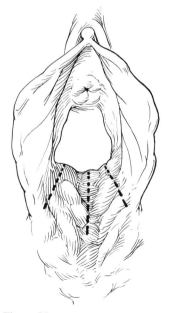

Figure 56
Proposed sites of vaginal incisions.

verse relationship, give sufficient diameter to the introitus (Fig. 57).

Vertical Z-plasty

A technique that incorporates a Z-plasty procedure involves the transplantation of two interdigitating triangular flaps. The length and arm of the Z are determined by the degree of the stenosis, but generally each is about 2 cm in length. The angles of the Z are also determined by the degree of stenosis, but they are usually about 60°. The length of the incision in a transverse direction is determined by the size of the angle (angles *A* and *B* on Fig. 58). As the angles (usually of equal size) increase, so does the transverse lengthening. The midpoint (in the anteroposterior direction) of the scar is identified (the most significant portion of contracture), and a transverse incision (the common limb of the Z-plasty) is made through to the vaginal wall. The appropriate and equal angle that will provide adequate diameter is determined by the common limb incision. The upper arm of the Z is extended into the vagina, and the lower arm is extended toward the perineum (Fig. 59*A*). If the maneuver is well planned, the flaps will fall into their new transposed positions. In fact, it is difficult for these to be replaced into their old relationships. Any bridge of scar tissue is removed, complete hemostasis is obtained, and the transposed flaps are approximated free of tension with 4–0 absorbable sutures (Fig. 59*B*).

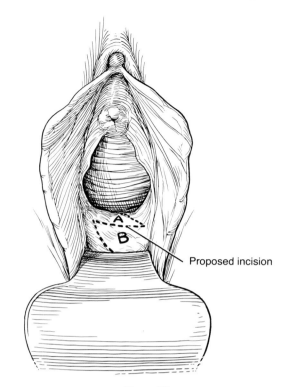

Proposed incision

Figure 58

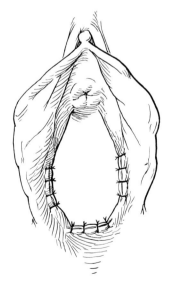

Figure 57
Transverse suture lines.

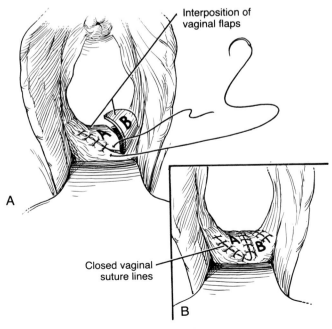

Interposition of vaginal flaps

Closed vaginal suture lines

Figure 59

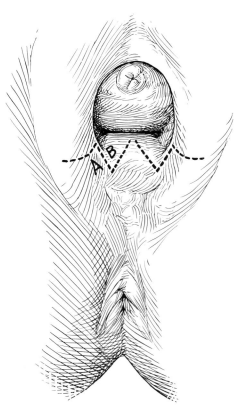

Figure 60

Transverse Z-plasty

An alternative approach is to make the Z-plasty on either side of the introital opening. This technique results in the absence of the suture line in the midline, and the increase in the introital diameter results from a duplication of the flaps at the 4- and 8-o'clock positions of the introitus (Fig. 60).

The incisions are cut into the subhymenal band for a distance of about 2 to 3 cm into the vaginal mucosa and onto the skin of the fossa navicularis. The tissues are mobilized and the subcutaneous tissues are approximated with several fine absorbable sutures, and the mucosa is closed with vertical mattress stitches of 4–0 delayed absorbable suture on a cutting needle. Care must be taken to approximate the apices of the incisions to gain as much transverse diameter as possible (Fig. 61A). Occasionally, "dog ears" of the hymenal and vestibular tissues result, and these need to be rounded off with scissors and an appropriate number of absorbable sutures to produce a smooth approximation of the vagina with the perineal skin (Fig. 61B).

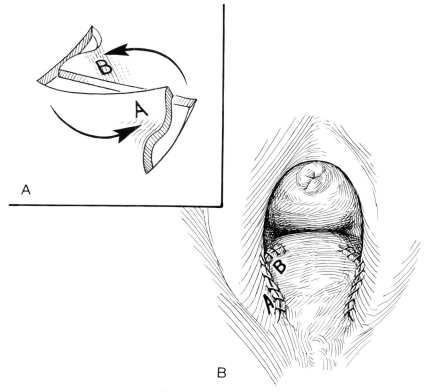

Figure 61
Transposed vaginal flaps.

Middle and Upper Vagina

Unilateral Flap

A lateral stricture of the vagina may result from a faulty posterior colpoperineorrhaphy (at the time of vaginal hysterectomy or posthysterectomy vaginal vault prolapse); this can result in a functionally short vagina and dyspareunia. Figure 62A depicts a contracture of the left side of the vagina. The stenotic opening into the upper segment of the vagina permits the passage of a small, curved forceps. Figure 62B shows this same narrowed contracture in a longitudinal view, emphasizing a thickened underlying scar and narrow canal connecting the lower with the upper vaginal segment. Figure 62C depicts the site of the incision and proposed perineal flap. Initially, with the use of a knife, the introital and vaginal extent of the scar is incised and undermined with Mayo scissors to open this portion of the contracture completely throughout the entire longitudinal length of scarred vagina. The approximate distance from the hymen to the apex of the vaginal incision is determined to aid in calculating the appropriate length of the hinged perineal flap to be developed just lateral to the labium majus on the side of the contracture (Fig. 63).

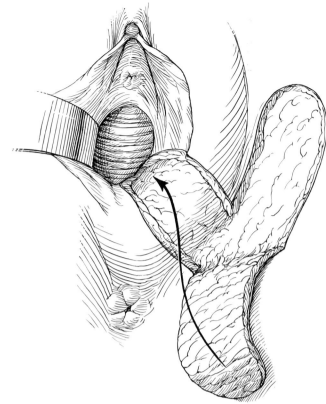

Figure 63
Mobilized vaginal wall and release of strictured vagina.

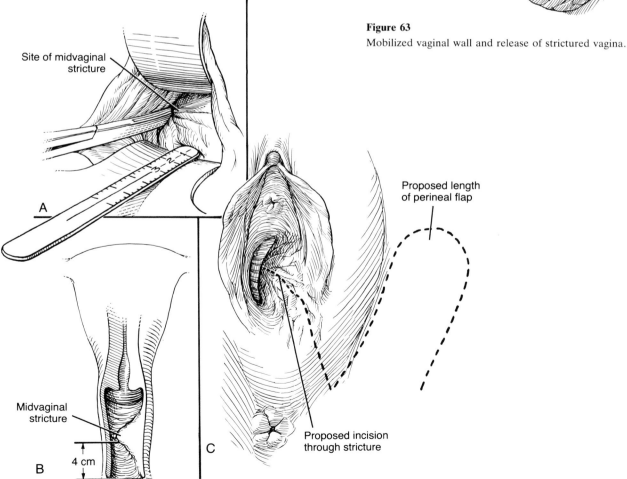

Site of midvaginal stricture

A

Midvaginal stricture

4 cm

B

C

Proposed length of perineal flap

Proposed incision through stricture

Figure 62

We prefer to make the distal end of the tongue flap round rather than pointed to avoid the potential slough of the most distal portion of the flap. We are careful to maintain the blood supply to the flap but have found that the length of the flap can be several times the width of the base. Careful hemostasis is obtained throughout the vagina, which will be the bed for the perineal flap. Not infrequently, some troublesome bleeding occurs if the lower portion of the levator muscles needs to be incised, but this can be controlled with appropriate cautery or fine-suture ligature. A small portion of the subcutaneous tissue is left on the tongue of the hinged flap, and this results in a soft pad at the site of the previous contracture (Fig. 64). With a Deaver retractor in the vagina to aid in exposure, the flap is placed, and the initial sutures inserted are those at the top of the vaginal incision. The tongue is fixed in place with fine, interrupted, vertical mattress sutures. The edges of the flap are approximated to the edges of the vagina. Care is taken to perform this step symmetrically in order to minimize distortion of the flap. A small suction catheter can be placed in the bed of the flap, and it is generally removed in 48 hours.

Bilateral Flap

Occasionally, a scar may result in contracture in the midvagina, most frequently after vaginal repair for vault prolapse or posterior colpoperineorrhaphy as part of a vaginal hysterectomy and repair. The resultant restriction produces a short vagina and significant dyspareunia. The approach taken is a vaginal incision through the point of the contracting scar, similar to that described for a unilateral flap, but it is performed bilaterally (Fig. 65). It is crucial that not only the skin of the contracture but also the underlying scar are completely incised and that the surrounding vaginal epithelium is freed in such a fashion that any remaining adhesion cannot be identified.

Both vaginal incisions are extended vertically through the entire length of the scar, and the underlying tissues are freed (Fig. 66), after which meticulous hemostasis is obtained. Once the vaginal incision and the bed are prepared, the flap is developed; the vaginal defect is then measured to determine the necessary length and width of the perineal flap. When making the perineal incision, we develop the flap

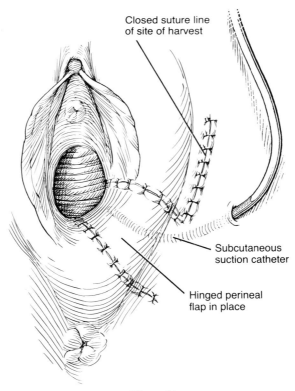

Closed suture line of site of harvest

Subcutaneous suction catheter

Hinged perineal flap in place

Figure 64

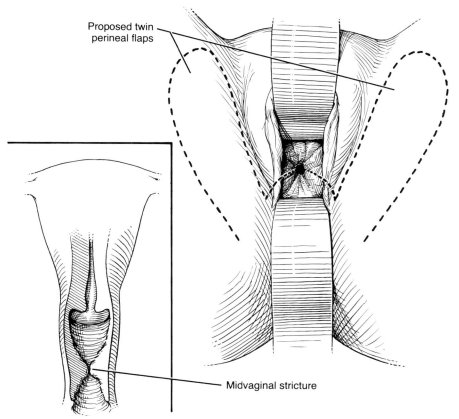

Proposed twin
perineal flaps

Midvaginal stricture

Figure 65

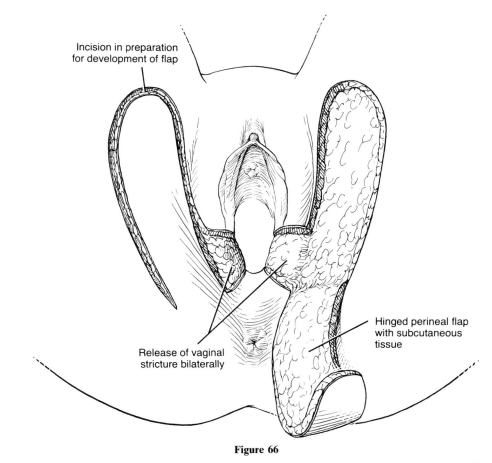

Incision in preparation
for development of flap

Release of vaginal
stricture bilaterally

Hinged perineal flap
with subcutaneous
tissue

Figure 66

43

approximately 1 cm longer than the vaginal incision to ensure that there will not be any tension on the longitudinal length of the flap.

The flap is then secured in position with 3–0 vertical mattress sutures that are placed first at the apex of the vagina and then on both edges of the flap to ensure symmetric placement. Beneath each flap, a suction catheter is run just short of the apex of the flap and is brought out on the perineum high enough so that the patient can sit in a chair and yet not sit on the drains or bend the catheters (Fig. 67). These are customarily removed in 48 hours. The resultant vagina and introitus should be of adequate diameter and totally free of any contracting band or scar.

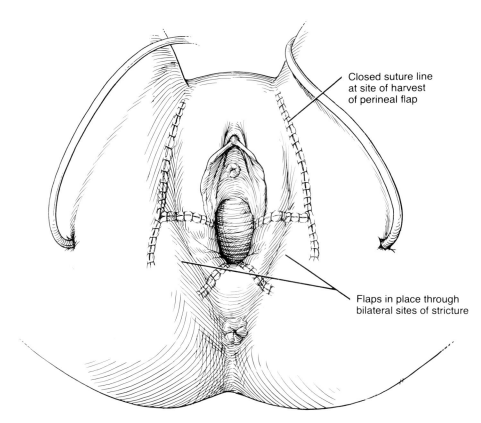

Closed suture line at site of harvest of perineal flap

Flaps in place through bilateral sites of stricture

Figure 67

Obliteration of the Vagina

Skin Graft Repair

Less common than stricture, but occurring with seemingly greater frequency, is the loss of the total length of the vagina except the distal 2 to 3 cm. This customarily occurs after vaginal hysterectomy and repair or after repair of posthysterectomy vaginal vault prolapse. The ruler in place in Figure 68 shows a vagina of 2 cm in depth, and the stippled line indicates the approximate area where the incision is made to develop the space for future reconstruction of the vagina.

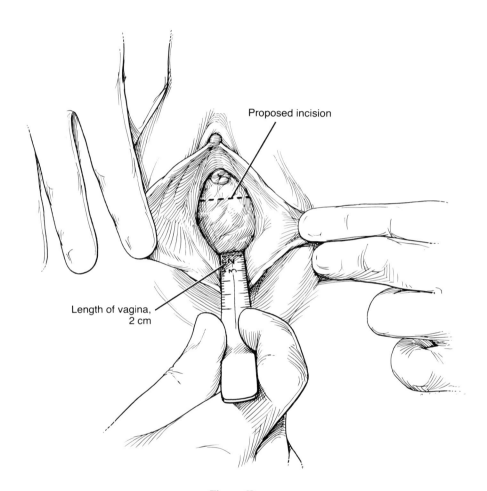

Proposed incision

Length of vagina, 2 cm

Figure 68

With the surgeon's left index finger in the rectum, traction is applied to the posterior vaginal wall, countertraction is applied on the upper edge of the vaginal incision, and sharp dissection proceeds with a Mayo scissors (Fig. 69A); space is developed by keeping the dissection immediately adjacent to the anterior wall of the rectum. Figure 69B shows the proper line of dissection and the proximity of it to the urethra, the bladder, and the rectum. Because of this, there is a risk of injury to these structures.

With continued traction on the cut edge of the vaginal lining and countertraction applied with the finger in the rectum, the proper line of dissection is immediately adjacent to the longitudinal fibers of the rectum (Fig. 70A). The Deaver retractor is used to elevate the urethra and the base of the bladder superiorly, and appropriate traction is applied on the rectum posteriorly to provide countertraction and aid in the maintenance of the proper line of dissection separating the base of the bladder from the lower rectal canal (Fig. 70B). The dissection is continued in the cephalad direction until the peritoneum of the back

of the bladder or the anterior surface of the sigmoid colon is encountered.

In Figure 71A, the space developed was 10 cm long. If hemostasis is adequate, a skin graft is harvested from the buttocks and placed over a condom-covered sponge-rubber mold. This phase of the operative procedure is the same as that used for agenesis of the vagina. However, frequently the dissection is associated with less than perfect hemostasis, and there is diffuse oozing from the muscular fibers of the anterior rectal wall or connective tissue beneath the base of the urethra, the bladder neck, and the bladder. Under these circumstances, we place a vaginal pack in the developed space (Fig. 71B). After 24 to 48 hours the patient is returned to the operating room, the pack is removed, and the vagina is inspected and irrigated. If hemostasis is adequate, we proceed with placement of a skin graft. We follow the same procedure as described for placement of the skin graft for agenesis of the vagina, fixing the graft in place by suturing the labia and underlying muscle with 0 delayed absorbable sutures.

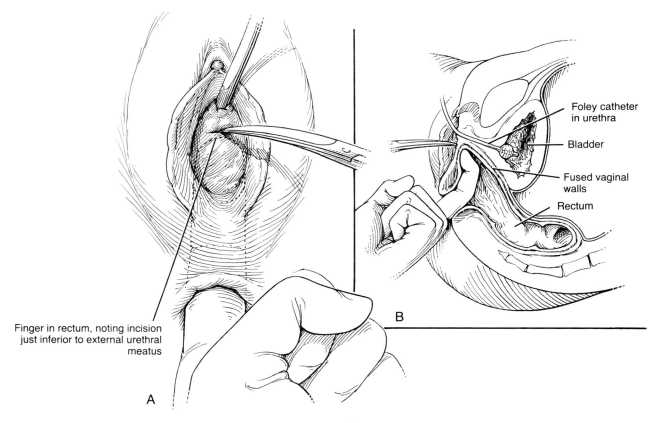

Finger in rectum, noting incision just inferior to external urethral meatus

A

Foley catheter in urethra

Bladder

Fused vaginal walls

Rectum

B

Figure 69

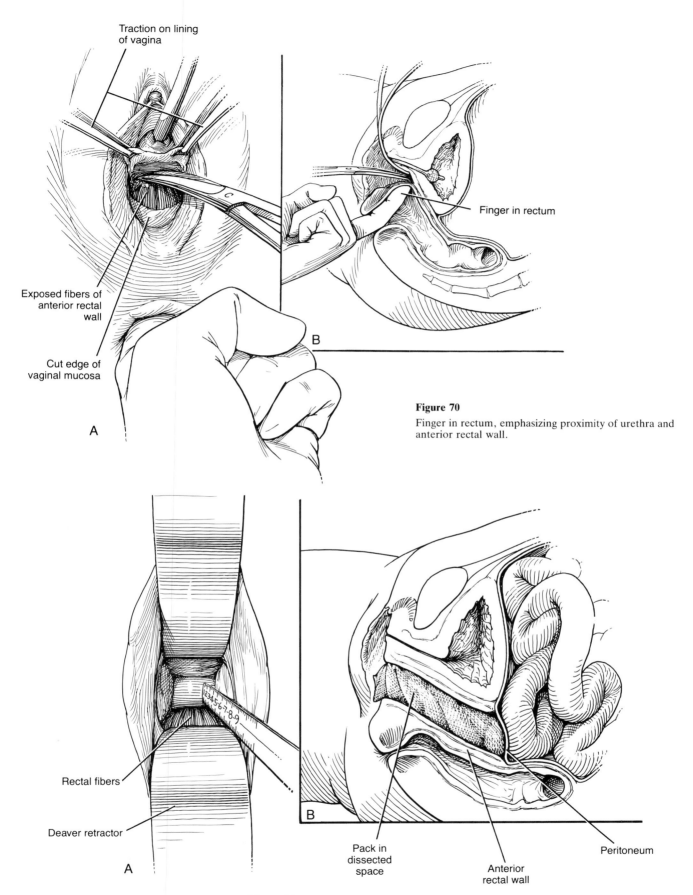

Traction on lining
of vagina

Exposed fibers of
anterior rectal
wall

Cut edge of
vaginal mucosa

A

B

Finger in rectum

Figure 70

Finger in rectum, emphasizing proximity of urethra and
anterior rectal wall.

Rectal fibers

Deaver retractor

A

B

Pack in
dissected
space

Anterior
rectal wall

Peritoneum

Figure 71

Dissected space of appropriate length *(A)*.

Skin Graft Repair with Omentum

An alternative approach is to use the omentum to line the developed space. The dissection to develop the space is the same as that already described. A pack is then placed in the space created between the anterior wall of the rectum, the posterior wall of the urethra and bladder, and the lateral levator muscles. Through a lower midline incision (Fig. 72A), the omentum is freed from the transverse colon, and its right side is left attached for appropriate blood supply (Fig. 72B). The resultant apron of omentum is then developed in a tube-like fashion (Fig. 72C) and sutured to the peritoneum at the back of the bladder along the right pelvic side wall, in front of the sigmoid

peritoneum posteriorly, about the previously placed pack (Fig. 73). This omentum serves as a housing and provides blood for the skin graft that will be placed to create the new vagina.

Careful hemostasis must be accomplished as the omentum is sutured about the pack, and care must be taken to ensure that the pack is not included in the suture line.

The tubular-shaped omentum pedicle is thus created (Fig. 74), and no attempt is made to fix it in place. Because the sigmoid colon fills the left side of the pelvis, the small bowel is prevented from becoming fixed and potentially obstructed deep in the pelvis.

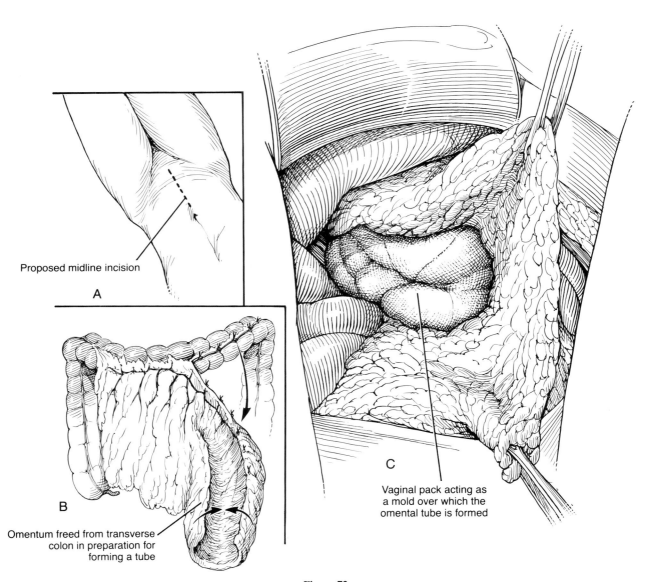

Proposed midline incision

A

B

Omentum freed from transverse
colon in preparation for
forming a tube

C

Vaginal pack acting as
a mold over which the
omental tube is formed

Figure 72

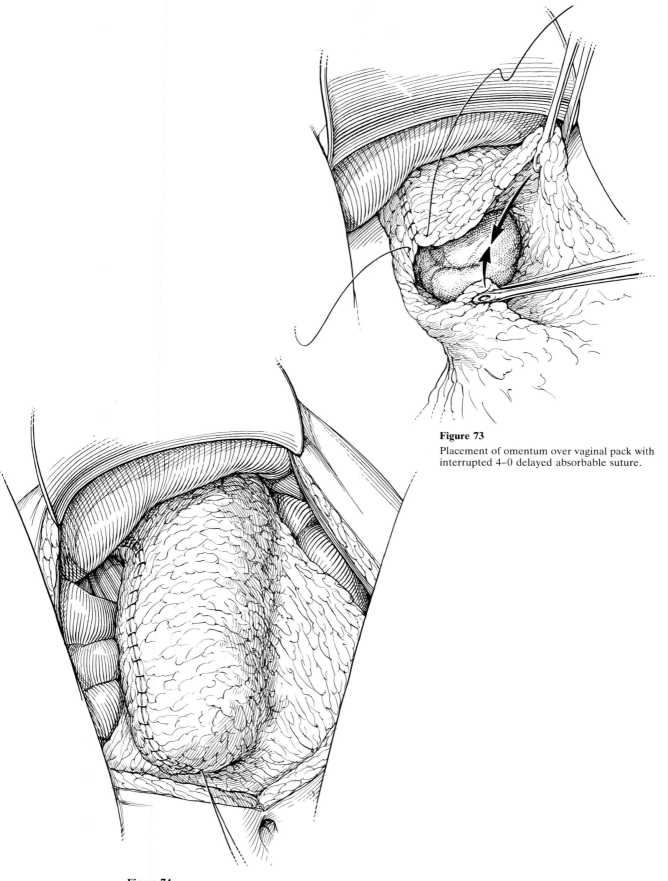

Figure 73
Placement of omentum over vaginal pack with interrupted 4–0 delayed absorbable suture.

Figure 74
Pack covered with tube of omentum.

If hemostasis is adequate, the third step of the procedure—that of placing the skin-covered sponge-rubber mold in the space—can be accomplished (Fig. 75). On occasion, we delay this step for 48 hours, at which time the patient is brought back to the operating room and skin is harvested from the buttocks, much as is done in the McIndoe procedure described on page 26. The pack is removed, and the space is irrigated and carefully inspected to ensure that adequate hemostasis has been obtained. The full length of the skin-covered sponge-rubber mold is then inserted as described for the McIndoe procedure (Fig. 76).

Eight to ten days later, the patient is returned to the operating room; the sponge-rubber mold is carefully removed, the vagina is irrigated and inspected, and a polyethylene mold covered with an antibiotic cream is inserted (Fig. 77). Twice a day this mold is removed, washed with soap and water, carefully dried, coated with antibiotic cream, and reinserted. Sexual relations can be reestablished 2 months after operation. When properly accomplished, this technique has been remarkably successful, resulting in a vagina of excellent depth, diameter, and pliability.

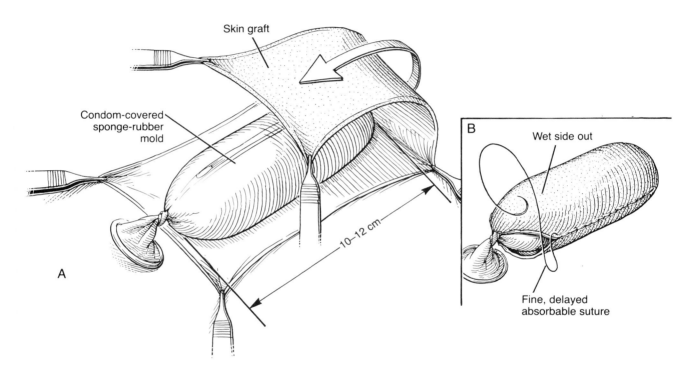

Figure 75

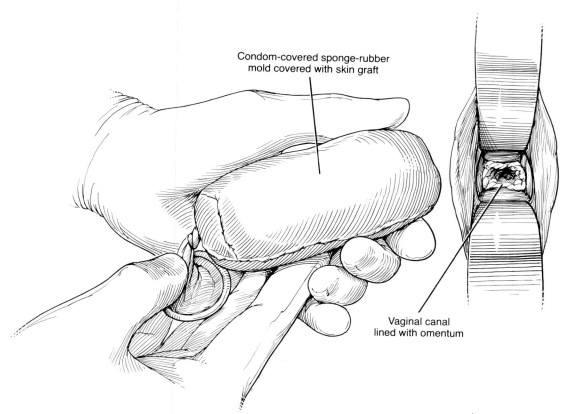

Condom-covered sponge-rubber
mold covered with skin graft

Vaginal canal
lined with omentum

Figure 76

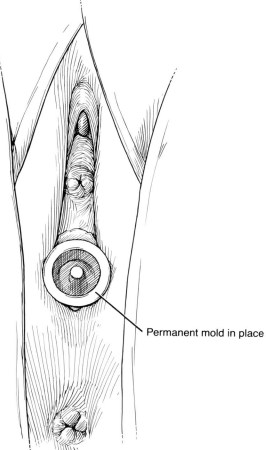

Permanent mold in place

Figure 77

Colon Replacement

Stricture and obliteration of the vagina usually develop after a combination of operation and radiation; they result in an extremely thick and firm scar of the introitus and entire vaginal length. The thick, white scar-laden tissue has a blood supply that is equally compromised, and it does not lend itself readily to the placement of a skin graft. Under these circumstances, we have used the sigmoid colon to replace the vagina. The introitus is an extremely thick band of cicatricial scar that requires bilateral Schuchardt-type incisions, generally carried out at the 4- and 8-o'clock positions (Fig. 78). These long and deep incisions are required to provide the space that will accept the sigmoid colon with its mesentery.

Once the perineal phase has been accomplished (extreme care is necessary to obtain hemostasis), the abdomen is opened through a lower midline incision, and the mesentery of the sigmoid is transilluminated to be sure that the segment of sigmoid that is to be the future vagina has an adequate blood supply (Fig. 79). Figure 80, a lateral view, depicts the approximate location of the sigmoid that will serve as the vagina. After the branches of the superior hemorrhoidal artery have been divided, the cleavage plane can be developed posterior to the rectum to free it from the hollow of the sacrum.

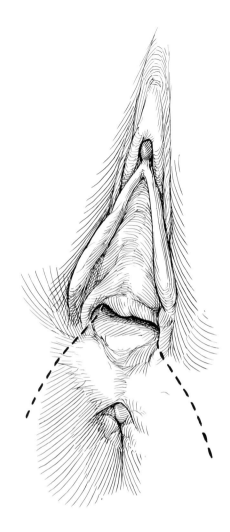

Figure 78
Proposed perineal incisions (dashed lines) for contracted introitus resulting from radiation.

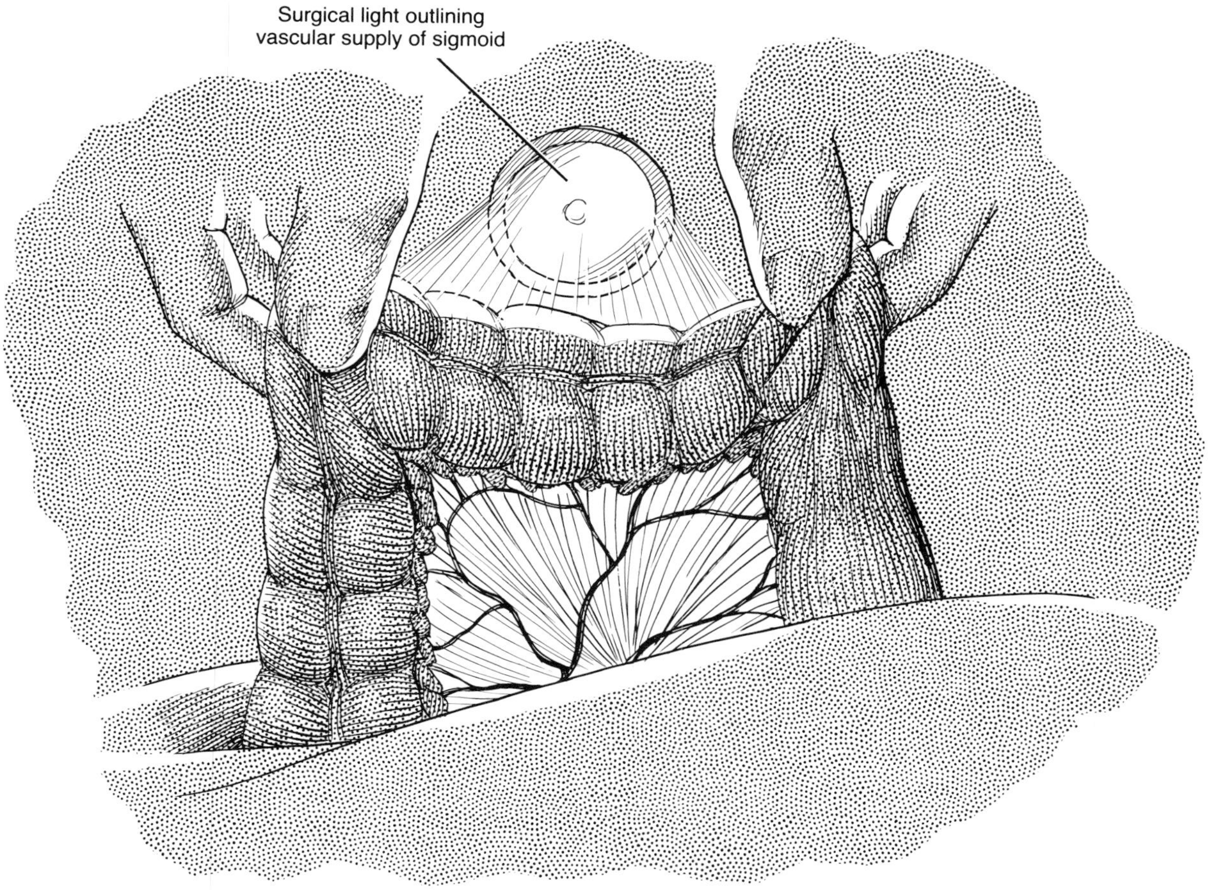

Surgical light outlining
vascular supply of sigmoid

Figure 79

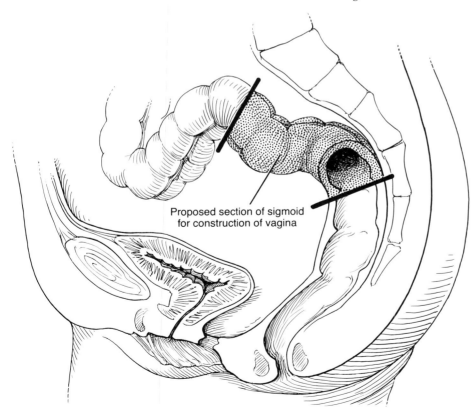

Proposed section of sigmoid
for construction of vagina

Figure 80

The sigmoid is transected 5 to 10 cm from its distal end, and care is taken to preserve the arterial and venous blood supply (Fig. 81A). An end-to-end anastomosis is accomplished from the superior edge of the mobilized rectum to the sigmoid (sigmoidal rec-

tostomy) with an inner layer of 3–0 delayed absorbable suture and an outer layer of interrupted 3–0 silk suture. The isolated segment of sigmoid with its mesentery lies parallel and reverse to the sigmoid (Fig. 81B). The sigmoid vagina is situated anterior to

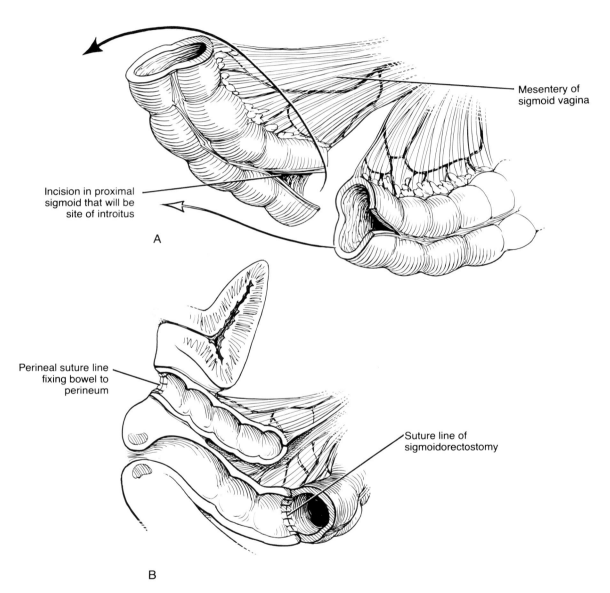

Mesentery of
sigmoid vagina

Incision in proximal
sigmoid that will be
site of introitus

A

Perineal suture line
fixing bowel to
perineum

Suture line of
sigmoidorectostomy

B

Figure 81

the sigmoidal rectal anastomosis (Fig. 82). The proximal end of the isolated segment is carried down to the introitus, where it is fixed in place with multiple interrupted 3–0 delayed absorbable sutures. The distal end of the segment of sigmoid that forms the apex of the new vagina is inverted with a single row of vertical mattress sutures with 3–0 delayed absorbable suture.

We prefer to place a large suction drain in the pelvis close to but not touching the colon anastomosis; it is brought out through a stab wound lateral to the midline incision and is customarily left in place for 4 to 6 days. The pelvis is cleanly reperitonealized, and everything except the inner end of the new vagina is retroperitoneal.

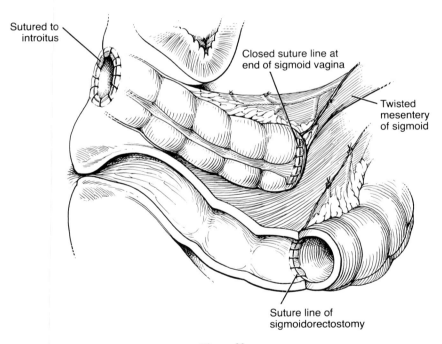

Sutured to introitus

Closed suture line at end of sigmoid vagina

Twisted mesentery of sigmoid

Suture line of sigmoidorectostomy

Figure 82

Gartner's Duct Cyst

Most wolffian duct cysts of the genital tract are related to the fallopian tube, ovary, uterus, broad ligaments, cervix, vagina, and vulva. Cystic tumors can appear anywhere along the embryonic distribution of the wolffian duct. Rarely, a Gartner duct cyst communicates with a ureter connected to a small, dysplastic, nonfunctioning kidney. In some cases, an ectopic ureter is dilated and may deform the vagina from one side, a finding suggesting a vaginal wall mass. The ectopic ureter must also be differentiated from a ureterocele, cystocele, and urethral diverticulum.

If a Gartner duct cyst in the vagina is small and asymptomatic, no treatment is indicated; however, large cysts are usually best excised by a vaginal approach. If the cyst is particularly large (sometimes elevating the base of the bladder and displacing the ureter or extending into the broad ligament), an abdominal approach may be indicated. An alternative procedure with a large Gartner duct cyst is marsupialization of the cyst from its vaginal surface into the vagina. The cyst in Figure 83 is relatively small, and an excision is performed. Figure 83A shows the proposed incision over a Gartner duct cyst located in the left vaginal fornix. Figure 83B shows the relative

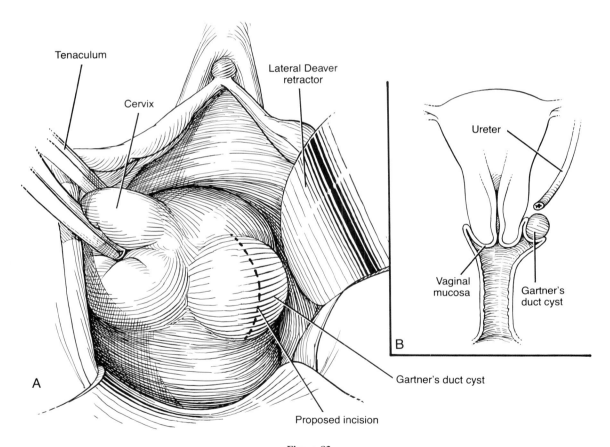

Figure 83

locations of the cervix, left vaginal fornix, Gartner's duct cyst, and left ureter. With countertraction on the vaginal wall and traction applied to the wall of the cyst, the adhesive connections between the cyst and the vagina are sharply divided (Fig. 84A). The

cyst is excised intact, and the suture line is closed with a single layer of interrupted 4–0 delayed absorbable suture incorporating a small portion of the underlying supportive tissues (Fig. 84B). The proximity of the ureter should always be kept in mind.

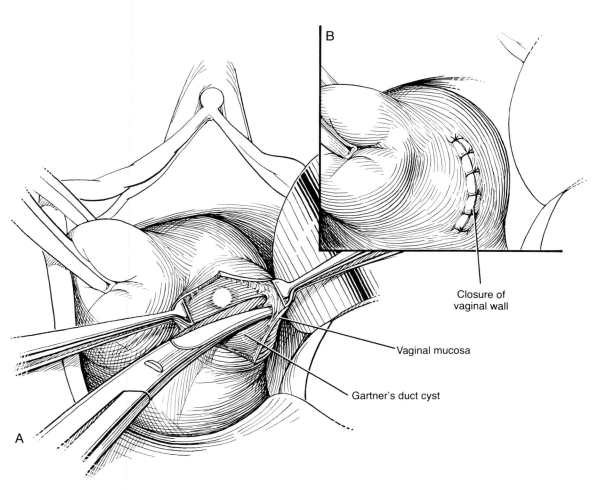

Closure of
vaginal wall

Vaginal mucosa

Gartner's duct cyst

Figure 84

Partial Excision of the Vagina

Focal areas of carcinoma in situ of the vagina may be treated by several different methods. For patients in whom partial excision is preferable, we have found it advantageous to use Schiller stain in addition to colposcopically directed biopsies to outline the area of involvement. Once this area is identified, an incision is made, generally in the 3-o'clock position, through the full thickness of the vaginal lining to ensure that the rim is adequate to provide for histologic confirmation of clearance of the underlying in situ lesion.

In Figure 85, after colposcopic examination, Schiller staining shows the involved (nonstaining) area at the apex of the vagina in a patient who had previously undergone hysterectomy for a similar lesion in the cervix.

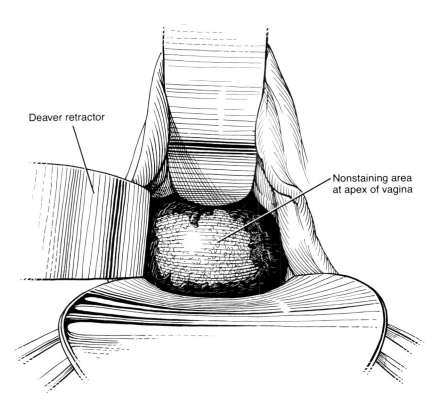

Deaver retractor

Nonstaining area at apex of vagina

Figure 85

In Figure 86*A*, forceps traction on the cut edge of the vaginal wall and countertraction on the normal vagina assist in sharp dissection of the vaginal wall from the underlying tissue. Figure 86*B* shows a simple single-layered closure including the lining of the vagina and underlying supporting tissues to ensure adequate hemostasis and prevent any dead space and fluid collection.

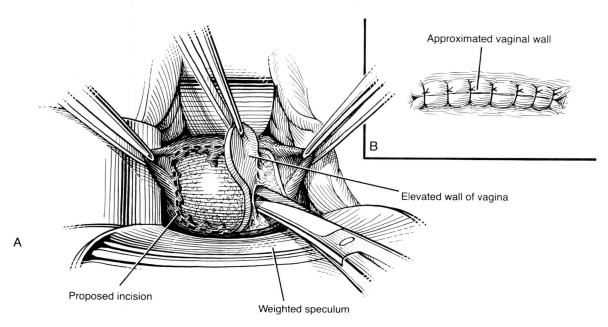

Approximated vaginal wall

B

Elevated wall of vagina

A

Proposed incision

Weighted speculum

Figure 86

Total Excision of the Vagina

Patients with multicentric areas of in situ carcinoma of the vagina may require a total vaginectomy.

An initial incision is made just inside the introitus (Fig. 87*A*), and the vaginal wall is incised, with a broad Allis forceps providing traction on the vaginal wall. Countertraction is applied to the wall of the vagina to facilitate dissection (Fig. 87*B*).

The surgeon may find it advantageous to insert the index finger in the vagina and hold the Allis forceps with the left hand and thus provide constant traction, which aids in maintaining accurate dissection and minimizing blood loss. The dissection is continued in a circumferential fashion all the way to the apex of the vagina (Fig. 88). Care must be taken that the corners of the vagina are completely excised and that

no "button" of tissue is inadvertently left that later could develop into invasive disease.

Once the entire vaginal lining has been removed, careful and complete hemostasis must be accomplished with cautery and the use of fine interrupted absorbable sutures (Fig. 89*A*). If function of the vagina is unnecessary, a vaginal pack can be inserted after the vaginectomy to aid in hemostasis. If a functional vagina is desirable and excellent hemostasis has been obtained, we obtain a split-thickness skin graft (Fig. 89*B*) and apply it over a condom-covered sponge-rubber mold, as is done for a McIndoe procedure. If there is doubt regarding hemostasis, it is preferable to leave a pack in the vagina and delay placement of the split-thickness skin graft for 1 to 2 days after the total vaginectomy. This delay ensures a dry, granulating bed for the graft and a better opportunity for full take of the skin graft.

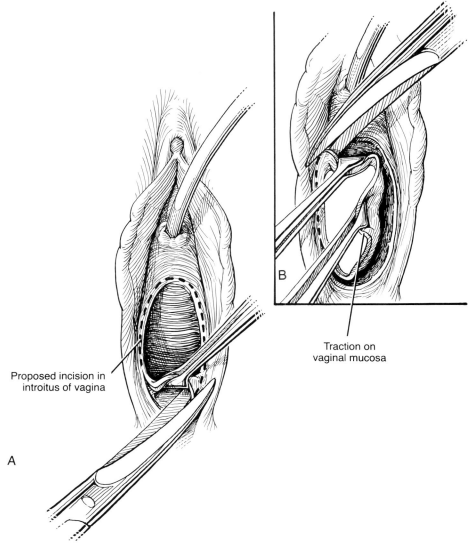

Proposed incision in
introitus of vagina

Traction on
vaginal mucosa

A

B

Figure 87

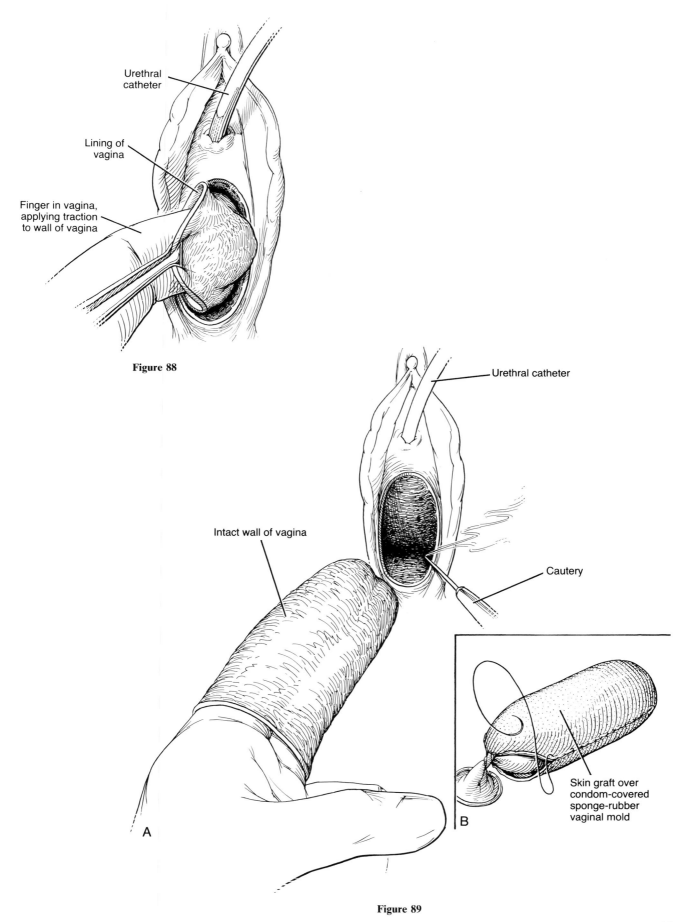

Urethral catheter

Lining of vagina

Finger in vagina, applying traction to wall of vagina

Figure 88

Urethral catheter

Intact wall of vagina

Cautery

Skin graft over condom-covered sponge-rubber vaginal mold

A

B

Figure 89

Tumor in the Rectovaginal Septum

Primary tumors of the rectovaginal septum are relatively uncommon, and their nature may be difficult to establish. Tumors in this area may arise from any of the constituent elements of the vagina, the rectum, or the rectovaginal fascia. In addition, because this area is the site of complex embryonic developments, neoplasms may be derived from embryonic remnants, congenital malformations, or misplaced tissue. The most common primary tumors in the rectovaginal septum are those of endometriosis, fibroma, or leiomyoma. Malignant tumors are usually secondary to extensions from adjacent organs such as the rectum, cervix, vagina, or vulva. Primary adenocarcinoma of the rectovaginal septum may arise from endometriosis

in the septum. Less commonly, leiomyosarcoma may arise as a primary tumor in the rectovaginal septum. On rectovaginal examination, the tumor mass is easily palpated within the septum (Fig. 90).

An incision is made in a vertical direction through the vaginal mucosa overlying the mass, and the mucosa is dissected off the anterior surface of the underlying tumor (Fig. 91A). With traction applied to the tumor and countertraction on the vaginal wall, sharp dissection adjacent to the tumor mass allows for its complete excision and minimizes the potential risks of entering the lumen of the rectum. Once the mass is excised and hemostasis is established, the vaginal wall may be closed with a single layer of fine delayed absorbable sutures (Fig. 91B).

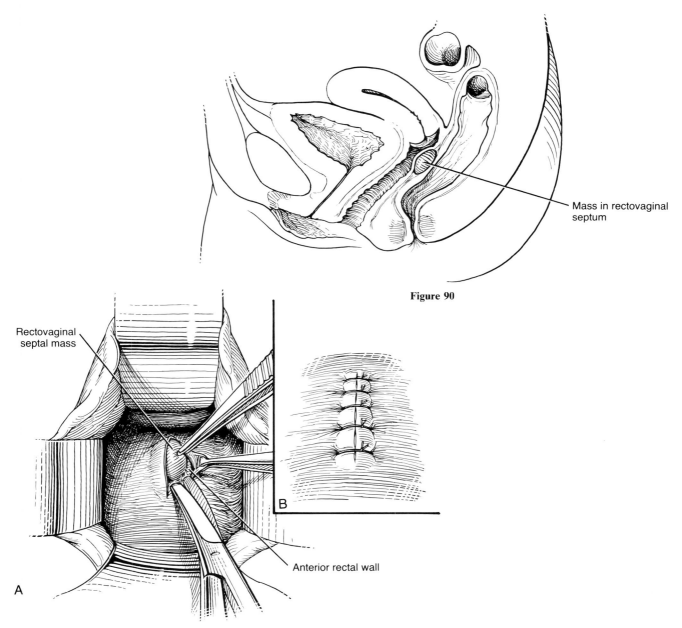

Mass in rectovaginal septum

Figure 90

Rectovaginal septal mass

Anterior rectal wall

A

B

Figure 91

Rectocele

Rectocele alone, without associated enterocele and cystocele, infrequently requires repair. Occasionally, a rectocele is large enough to protrude through the vaginal orifice. It may permit accumulation of stool, making evacuation difficult and requiring reduction of the rectocele (posterior vaginal wall) into the rectum to expedite expulsion of feces (Fig. 92). A posterior colpoperineorrhaphy will correct these symptoms.

Two tenacula (Henrotin vulsellum clamps) are appropriately placed on the right and left posterior labia (the lateral wings of the weighted speculum may produce a groove in the introitus at pressor sites), where their approximation will result in a normal-sized introitus (Fig. 93). These forceps form the base of a triangle, the apex of which is far up on the posterior wall of the vagina, to aid in correction of the entire rectocele and to exclude the presence of an enterocele.

The dissection is initiated with incision of the skin of the perineum, exposing the underlying soft tissue and perineal muscles. The width of the incision is determined by the size of the introitus and the need to preserve a functional vagina.

Traction applied to the perineal skin aids in exposing the proper plane of dissection, which is best accomplished with sharp dissection (we prefer the use of

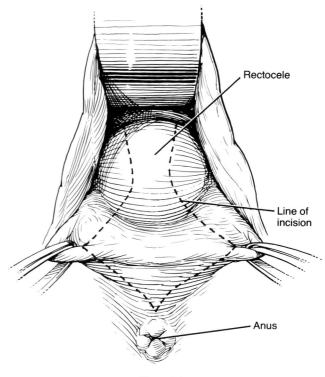

Figure 93

Mayo scissors) and freeing the rectum posteriorly from the posterior vaginal wall. Approximately 3 to 4 cm inside the introitus, the attachments in the rectovaginal space are easily separated with a spreading action of the Mayo scissors (Fig. 94).

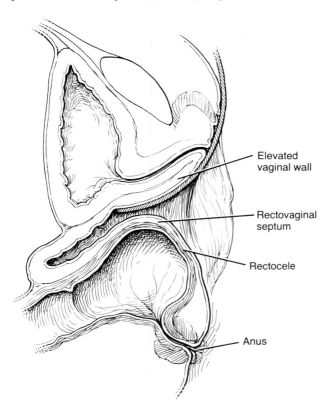

Figure 92

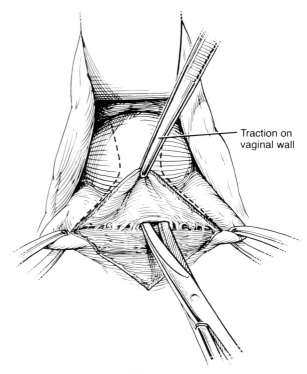

Figure 94

In an alternating manner, initially on the patient's left (Fig. 95A) and then on the patient's right (Fig. 95B), the vaginal wall is placed under appropriate traction and a symmetric and appropriate-sized strip of posterior vaginal wall is excised in a bloodless fashion. This resection is continued in the rectovaginal septum superiorly to a distance that permits complete correction of the entire rectocele. This may necessitate dissection to the posterior fornix or scar at the site of previous hysterectomy. It must be absolutely certain that there is no enterocele above what is initially interpreted as a pure rectocele.

Repair of the rectocele is begun at the apex by passing a 3–0 delayed absorbable suture through the edge of the vaginal wall and incorporating appropriate portions of the rectovaginal fascia, after which it is tied in the midline (Fig. 96). As each interrupted suture is placed, the surgeon depresses the anterior rectal wall with the left index and middle fingers, which serve as a guide in the placement of the intervening sutures in the rectovaginal fascia. As each suture is tied in the midline, the diameter of the vagina is evaluated to ensure that there is not overzealous

approximation of the fascia, which creates a tense, transverse bar with resultant narrowing that may create dyspareunia. As the vaginal wall and underlying supporting tissues are approximated, we proceed to the lower aspects of the vagina. With cephalad traction on the cut edge of the posterior vaginal wall and counterpressure on the anterior wall of the rectum, the tissues are separated off the medial and superior surfaces of the levator muscle with Mayo scissors. While this step is accomplished bilaterally, there may be some bleeding from the venous plexus about the muscle. No specific measure to control the bleeding is attempted at this point because the bleeding will subside when the levator muscles are approximated in the midline. The anterior rectal wall is depressed and pushed medially with the surgeon's left index and middle fingers (Fig. 97A) to expose the medial edge of the levator muscle. This maneuver permits an appropriately deep placement of monofilament, delayed absorbable suture through the muscle but protects the anterior rectal wall and thus prevents placement of the suture into the rectal lumen (Fig. 97B).

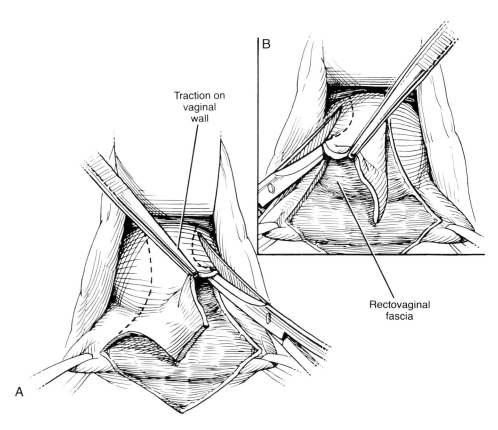

Traction on vaginal wall

Rectovaginal fascia

Figure 95

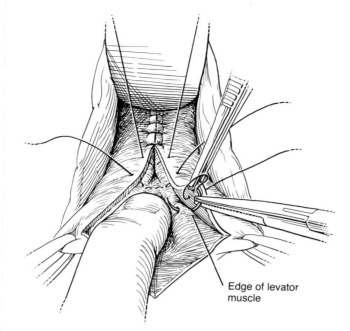

Figure 96

Single-layer closure of lining of vagina and underlying rectovaginal fascia.

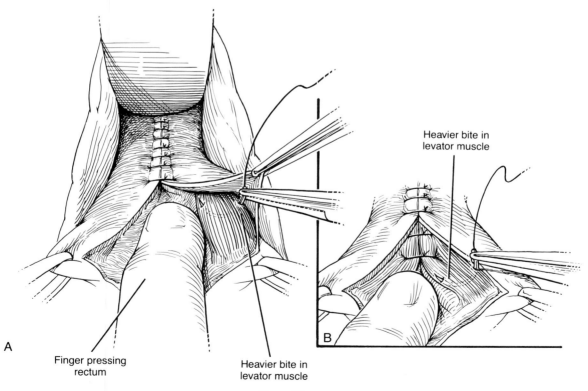

Figure 97

After placement of the suture through the medial edge of the left levator muscle, the intervening rectovaginal fascia is incorporated with this same suture, which is then passed through the medial edge of the right levator muscle as the surgeon depresses the anterior rectal wall down and to the patient's left. Again, the aperture of the vaginal introitus is evaluated to ensure that appropriate support has been developed without adversely compromising the vaginal diameter. If the approximation of the levator muscles is too high and tight, a transverse bar or ridge may result in dyspareunia. After placement of two to four sutures in the levator muscles, the edges of the vagina are approximated (over the muscle) in the midline with interrupted 4–0 delayed absorbable suture, each suture incorporating a small portion of the underlying levator muscle to avoid any dead space (Fig. 98*A*).

A perineorrhaphy is then accomplished in a similar fashion with approximation of the perineal muscles and subcuticular closure of the skin (Fig. 98*B*), the

surgeon again being careful that this does not compromise the vaginal lumen or result in a "dashboard" perineum. With appropriate retraction, the entire operative field is carefully inspected, beginning at the apex, to ensure that adequate hemostasis has been obtained. The anterior and posterior vaginal walls are carefully inspected, and if there is any evidence of significant ooze, appropriate sutures are placed.

Once hemostasis is accomplished, the anterior vaginal wall is elevated with the Deaver retractor to provide for easy insertion of a vaginal pack. We use this pack to provide some support to the repair in the event that the patient experiences any coughing or vomiting during the immediate postoperative period. It may also aid in compression to the operative sites to reduce any venous ooze. Because the vaginal pack is between two hollow organs (bladder and rectum), it cannot be so tightly packed that it would significantly alter bleeding from a sizable arterial vessel. A no. 16 Foley catheter is inserted through the urethra, and the bladder is emptied and the urine inspected.

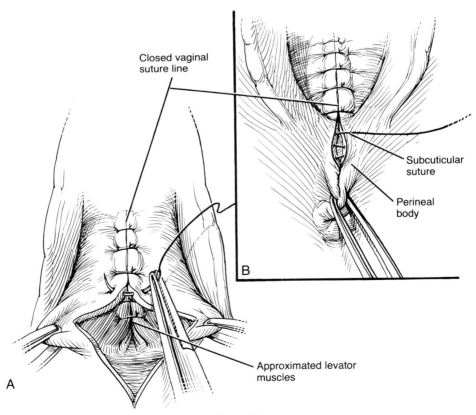

Closed vaginal suture line

Subcuticular suture

Perineal body

Approximated levator muscles

A

B

Figure 98

Repair of Enterotomy

When the posterior vaginal wall is separated in the rectovaginal space (Fig. 99A), it is possible to incise the rectal wall and create a rectostomy, which is easily recognized (Fig. 99B). In this situation, the appropriate plane is developed just superficial (closer to the vaginal wall) to the prior incision, and resection of the prescribed wedge of posterior vaginal wall proceeds. Repair of the rectocele is begun in the customary fashion at the apex of this resection and continued down to the area of the enterotomy. Completing the repair down to this area provides hemostasis (and thus visibility) for repair of the rectostomy and also indicates whether any mobilization of the posterior vaginal wall from the anterior wall of the rectum is necessary to facilitate a tension-free closure

of the rectostomy (Fig. 99C). Closure of the rectostomy is done in a vertical or transverse fashion, depending on its shape. The initial layer of sutures is placed in an extramucosal location, either running or interrupted, with 3–0 delayed absorbable suture. The initial suture line runs just distal to the edges of the rectostomy.

A second layer of sutures placed in a similar extramucosal location is placed such that when they are tied, the initial suture line is inverted (Fig. 99D). The second suture line extends just distal to the most distal sutures of the initial suture line. The posterior colpoperineorrhaphy is then accomplished in the customary fashion over the two-layer closure of the rectostomy.

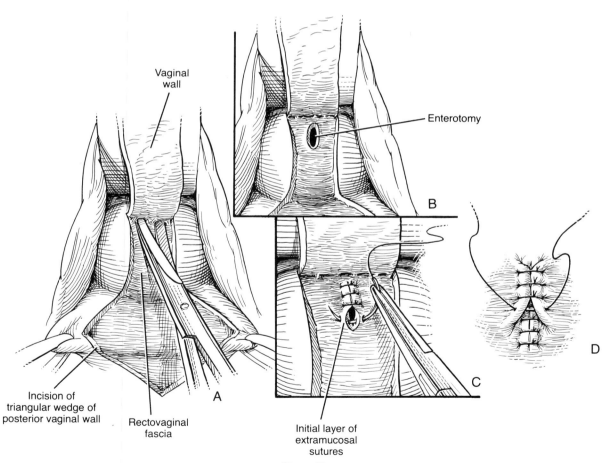

Vaginal wall

Enterotomy

Incision of triangular wedge of posterior vaginal wall

Rectovaginal fascia

Initial layer of extramucosal sutures

A

B

C

D

Figure 99

Enterocele and Rectocele

Enterocele is herniation of the pouch of Douglas in the rectovaginal septum, thus presenting as a bulging mass in the posterior fornix and upper posterior vaginal wall (Fig. 100*A*). Enterocele is usually one facet of the other associated relaxations, consisting of cystocele, rectocele, and posthysterectomy vaginal vault prolapse. Occasionally, a sizable enterocele, generally associated with a rectocele, develops behind a well-supported vaginal apex and anterior vaginal wall (Fig. 100*B*). This possibly represents a neglected or unrecognized enterocele present at the time of previous hysterectomy.

An uncommon variation of simple enterocele is the combination of an enterocele in the vagina with a sliding prolapse of the anterior rectal wall (Fig. 100*C*). This develops from intra-abdominal pressure exerting a force on the anterior wall of the rectum, which results in eversion of the anterior rectal wall. The patient frequently complains of obstipation (partial obstruction) with prolapse of a mass out of the rectum (rectal enterocele) and vagina (vaginal enterocele). This condition can be demonstrated by examining the standing patient during a Valsalva maneuver.

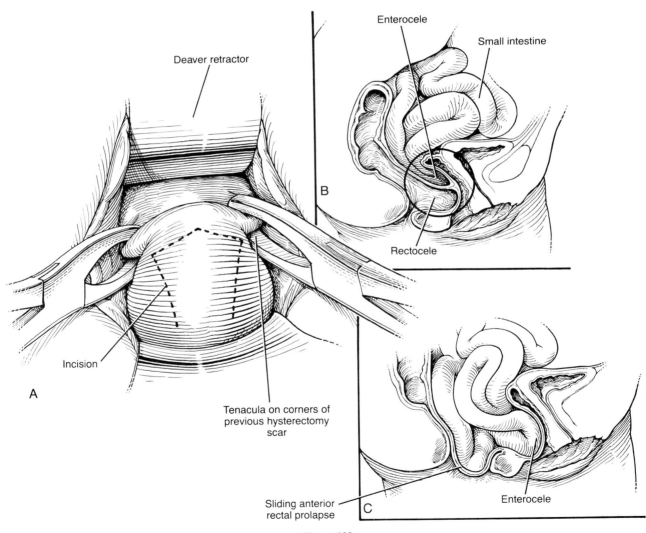

Figure 100

At operation the surgeon may insert a finger in the pouch of Douglas and evert the anterior rectal wall (Fig. 101). We expect that a rectal enterocele is more common than generally appreciated because the rec- tal wall prolapse remains hidden behind a snug anal sphincter. Correction of the enterocele, as will be demonstrated, corrects the rectal and vaginal pro- lapse.

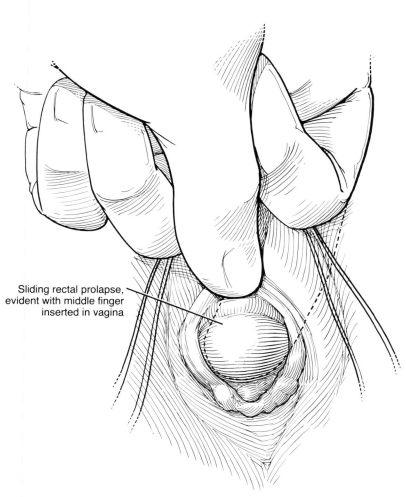

Sliding rectal prolapse, evident with middle finger inserted in vagina

Figure 101

The basic principles used for correction of posthysterectomy vaginal vault prolapse apply to correction of this simpler form of vaginal prolapse. Tenacula are placed on the corners of the previous hysterectomy scar, which is well supported high in the vagina (Fig. 100*A*). A transverse incision is made through the vaginal mucosa behind the hysterectomy scar, and the appropriate-sized wedge of posterior vagina (determined by the size of the enterocele and the need for a functional vagina) is reflected inferiorly and placed under the tongue of the weighted speculum (Fig. 102). A Deaver retractor is used to elevate the bladder superiorly (to provide countertraction on the scar), and the surgeon retracts the inferior wall of the enterocele, which is carefully entered with use of Mayo scissors (Fig. 103).

The surgeon places the index finger in the enterocele to mobilize the anterior wall of the rectum and sigmoid (Fig. 104). With sharp dissection in the proper plane, which is essentially bloodless, the longitudinal muscle fibers of the rectum and sigmoid are

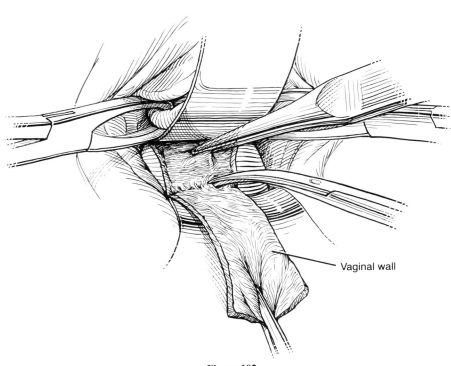

Vaginal wall

Figure 102

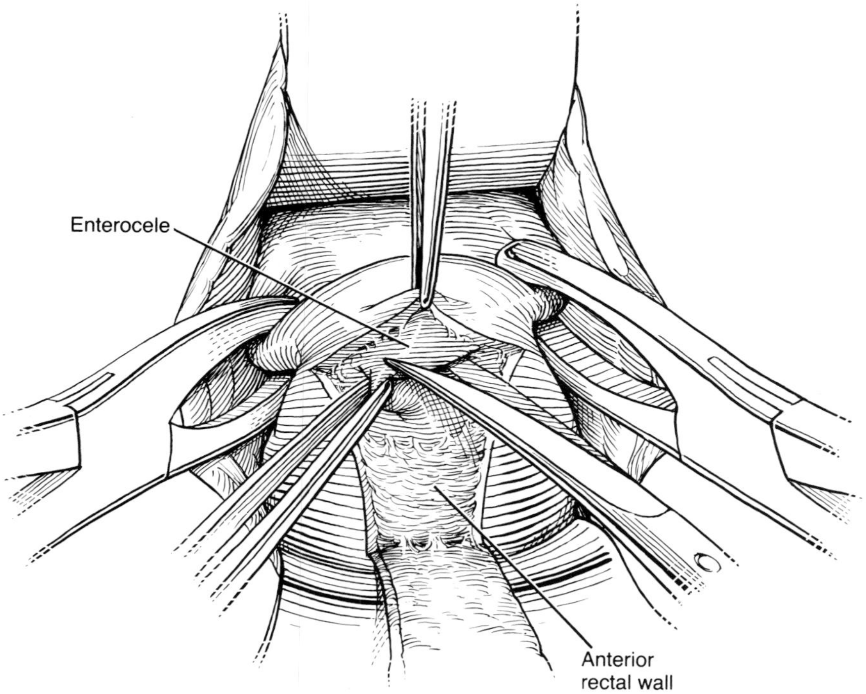

Enterocele

Anterior
rectal wall

Figure 103

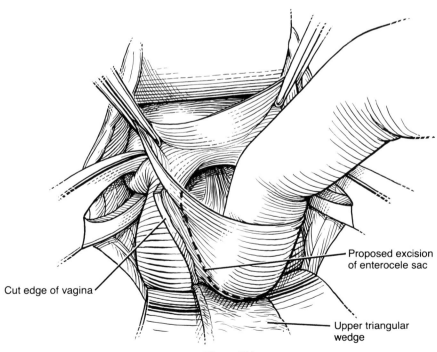

Cut edge of vagina

Proposed excision
of enterocele sac

Upper triangular
wedge

Figure 104

exposed. The redundant peritoneum is excised. Placement of the internal and external McCall sutures is described in detail on page 85. One to three internal McCall sutures are placed (Fig. 105*A* and *B*); when tied, they pull the uterosacral and vaginosacral ligaments and pararectal fascia across the midline, obliterating the pouch of Douglas. One to three external McCall sutures are placed, starting through the vagina, in a similar fashion (Fig. 105*C*), after which the pelvis is reperitonealized at a level superior to all sutures previously placed. This reperitonealizing suture is also brought out through the edges of the posterior vaginal wall created by the reflected wedge of posterior vagina. The reperitonealizing and McCall sutures are tied in the reverse order in which they were placed; this method obliterates the posterior cul-de-sac and creates a thick bar of supporting tissues to prevent recurrence of the enterocele. The apex of the vault is closed in a transverse fashion, after which a vaginal sponge is inserted in the apex and a Deaver retractor is applied to the sponge to elevate the vagina.

The perineorrhaphy is then begun, and the wedge of posterior vagina is separated from the underlying rectovaginal fascia in the same fashion in which a posterior colpoperineorrhaphy is accomplished for treatment of rectocele. The incision is continued in the superior direction until it meets the upper triangular wedge of posterior vagina, which has been under the weighted speculum (Fig. 106). The posterior colpoperineorrhaphy is then accomplished in the same manner described for rectocele.

With 3–0 delayed absorbable suture, the edges of the vaginal wall and the underlying rectovaginal fascia are closed with a single layer of interrupted suture (Fig. 107). As each suture is tied in the midline, the diameter of the vagina is evaluated to be sure that there will be adequate room for vaginal function. At the appropriate level, the underlying levator muscle is approximated as a separate layer, after which the overlying vaginal mucosa is closed with interrupted sutures (Fig. 108). Again, the aperture of the vaginal

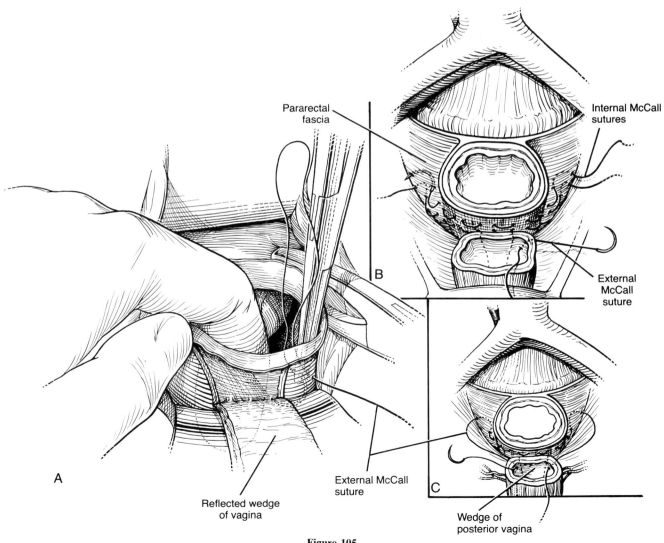

Pararectal fascia

Internal McCall sutures

External McCall suture

B

Reflected wedge of vagina

External McCall suture

A

C

Wedge of posterior vagina

Figure 105

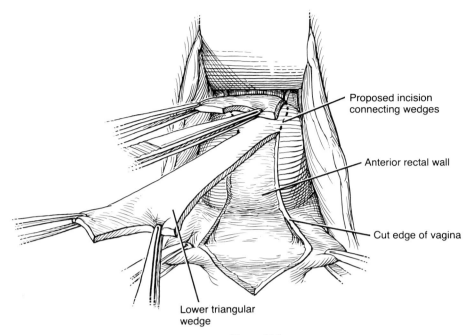

Proposed incision
connecting wedges

Anterior rectal wall

Cut edge of vagina

Lower triangular
wedge

Figure 106

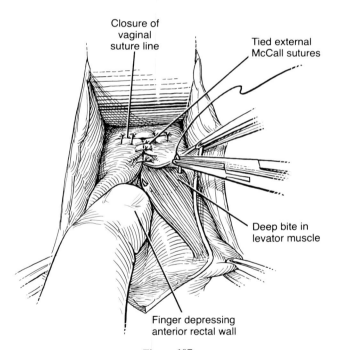

Closure of
vaginal
suture line

Tied external
McCall sutures

Deep bite in
levator muscle

Finger depressing
anterior rectal wall

Figure 107

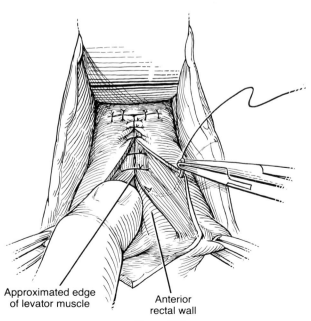

Approximated edge
of levator muscle

Anterior
rectal wall

Figure 108

canal is evaluated to ensure that appropriate support has been developed without adversely compromising the vaginal diameter. The procedure is continued in an inferior fashion with increasingly larger portions of the levator muscle approximated as the introitus is approached (Fig. 109). At completion, it is apparent that the apex of the vagina is well supported and that the patulous diameter of the vagina is corrected with excellent support from the transverse suture line all the way to the introitus (Fig. 110).

Figure 111, a lateral view, shows that the upper two thirds of the vagina is pulled far cephalad and posterior such that in the standing position the upper vagina is parallel to the floor, lying on the underlying levator plate. The suture line extends from the apex of the vagina along the posterior wall all the way to the introitus. The well-supported anterior vaginal wall and suburethral areas are not involved with the operative correction of pure enterocele-rectocele.

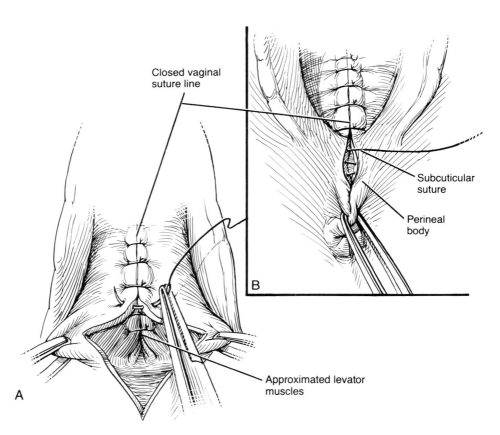

Figure 109

Closed vaginal suture line

Subcuticular suture

Perineal body

Approximated levator muscles

A

B

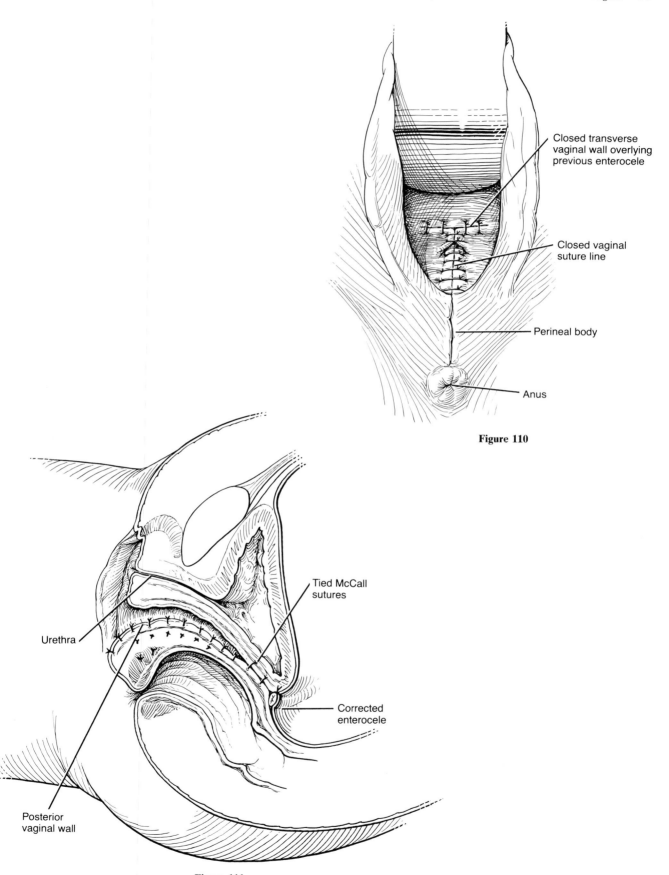

Closed transverse
vaginal wall overlying
previous enterocele

Closed vaginal
suture line

Perineal body

Anus

Figure 110

Tied McCall
sutures

Urethra

Corrected
enterocele

Posterior
vaginal wall

Figure 111

Complete Posthysterectomy Vaginal Vault Prolapse

Vaginal Repair

Prolapse of the vagina after hysterectomy remains a distressing complication for the patient and her surgeon. Hysterectomy is a common operation; as patients live longer and have more active lives, prolapse of the vagina can be expected to become more frequent. Additional factors, such as the adequacy of pelvic support before hysterectomy, the operative findings (cervical or broad ligament fibroids, presence of a potential enterocele), the hysterectomy technique, and the patient's postoperative course, in addition to specific factors of inheritance, have an influence on the development of prolapse of the vagina. The same etiologic factors resulting in uterine procidentia or prolapse of the cervical stump are also present and can result in posthysterectomy vaginal vault prolapse. We prefer to correct prolapse of the

vagina with a vaginal approach, using the same supporting tissues commonly used for repair of procidentia. The objective is to restore the vagina to its normal axis by fixing the apex back on the uterosacral (and vaginosacral) ligaments and pararectal fascia. Further, patients with advanced and generalized prolapse of this type require excision of the enterocele sac with obliteration of the posterior cul-de-sac, fixation of the vault to the pararectal fascia, and support from below by wide dissection and repair of the full length of the anterior and posterior vaginal walls and perineum. Although an overall plan for operation is needed, it is never routine but, rather, requires the surgeon to tailor the operation extemporaneously to the particular needs of the patient and the degree of pelvic relaxation.

Tenacula are placed on the corners of the old hysterectomy scar. Occasionally one corner of the vault has better support than the other; if so, the tenacula have to be adjusted by moving them superiorly or inferiorly on the corner (lateral) supporting tissues (Figs. 112*A*

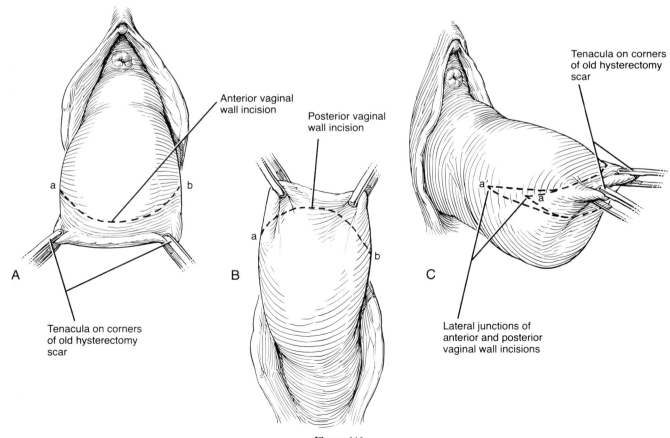

Anterior vaginal wall incision

Posterior vaginal wall incision

Tenacula on corners of old hysterectomy scar

A

B

C

Tenacula on corners of old hysterectomy scar

Lateral junctions of anterior and posterior vaginal wall incisions

Figure 112

and 113). An elliptic incision is made through the anterior vaginal mucosa (*a–b* in Figs. 112*A* and 113). A similar incision is made in the vaginal mucosa posterior to the hysterectomy scar (Fig. 112*B*). The vaginal depth is governed by the point of junction of these two incisions on the lateral wall of the vagina at the 3- and 9-o'clock positions (Fig. 112*C*) (a larger

vagina results if the corner is at *a* and *b*, and a shorter vagina results if the corners are at *a'* and *b'*) of the posterior incision. The vaginal depth can be determined by measuring the distance from the corner (*a* and *a'* or *b* and *b'*, the future corner of the apex of the vagina) to the introitus.

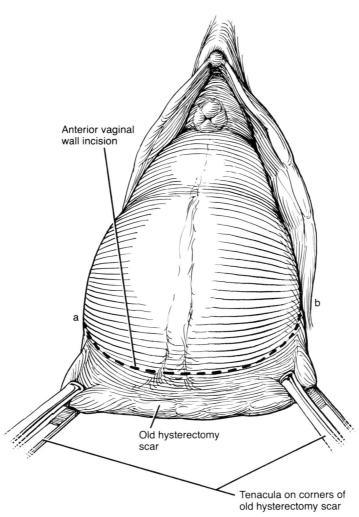

Anterior vaginal wall incision

Old hysterectomy scar

Tenacula on corners of old hysterectomy scar

Figure 113

With elevation and traction of the tenacula on the corners of the scar and countertraction on the cut edge of the posterior vaginal wall with Mayo scissors, the vagina is separated from the underlying enterocele sac and reflected off the enterocele and anterior rectal wall in order to narrow the vault and provide access to the lateral fascial supports of the vagina and the pararectal area (Fig. 114). The width of the reflected vaginal wedge is determined by the size of the prolapse and the need to preserve a functional vagina. If vaginal function is not important, this wedge may include most of the posterior vaginal wall (Fig. 115) with a similar-sized resection of the anterior vaginal wall in repair of the cystocele. This type of wedge narrows the inlet (apex) to the vagina to a tightened cone coupled with obliteration of the pouch of Douglas; it thus reduces the opportunity for development of recurrent enterocele. After the posterior vaginal wall is turned down and placed under the tongue of

the weighted speculum, the enterocele sac is entered at the appropriate location behind the old hysterectomy scar (Fig. 116). The scar usually represents the junction of the bladder anteriorly with the enterocele and the anterior rectal wall posteriorly. For this reason, we generally enter the enterocele approximately 1 cm behind the old scar, being aware that a large cystocele can be protruding behind the old transverse hysterectomy scar, which would lend itself to potential injury. Entering the enterocele sac is rarely difficult. It can be recognized by observation of its typical and obvious difference from the muscular fibers that represent the anterior rectal wall or those of the posterior wall of the bladder. The peritoneum of an enterocele sac is easy for the surgeon to palpate between the index finger and thumb; this further identifies the appropriate site at which to enter the sac.

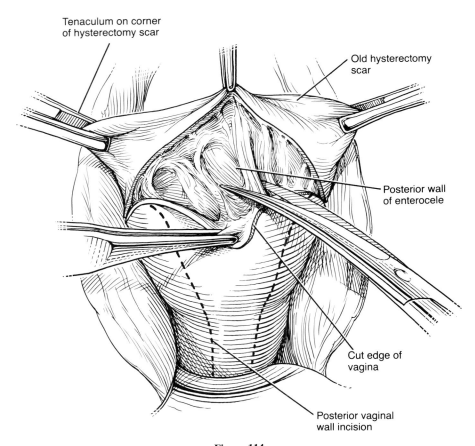

Tenaculum on corner
of hysterectomy scar

Old hysterectomy
scar

Posterior wall
of enterocele

Cut edge of
vagina

Posterior vaginal
wall incision

Figure 114

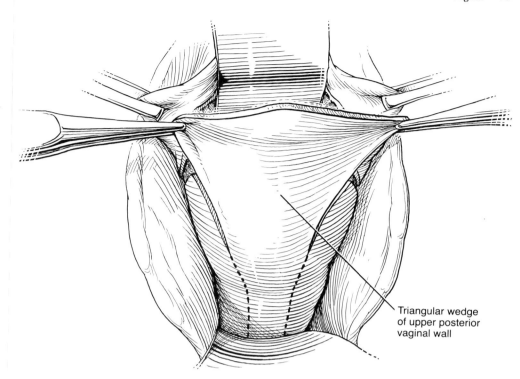

Triangular wedge
of upper posterior
vaginal wall

Figure 115

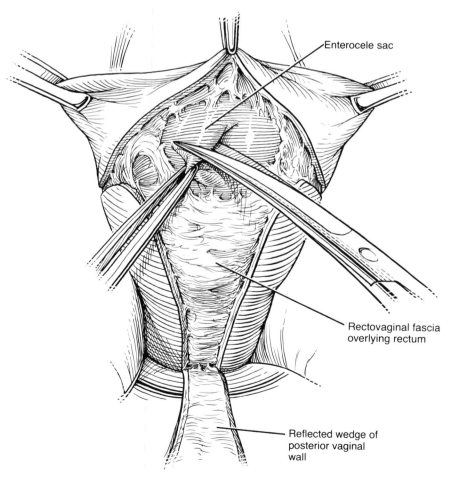

Enterocele sac

Rectovaginal fascia
overlying rectum

Reflected wedge of
posterior vaginal
wall

Figure 116

Any adhesions in the enterocele sac are freed to facilitate later resection of the peritoneum of the sac. The index finger of the surgeon's left hand is then introduced through the peritoneum of the posterior enterocele, applying traction to the peritoneum covering the posterior surface of the bladder; this technique aids in appropriate dissection as the attach-ments of the peritoneum and bladder are freed from the back of the hysterectomy scar (Fig. 117). The tissues are sharply dissected with Mayo scissors; with appropriate traction (cephalad direction) of the anterior vaginal wall, bladder, and peritoneum, the anterior cul-de-sac may be entered.

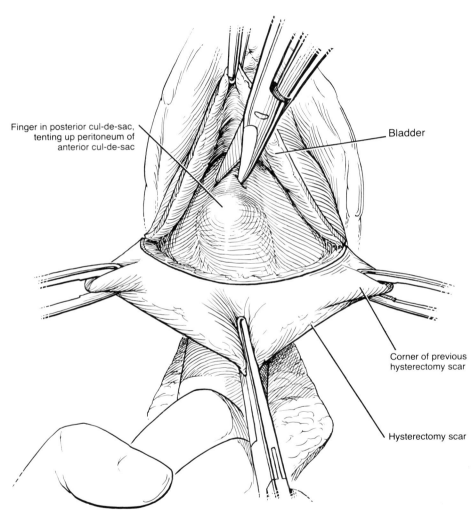

Finger in posterior cul-de-sac, tenting up peritoneum of anterior cul-de-sac

Bladder

Corner of previous hysterectomy scar

Hysterectomy scar

Figure 117

With a Deaver retractor inserted in the anterior cul-de-sac to elevate the bladder and the lower segment of the ureter and with tenacula placed on the corners of the hysterectomy scar, the attenuated remnants of the uterosacral-cardinal ligament complex are placed on tension (Fig. 118). A Deaver retractor is placed in the 3-o'clock position (patient's left vaginal fornix). The vaginal mucosa over the lateral supporting ligaments and pillar of the bladder (and lower ureter) is further mobilized (cephalad and lateral directions) by the gauze-covered right index finger of the surgeon. The ligamentous tissue thus exposed represents the most cephalad portion of the uterosacral-cardinal ligament complex remnant. The most inferior aspect (which represents the remnant of the uterosacral ligament) is clamped with a Heaney clamp (far superior) immediately adjacent to the cut edge of the vagina (Fig. 118). It is cut and tied with 2–0 delayed absorbable suture and tagged with a straight Kocher clamp.

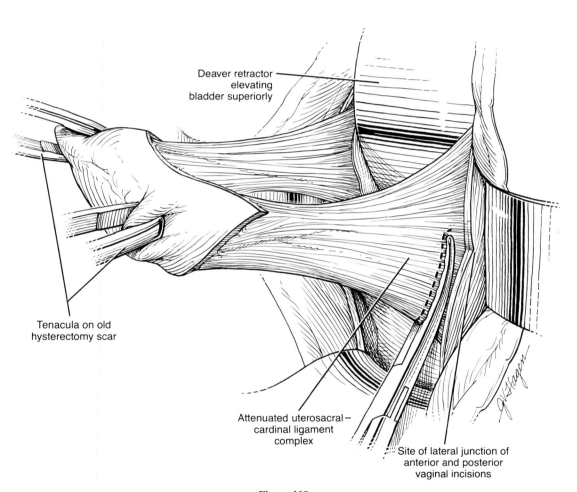

Deaver retractor elevating bladder superiorly

Tenacula on old hysterectomy scar

Attenuated uterosacral–cardinal ligament complex

Site of lateral junction of anterior and posterior vaginal incisions

Figure 118

The technique of the ties (Fig. 119) on the ligament is as follows. With a heavy no. 6 Mayo needle, a suture ligature of 2–0 delayed absorbable suture is passed through the tissue behind the Heaney clamp in the middle of the ligament, after which a single tie is placed on its inferior segment. This suture is then continued around the superior end of the pedicle and again tied. The clamp is slowly opened to permit the knot to tighten down on the tissue and thus prevent its retraction. Two additional knots are placed on the same suture. The suture is left long and clamped with a straight clamp (a straight clamp denotes the sacral ligament). The same maneuver is performed on the cardinal ligament, which is tagged with a curved forceps to denote it.

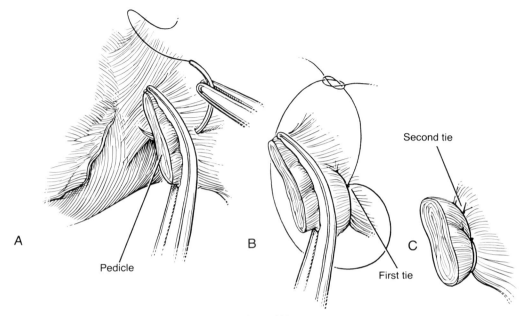

Pedicle

Second tie

First tie

A B C

Figure 119

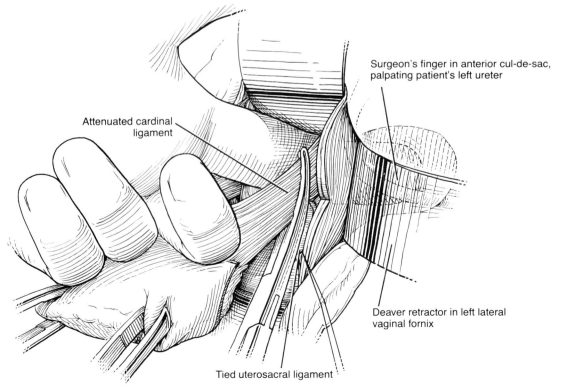

Attenuated cardinal ligament

Surgeon's finger in anterior cul-de-sac, palpating patient's left ureter

Deaver retractor in left lateral vaginal fornix

Tied uterosacral ligament

Figure 120

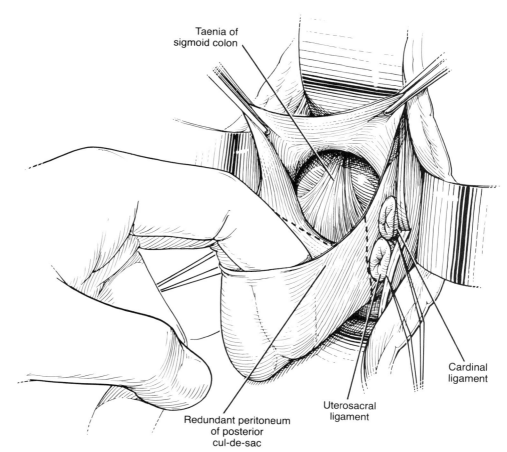

Figure 121

Before a Heaney clamp is placed on the remaining segment of the lateral supporting tissues (remnant of the cardinal ligament), the surgeon introduces the left index finger through the anterior cul-de-sac and palpates the lower segment of the ureter between the left index finger and the Deaver retractor in the 2- to 3-o'clock position in the lateral fornix (Fig. 120). Occasionally it is necessary to move the retractor superiorly or inferiorly to localize the lower segment of ureter. Once it is identified, the Heaney clamp can be applied far superiorly, usually immediately adjacent to the cut edge of the vagina across the remaining, supporting tissues, which are clamped, cut, and tied behind the forceps in a way that does not distort the ureter located 1 cm laterally and superiorly. A similar procedure is then accomplished on the patient's right side. The surgeon then places the left index and middle fingers inside the sac; with appropriate elevation of the sac with countertraction on the rectosigmoid, the peritoneum is further mobilized off the anterior wall of the sigmoid with Mayo scissors to remove the peritoneum of the pouch of Douglas completely (Fig. 121). The redundant peritoneum is resected and discarded (Fig. 122).

If there is sufficient relaxation, the cut edge of the anterior peritoneum overlying the posterior wall of the bladder can be grasped and separated from the bladder, and the peritoneum can be excised in a similar fashion.

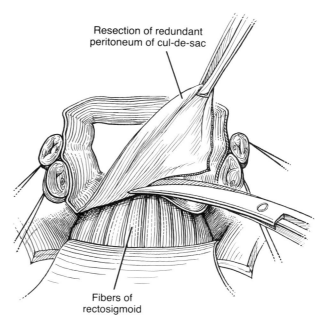

Figure 122

To this point, the peritoneum of the pouch of Douglas has been excised sufficiently superiorly so that the muscularis of the rectosigmoid can be identified and sufficiently laterally to the point of exposure of the uterosacral and cardinal ligaments. The latter have been clamped far superiorly to provide every possible support for these ligaments, which are frequently attenuated (Fig. 123).

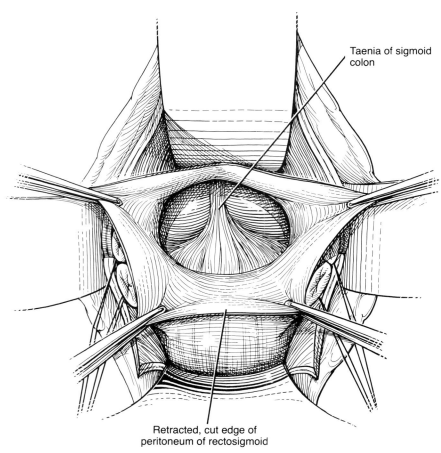

Taenia of sigmoid colon

Retracted, cut edge of peritoneum of rectosigmoid

Figure 123

Attention is now directed to placement of the McCall sutures, which we choose to divide into internal and external types. An internal McCall suture is placed as follows. With one Deaver retractor elevating the bladder superiorly in the 12-o'clock position and a second Deaver retractor in the 3-o'clock position, the surgeon introduces the left index finger in the posterior cul-de-sac, applying tension in a caudal and lateral direction (toward the patient's right side) to

expose the pararectal fascia in the left lateral position of the rectum (Fig. 124*A*). With a 0 monofilament delayed absorbable suture and a large needle, a deep bite of the pararectal fascia is obtained, and small bites are continued across the anterior surface of the rectum, where a similar portion of the pararectal fascia on the right side of the sigmoid is obtained. This suture is tagged, and a similar suture is placed just cephalad to this suture (Fig. 124*B*).

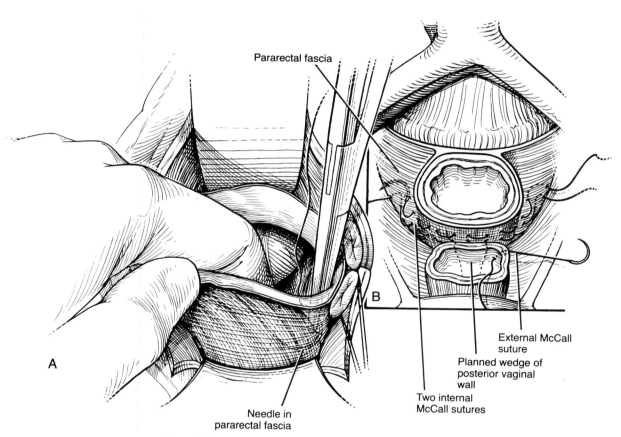

Pararectal fascia

B

A

External McCall suture

Planned wedge of posterior vaginal wall

Two internal McCall sutures

Needle in pararectal fascia

Figure 124
Surgeon's left index finger depressing side of sigmoid colon *(A)*.

An external McCall suture is now placed by engaging the full thickness of the posterior vaginal wall at the junction of the transverse incision and the vertical incision of the posterior vaginal wall created by the posterior wedge. The suture is passed through the peritoneum overlying the rectosigmoid, following which the same pararectal fascia is exposed by downward and right lateral displacement of the rectosigmoid. The tissues in front of the sigmoid are then incorporated in this running suture. When it reaches the right pararectal fascia, a similar portion is included in the needle by caudal and lateral (toward the patient's left side) displacement of the rectosigmoid to expose the pararectal fascia. This suture then is continued out through the peritoneum and the posterior vaginal wall, where it is tagged. The pararectal tissue incorporated in the McCall suture is the same uterosacral and vaginal sacral tissue that is cut during a radical hysterectomy (Fig. 125). The number of internal and external McCall sutures is determined by the size of the enterocele and the redundancy of

the upper vagina. When the McCall sutures are tied, they serve to close the peritoneum above the previous enterocele at a high level. This medial approximation of pararectal and endopelvic fasciae creates a thick block of tissue under the floor of the cul-de-sac and broad approximation of the fascia supports. One to three external McCall sutures are placed, the number again being determined by the degree of relaxation. A reperitonealizing suture is placed superior to all these sutures to obliterate the sac at an even higher level and bring the peritoneum of the anterior wall of the rectosigmoid to the posterior wall of the bladder (Fig. 126A).

The vault is now inspected to ensure perfect hemostasis. Closure of the vault is begun at the 3-o'clock position in the left vaginal fornix. A full thickness of the vagina is incorporated with 3–0 delayed absorbable suture, following which the needle is inserted proximal to the tie in the uterosacral ligament and distal to the cardinal ligament remnant (Fig. 126B).

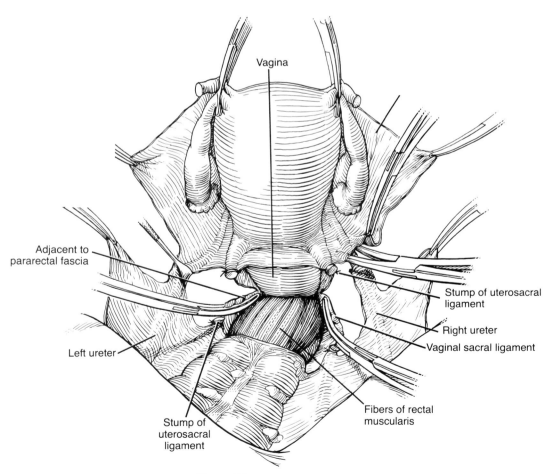

Figure 125
Dissection of radical hysterectomy.

It is continued through the full thickness of the anterior vaginal wall and tied. This closure of the vaginal cuff continues from a lateral to a medial direction and is usually accomplished with two to three sutures on each side.

Frequently, the rather flimsy uterosacral and cardinal ligaments that were originally attached to the prolapsed vagina have either retracted or become so attenuated and elongated by the descending vaginal vault as to be of little value in its future repair. However, the uterosacral-cardinal ligament complex located far superior to these distal remnants (lateral condensations of endopelvic fascia and adjacent ureters) can be identified and can be of significant value

for future repair. The paravaginal and pararectal fascial tissues may be of far greater importance for providing vaginal support and have been undisturbed or unaltered in any way by the previous hysterectomy or operative repairs for pelvic relaxation. Of equal importance are the levator muscles and their supporting fasciae, which are of value for future repair. Up to this point, attention has been focused on the use of the endopelvic fascia and its condensations, the uterosacral and cardinal ligaments, and the pararectal fascia to place the upper vagina far posteriorly in the presacral position (posterior pelvic location). This technique is greatly enhanced by high resection of the peritoneum of the enterocele sac with a high ligation.

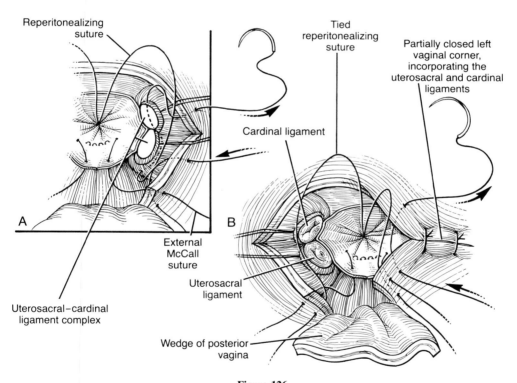

Figure 126

Attention is now directed to repair of the cystocele, for which a modified Kennedy technique and an appropriate posterior colpoperineorrhaphy are preferred. Both are done in a fashion similar to that described under Vaginal Hysterectomy for Uterine Procidentia, page 131. Figure 127 shows the tissues resected at the time of posthysterectomy vaginal vault prolapse. Part *A* shows the old transverse hysterectomy scar with its underlying attenuated attached remnants of the uterosacral and cardinal ligaments. Part *B* shows the right and left segments of the vaginal mucosa resected from the cystocele. Part *C* shows the wide upper vaginal wall resected from the redundant posterior vaginal wall with a long continuous segment all the way to the introitus. As seen in the lateral view (Fig. 128), the apex of the vagina is directed cephalad and posterior toward the hollow of the sacrum, where the posterior cul-de-sac is obliterated by the approximation of the pararectal fascia. The anterior vaginal wall is well supported by approximation of the underlying cervicopubic fascia. The posterior vaginal wall from the point of the tied McCall sutures all the way to the introitus is well supported by approximation of the vagina and underlying rectovaginal fascia and, at an appropriate level, approximation of the levator muscles.

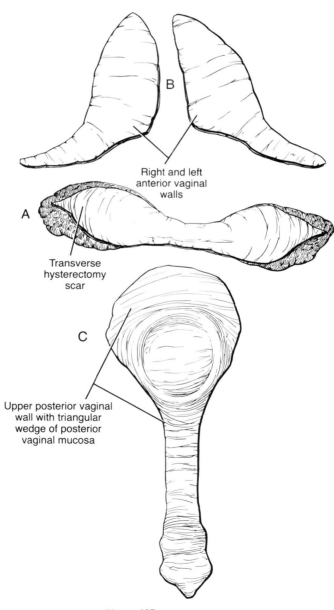

Right and left
anterior vaginal
walls

Transverse
hysterectomy
scar

Upper posterior vaginal
wall with triangular
wedge of posterior
vaginal mucosa

Figure 127

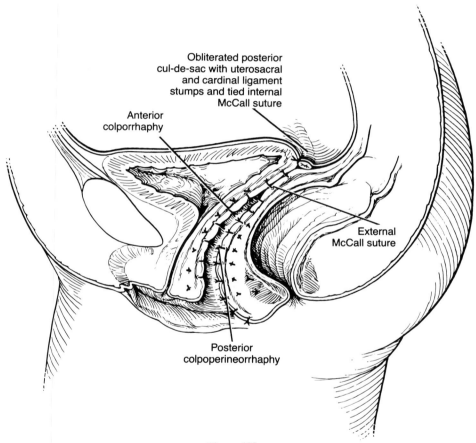

Obliterated posterior
cul-de-sac with uterosacral
and cardinal ligament
stumps and tied internal
McCall suture

Anterior
colporrhaphy

External
McCall suture

Posterior
colpoperineorrhaphy

Figure 128

Abdominal Repair

The need to preserve vaginal function in patients with recurrent prolapse of an already shortened and narrowed vagina (because of previous failed vaginal repairs) is the single most important indication for choosing an abdominal approach for posthysterectomy vaginal vault prolapse. In this limited group of patients (approximately 10% to 15% of patients with prolapse), we prefer an abdominal operation, which restores the vagina to its normal axis with the use of autogenous fascia or prosthetic material (Dacron, Teflon, Marlex, Gore-Tex).

The preoperative placement of vaginal packing in the already prepared vagina aids in demarcating the apex of the vagina from the posterior wall of the bladder (Fig. 129A). With the patient in a steep Trendelenburg position, an abdominal incision is made beginning at the level of the promontory; the peritoneum is incised, and the incision is continued toward the right pelvis just inferior to the right ureter and anteriorly over the top of the vagina to the left pelvis just inferior to the left ureter in front of the sigmoid to connect to the starting point (Fig. 129B). The entire enterocele sac (peritoneum of the pouch of Douglas) is excised as a wide sheet (Fig. 129C). Perfect hemostasis is easily obtained with light cautery or fine sutures, as required. Tenacula are placed on the corners of the vagina, and traction is applied in a posterior and a cephalad direction. The bladder is freed in the avascular space from the anterior surface of the vagina far inferiorly to expose a long segment of the anterior surface of the vagina, which will serve as the site of fixation of the suspending graft. The lateral pillars of the bladder are mobilized sufficiently such that there is no possibility of compromising the intramural portion of the ureters coursing from the lateral pelvic wall to enter the bladder (Fig. 130).

The graft is fixed to the anterior surface of the vagina with three rows of interrupted 3–0 nylon suture. The graft is then pulled posteriorly (but not taut) in such a way that the upper half of the vagina assumes a position parallel to the underlying levator muscles. The point at which the mesh fits on the sacrum free of tension (if the graft is under tension the patient may have pelvic pain or the change in the angular relationship of the urethra and bladder may result in urinary incontinence) is sutured with interrupted nylon sutures to the presacral fascia (Fig. 131). Generally, this point is in the area of S-1 to S-3. Again, the operative area is carefully inspected to ensure perfect hemostasis. Because all of the peritoneum of the

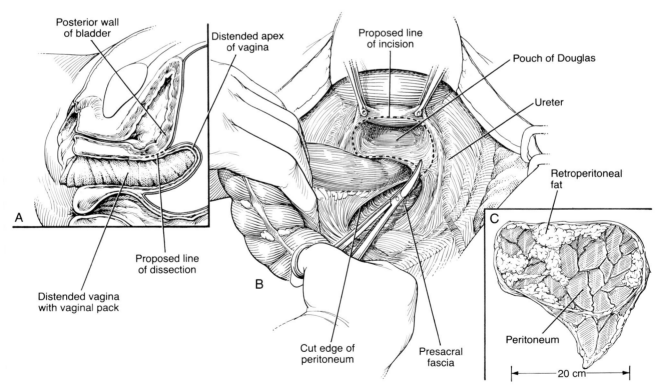

Posterior wall of bladder

Distended apex of vagina

Proposed line of incision

Pouch of Douglas

Ureter

Retroperitoneal fat

A

Proposed line of dissection

Distended vagina with vaginal pack

B

Cut edge of peritoneum

Presacral fascia

C

Peritoneum

20 cm

Figure 129

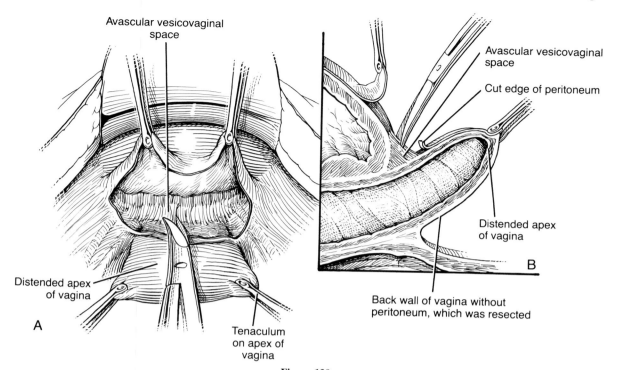

Avascular vesicovaginal
space

Avascular vesicovaginal
space

Cut edge of peritoneum

Distended apex
of vagina

Distended apex
of vagina

Tenaculum
on apex of
vagina

Back wall of vagina without
peritoneum, which was resected

A

B

Figure 130

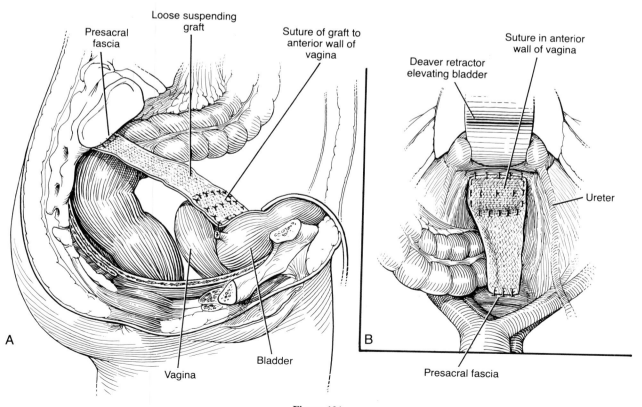

Presacral
fascia

Loose suspending
graft

Suture of graft to
anterior wall of
vagina

Deaver retractor
elevating bladder

Suture in anterior
wall of vagina

Ureter

Vagina

Bladder

Presacral fascia

A

B

Figure 131

pelvis inferior to the ureters has been excised, the sigmoid colon is freed from the left pelvis, brought across the pelvis, and fixed to the right pelvic side wall, the back of the bladder, and the left pelvis, and a suction catheter is brought out inferior to the sigmoid through a stab wound lateral to the midline incision (Fig. 132). This maneuver not only extraperitonealizes the graft but also allows any intra-abdominal pressure to be exerted immediately on the colon and its mesentery. Rarely, and usually after some months or years, patients with a permanent synthetic graft experience bloody or foul vaginal discharge. Examination might reveal an exposed segment of the previously placed graft (Fig. 133). We have found it necessary to use an abdominal approach to excise the entire graft and close the vaginal defect with 3–0 delayed absorbable sutures. The vaginal walls are sutured to the pararectal fascia with 2–0 delayed absorbable sutures. However, no graft material is used, and the support has proved satisfactory.

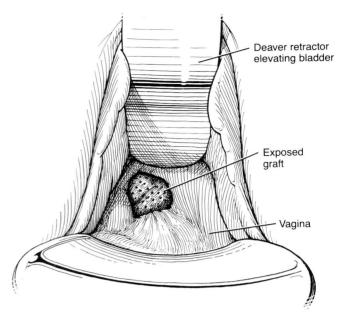

Figure 133

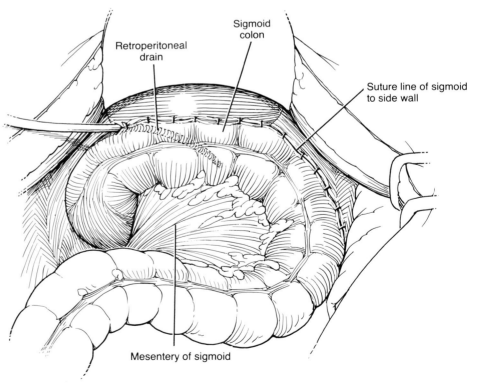

Figure 132

Ruptured Enterocele

Prolapse of the vagina after hysterectomy is occurring with greater frequency. Given sufficient time, peristalsis of the contents (small intestine) may be readily seen through the thin, attenuated enterocele. Because of rubbing and the trauma of exposure, ulceration of the vaginal mucosa may result, and, rarely, rupture of the enterocele ensues. The treatment of the subsequent evisceration must be individualized, depending on the condition of the patient, the degree of

trauma to the intestine, and the need to preserve a functional vagina.

Vaginal Repair

In Figure 134, the evisceration had been present for a short time, and the intestine in this elderly patient with multiple medical problems had been exposed to minimal trauma. The exposed bowel was vigorously irrigated with a warm saline solution, and the vaginal defect was enlarged to permit further inspection of

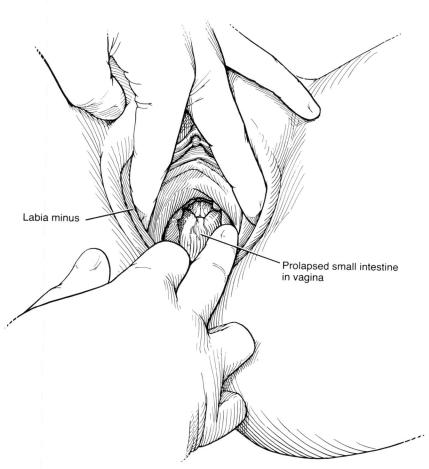

Figure 134

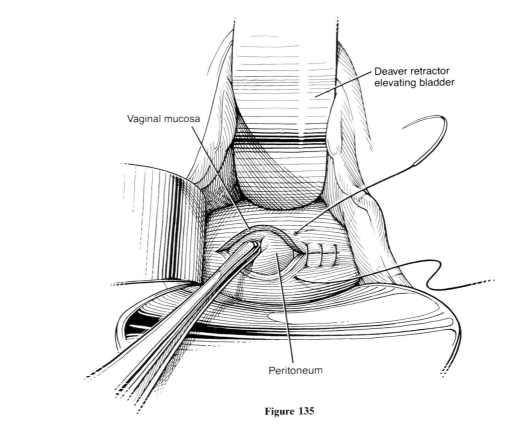

Figure 135

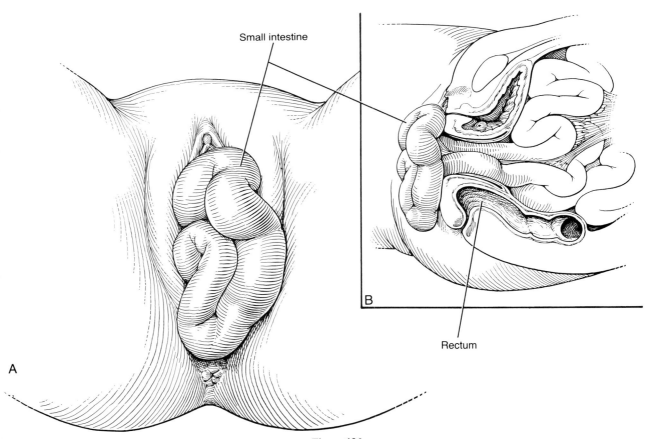

Figure 136

the adjacent intestine, which had been incarcerated in the neck of the hernial defect. After adequate exposure and examination, the intestine was easily replaced in the abdominal cavity, and three internal McCall sutures were placed. The pelvis was reperitonealized, severely narrowing and coning down the apex of the vagina by high approximation of the levator muscles (Fig. 135).

Abdominal Repair

In another patient, the prolapse of the intestines was considerably greater, resulting in an incarcerated, edematous mass at the introitus as a result of prolapse through a tight ring at the apex of the vagina (Fig. 136). The intestine was bathed with warm saline and covered with moist saline towels, while, through a lower midline incision, gentle traction on the intestine permitted reduction of the small bowel into the abdominal cavity (Fig. 137). The bowel again was inspected and its blood supply carefully assessed, and prompt return of the normal color and peristalsis was noted. In this patient, the enterocele sac was excised from above along with a generous portion of the upper vagina, which was closed primarily. The vagina was then fixed with permanent sutures to the hollow of the sacrum by a wide strip of fascia harvested from the anterior abdominal wall.

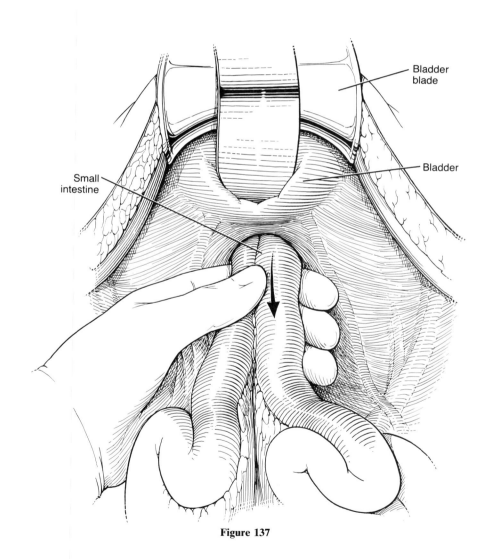

Figure 137

Cervix

Cerclage

Cervical incompetence is the premature, painless dilatation and effacement of the cervix in the absence of uterine contractions (Fig. 138). Its cause is unknown and probably is multifactorial. When possible, we prefer the modified Shirodkar operation for the management of this condition.

Traction is applied to the anterior and posterior lips of the cervix with ring forceps (Fig. 139). A transverse incision is made into the anterior wall of the cervix, approximately 3 cm in length. The vaginal wall is elevated with sharp dissection, and the posterior wall of the bladder is separated from the underlying isthmus of the cervix. The bladder is elevated superiorly to the level of the internal os. Complete hemostasis is obtained with light cautery or fine suture ligatures. A second incision is made in the posterior wall of the cervix, after which the vaginal wall is elevated in a similar fashion and to a level parallel to that in the anterior vaginal wall.

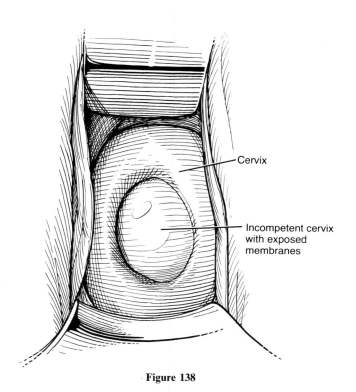

Figure 138

Cervix

Incompetent cervix with exposed membranes

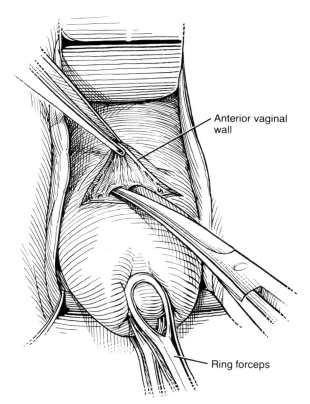

Anterior vaginal wall

Ring forceps

Figure 139

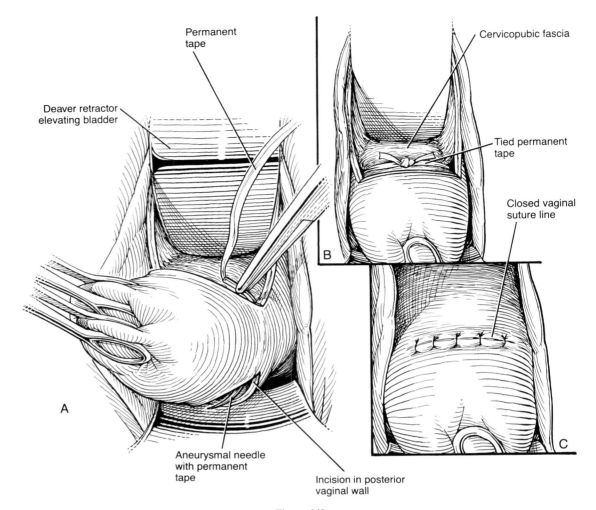

Figure 140

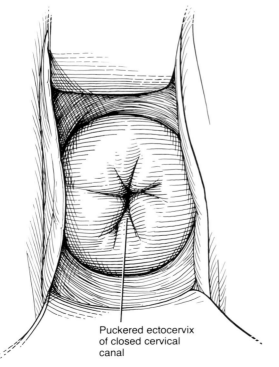

Figure 141

A large aneurysmal needle introduces a nylon suture within the left lateral wall of the cervix; the needle enters at the left corner of the anterior incision (junction of vaginal mucosa and cervix) and comes out the edge of the posterior incision (Fig. 140*A*). Traction on the needle delivers the "swaged-on" permanent tape through the canal made by the needle. The same needle now enters the incision at the right posterior lateral wall of the cervix, coming out the right corner of the anterior incision. The suture (at the level of the internal os, 3 to 5 cm from the external os) is tightened and tied (Fig. 140*B*), and a short tail is left on the knot. Perfect hemostasis is ensured, and the vaginal wall is approximated (anterior and posterior vaginal incisions) with 3–0 delayed absorbable suture (Fig. 140*C*). When tightened, the cerclage suture gives a puckered appearance to the external os of the cervix (Fig. 141).

Conization

Cold-knife conization of the cervix consists of removal of a cone-shaped wedge of tissue from the cervix uteri. Care is taken during the vaginal preparation that the cervix not be touched, so as to prevent any denuding of the cervical epithelium. With tenacula placed in the 3- and the 9-o'clock positions, the cervix is exposed, and Lugol stain is applied to the cervix and the upper vagina. A circular incision is made with a no. 11 blade, beginning in the 1-o'clock position, outside the nonstaining area, with the tip of the blade directed toward the endocervical canal (Fig. 142 *A*). To be sure that the specimen will be adequate, a sufficient portion of the uninvolved endocervical epithelium above the potential lesion and the uninvolved ectocervix lateral to any potential lesion on the portio must be included.

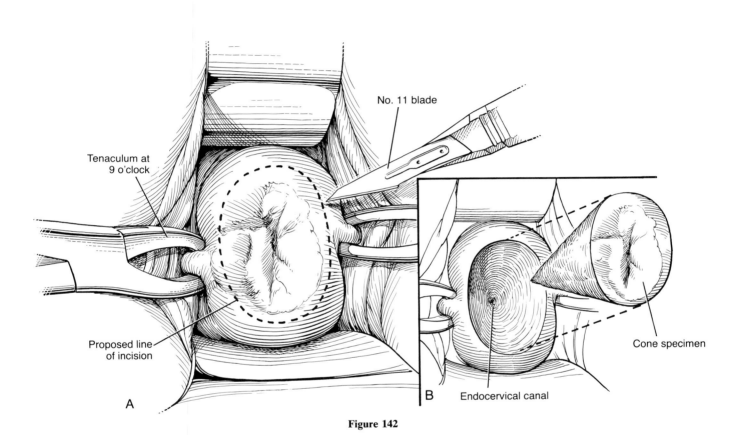

Tenaculum at
9 o'clock

No. 11 blade

Proposed line
of incision

Cone specimen

Endocervical canal

A

B

Figure 142

The size of the specimen varies. Generally, in young patients the lesions are on the portio, so the cone may have a broad base and the tip consists of a wide angle. In older women, the squamocolumnar junction may be located at a higher position in the endocervical canal; the cone specimen, therefore, includes a larger portion of the endocervix and the angle is sharper (Fig. 142*B*). The specimen should consist of a single en bloc portion of the portio and endocervix. The specimen then is incised in the 12-o'clock position to assist the pathologist in accurate interpretation of the frozen-section specimen. A dilation and curettage procedure is then performed, after which sutures are placed in the cervix to obtain complete hemostasis. To facilitate future study of the cervix and endocervical area, we do not draw the surrounding vaginal epithelium into the cervix. Light cautery is applied to the uppermost aspects of the endocervix, after which simple interrupted sutures are placed through the vaginal epithelium to include a portion of the endocervical canal, and they are then tied lateral to the incision (Fig. 143). These four sutures result in excellent hemostasis and a cervix that looks essentially normal once the sutures dissolve and healing is complete. This procedure also permits accurate study of the cervix, and the endocervix is not hidden from future colposcopic evaluation.

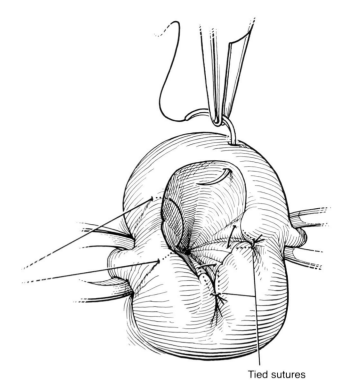

Tied sutures

Figure 143

Prolapse of Cervical Stump

Supracervical hysterectomy is done less frequently now than it was in the past. However, there continue to be very select and appropriate indications for supracervical hysterectomy, which leaves a cervix that may later need to be removed. It is important to understand how supracervical hysterectomies are initially accomplished, because later excision of the stump can be more logically and safely accomplished. As a rule with supracervical hysterectomy, a wedge-shaped (conization-type maneuver as described previously) incision has been made so as to form flaps of the cervical tissue that, when sutured together, obliterate the raw surfaces of the remaining cervical stump. Occasionally, the maneuver is accomplished in such a fashion as to essentially core out the cervix and endocervical canal, and a thin shell of cervical tissue is left. A more rapid method of supracervical hysterectomy is simply to cut across the cervix and establish hemostasis with placement of interrupted sutures; this procedure thus obliterates the endocervical canal.

Regardless of the method chosen, after hemostasis is obtained, generally the bladder peritoneum is brought over the top of the stump of the cervix and sutured to the posterior wall of the remaining cervix and posterior cul-de-sac. Occasionally, the sigmoid is brought over the peritoneal closure and sutured to the peritoneum covering the back of the bladder. With this understanding, if one is removing a prolapsed or retained cervical stump transvaginally, a circular incision is made through the vaginal wall and carried laterally (Fig. 144A) in an appropriate fashion, depending on the degree of prolapse, much like that carried out for vaginal hysterectomy (Fig. 144B). The anterior vaginal wall is separated from the underlying cervical stump in the same way as one would enter the anterior cul-de-sac with vaginal hysterec-

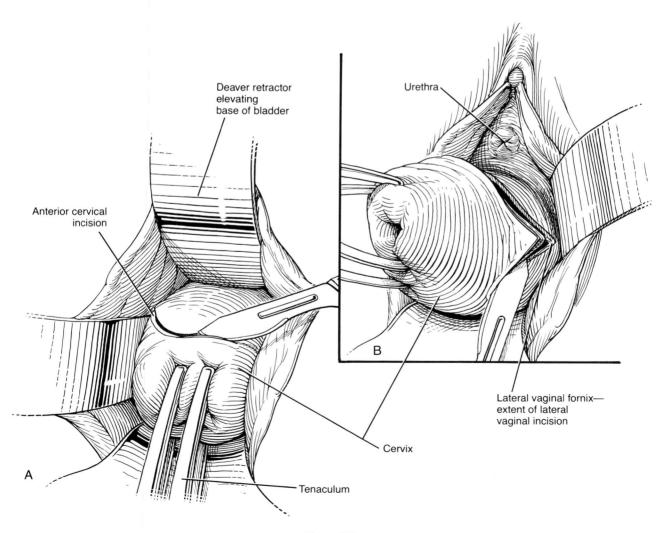

Figure 144

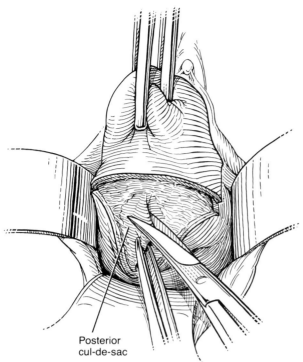

Posterior
cul-de-sac

Figure 145

tomy. If the anterior cul-de-sac cannot be entered because of adhesions, the cervix is then drawn anteriorly and the posterior cul-de-sac is entered (Fig. 145). It is preferable to enter the abdominal cavity (especially if there is prolapse) to manage the real or potential enterocele.

The cul-de-sac and the superior surface of the cervical stump are palpated, and any adhesions are sharply or bluntly mobilized. The surgeon then introduces the left index finger through the posterior cul-de-sac over the superior surface of the retained stump and, with a Deaver retractor elevating the bladder superiorly, cuts the peritoneum and enters the anterior cul-de-sac with sharp dissection under direct vision (Fig. 146).

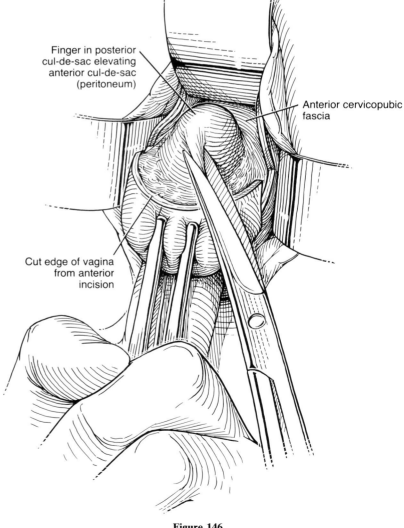

Finger in posterior
cul-de-sac elevating
anterior cul-de-sac
(peritoneum)

Anterior cervicopubic
fascia

Cut edge of vagina
from anterior
incision

Figure 146

The Deaver retractor is then inserted in the anterior cul-de-sac, lifting the bladder and ureters superiorly (Fig. 147).

The vaginal walls are mobilized laterally to facilitate high placement of a Heaney clamp on the remnants of the uterosacral-cardinal ligament complex (Fig. 148). The Heaney clamp is placed far laterally, immediately adjacent to the cut edge of the vagina, where it is clamped, cut, and suture-ligated. The

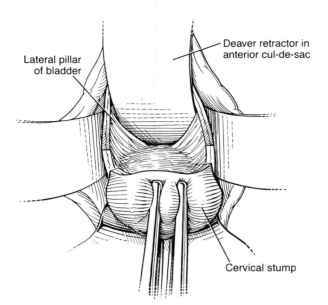

Figure 147

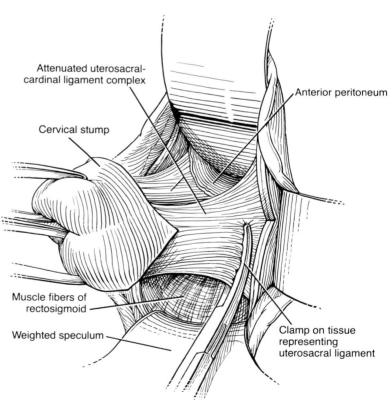

Figure 148

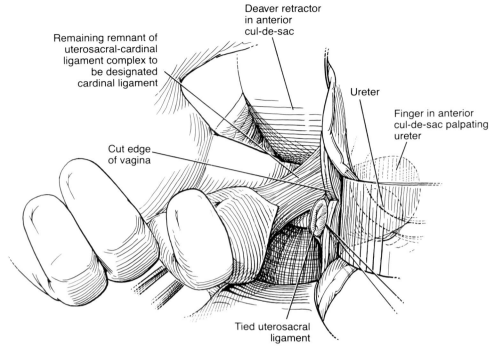

Remaining remnant of
uterosacral-cardinal
ligament complex to
be designated
cardinal ligament

Deaver retractor
in anterior
cul-de-sac

Ureter

Finger in anterior
cul-de-sac palpating
ureter

Cut edge
of vagina

Tied uterosacral
ligament

Figure 149

ureter is palpated in the same fashion as for a vaginal
hysterectomy—the left index finger is introduced
through the anterior cul-de-sac, and the left ureter is
palpated between the tip of the finger and the Deaver
retractor in the 3-o'clock position (Fig. 149). Once
the location of the ureter is established, a clamp can
be safely placed high on the remnant of the cardinal
ligament. A similar maneuver is accomplished on the
patient's right side.

The excess peritoneum of the posterior cul-de-sac and
enterocele sac is excised (Fig. 150), and one to three

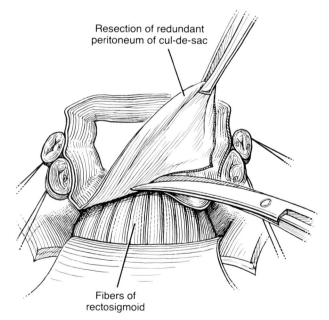

Resection of redundant
peritoneum of cul-de-sac

Fibers of
rectosigmoid

Figure 150

internal McCall sutures are placed (the number is determined by the size of the enterocele present) (Fig. 151). (Details of the technique are reviewed on page 85.) An external McCall suture is placed in the same fashion as for a vaginal hysterectomy with or without procidentia. Once the pelvis is reperito-

nealized, the vagina is closed in the same way as is accomplished for a vaginal hysterectomy. The anterior or posterior vaginal wall is appropriately repaired, depending on the degree of vaginal wall relaxation.

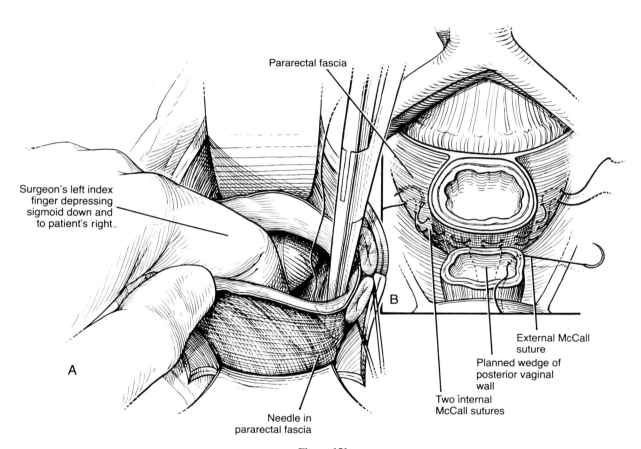

Pararectal fascia

Surgeon's left index finger depressing sigmoid down and to patient's right

Needle in pararectal fascia

External McCall suture

Planned wedge of posterior vaginal wall

Two internal McCall sutures

A

B

Figure 151

Cervical Stump: Abdominal Excision

Occasionally, because of either high fixation of the cervical stump or other intra-abdominal abnormality, one may want to remove the cervical stump through an abdominal incision (Fig. 152 A). Preoperatively, a vaginal pack is placed to assist in elevating the cervical stump into the abdominal cavity; it also aids in delineation of the cervical stump from the bladder. The vaginal pack and the firm body of the cervical stump can then be palpated, and a vulsellum tenaculum is placed on the apex to assist in applying traction (Fig. 152B). With cephalad traction on the cervical stump, the peritoneal reflection from the back of the bladder is incised; the bladder is sharply dissected from the anterior surface of the isthmus and lower portion of the cervix. The peritoneum lateral to the cervix may be incised and the ureter identified and palpated before the placement of Kocher forceps on the remaining portion of the cardinal ligament and its enclosed uterine artery (Fig. 153). The ligament is cut, first on the right side, and then a similar procedure is done on the left side. The vagina is entered in the same way as for an abdominal hysterectomy. The cervical stump is removed, and four vulsellum forceps are placed on the vaginal cuff to elevate and expose the entire circumference of the vaginal vault.

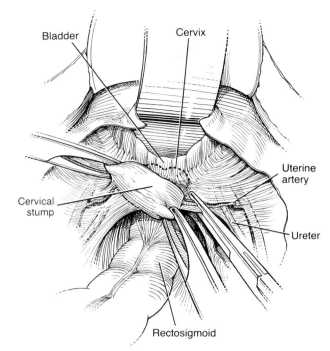

Figure 153

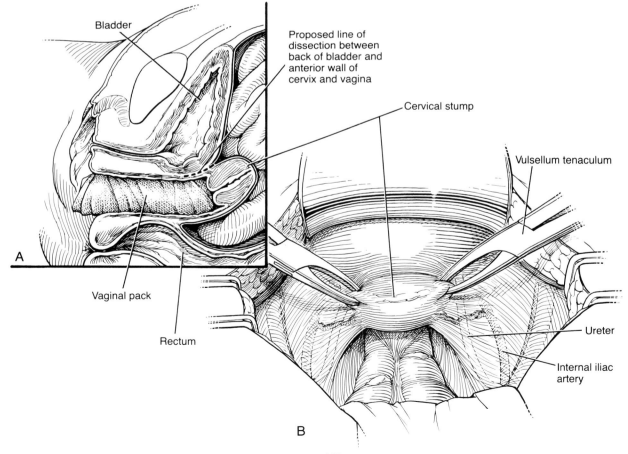

Figure 152

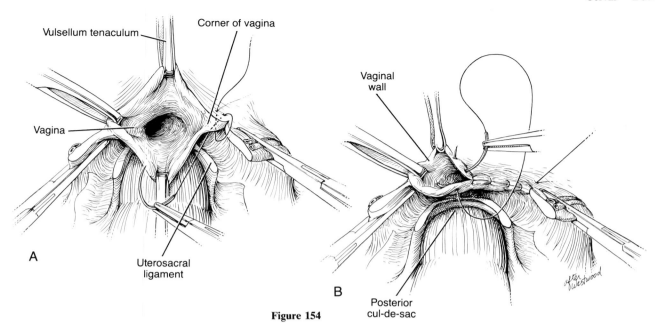

Figure 154

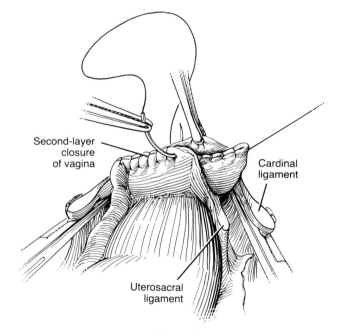

Figure 155

Accurate closure of the vagina is thereby facilitated while constant visualization of the bladder base and the rectum is maintained. The closure of the vaginal vault provides satisfactory hemostasis, affected by continuous suture of atraumatic 2–0 polyglycolic acid suture. The suture is started with a right vaginal "angle" stitch placed so that the small vaginal branch or branches of the uterine artery are ligated in addition to attaching lateral supporting tissues from the base of the cardinal ligament to the vaginal angle (Fig. 154*A*). The suture is continued toward the left side, each bite placed "submucosally" in the submucosa so that the squamous edges are actually approximated and inverted into the vagina (Fig. 154*B*). The suture into the vaginal wall is not exposed to the contamination therein. A generous portion of the left uterosacral ligament is included, following which the needle passes laterally to the vaginal fornix angle, through the lateral supporting tissues at the base of the cardinal ligament, and under the small vaginal vessels that can be noted there.

Anteriorly, the suture also includes a layer of the cervicopubic fascia that was previously prepared (Fig. 155). The angle suture is securely locked in this position, and the suture is then returned across the vaginal vault, which includes the underlying endopelvic fascia posteriorly, small bites of the top of the previously closed vagina, and the cervicopubic fascia anteriorly. When the right vaginal angle is reached, a secure bite is obtained of the right uterosacral ligament, vaginal angle, and cervicopubic fascia anteriorly. This suture is tied to the previously tagged suture and cut. A two-layer closure of the vaginal vault is accomplished with a single continuous suture that restores the continuity of the endopelvic fascia, the cervicopubic fascia anteriorly, the peritoneum (endopelvic fascia) and the uterosacral ligaments posteriorly, and the base of the cardinal ligament laterally.

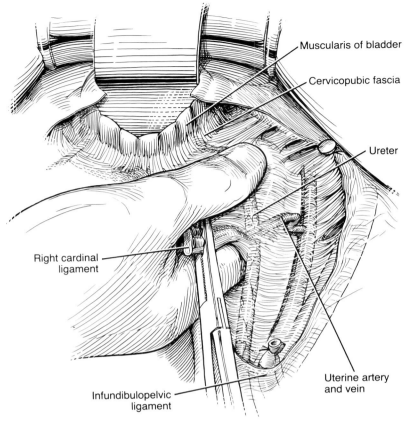

Figure 156

The previously placed Kocher clamp containing the upper portion of the cardinal ligament is now elevated toward the midline by the first assistant. The ureter is then palpated between the surgeon's index finger and thumb as it courses through the cardinal ligament toward the bladder (Fig. 156). This step provides a second check on the location of the ureter before the cardinal ligament is tied to the corner of the vagina.

The upper portion of the cardinal ligament containing the uterine artery is now attached securely to the vaginal angle and ligated (Fig. 157). To accomplish this, the needle first enters the peritoneum, the right uterosacral ligament, and the right angle of the vagina just lateral to the suture used to close the vaginal vault. This same procedure is accomplished on the opposite side. At this time, the pelvis should be completely inspected and meticulous hemostasis ensured.

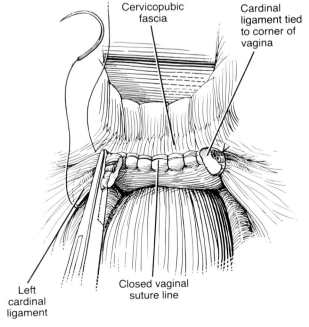

Figure 157

Uterus

Dilatation and Curettage

After the usual preparation and draping with the patient in the lithotomy position, a pelvic examination is performed, and the vulva, vagina, and cervix are carefully examined. A vulsellum tenaculum is placed on the anterior lip of the cervix to expose the external cervical os (Fig. 158A). A uterine probe may be inserted through the external cervical os into the uterine cavity to measure its depth. Care should be taken that this is extended into the uterine fundus in the proper direction to minimize the potential for

perforation. The probe is removed, and the cervical canal is dilated sufficiently to permit the easy passage of the curet. The curet is introduced into the endometrial cavity, and a systematic and complete curettage is accomplished (Fig. 158B). During curettage of the endometrial cavity, special attention is paid to the cornua. Once the tissue has been obtained for histologic study, the endometrial cavity is again explored with a polyp forceps to ensure that an endometrial or endocervical polyp or fibroid has not been overlooked. Frozen-section diagnosis is immediately obtained before proceeding with hysterectomy.

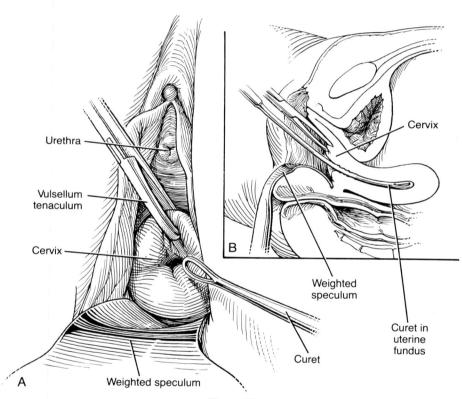

Figure 158

Vaginal Hysterectomy: Simple

With a weighted speculum in the vagina against the posterior vaginal wall, the anterior vaginal wall is lifted with a Deaver retractor (12-o'clock position). Deaver retractors are also placed on either side of the vagina to retract it laterally in the 3- and the 9-o'clock positions (Fig. 159). Traction is applied by placement of vulsellum tenacula on the distal edges of the anterior and posterior lips of the cervix. With a scalpel, an incision is made through the vaginal mucosa, the cut edges of which will retract superiorly because of the countertraction applied by the Deaver retractor superiorly and by the tenacula inferiorly. This incision should be sufficiently close to the distal end of the cervix such that there is no potential for injury to the bladder, which is reflected onto the anterior surface of the lower uterine segment. The incision is continued laterally from the 9-o'clock position to the 12-o'clock position to the 3-o'clock position. The superior extension of the lateral extent of the incision is dictated by the degree of descensus and the limitations of vaginal shortening.

With appropriate traction on the cervix being applied by the assistant, the surgeon picks up the cut edge of the vaginal mucosa and, using Mayo scissors with the points directed toward the endocervical canal, creates the plane of dissection between the bladder anteriorly and the anterior uterine wall posteriorly (Fig. 160). We prefer to use sharp dissection in developing this plane, progressing from the lower uterine segment superiorly.

At the appropriate level, the surgeon may insert the index finger against the lower uterine segment and feel the typical, silky, smooth fold of peritoneum of the anterior cul-de-sac (Fig. 161A). The anteriorly placed Deaver retractor is now inserted under the cut edge of the anterior vaginal wall and bladder, and it is lifted superiorly; this maneuver thus opens the incision to permit direct visualization of the fold of the peritoneum, which may be incised accurately and safely. The vesicouterine fold of peritoneum marks the anterior cul-de-sac and is identified as a concave line against the uterine wall (Fig. 161B). The two layers of peritoneum frequently move over each other to aid further in identification of the vesicouterine fold.

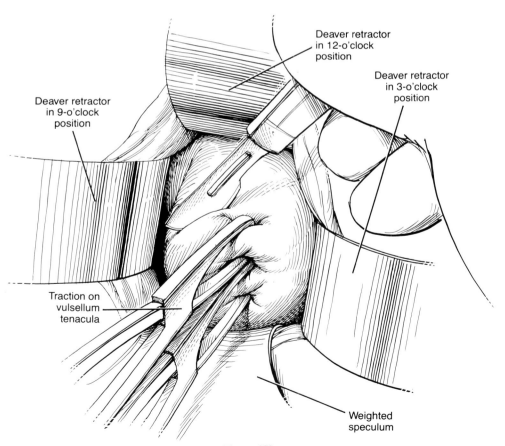

Deaver retractor in 12-o'clock position

Deaver retractor in 3-o'clock position

Deaver retractor in 9-o'clock position

Traction on vulsellum tenacula

Weighted speculum

Figure 159

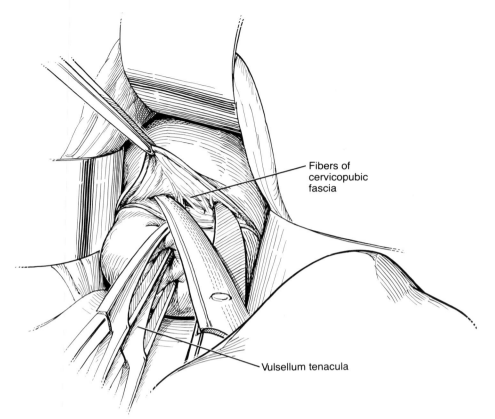

Fibers of
cervicopubic
fascia

Vulsellum tenacula

Figure 160

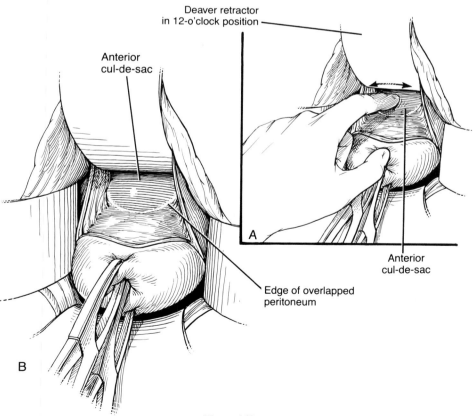

Deaver retractor
in 12-o'clock position

Anterior
cul-de-sac

Anterior
cul-de-sac

A

Edge of overlapped
peritoneum

B

Figure 161

The peritoneum is picked up with tooth forceps, and a Mayo scissors, with the points directed toward the uterus, is used to incise between the forceps and the uterine wall (Fig. 162). The incision of the anterior cul-de-sac is seen in lateral view (Fig. 163). The Deaver retractor beneath the cut edge of the anterior vaginal wall and base of the bladder is lifted superiorly; the forceps is used to pick up the peritoneum, which is incised with scissors between the forceps and the anterior wall (Fig. 163).

The peritoneal opening is made sufficiently large to accommodate a Deaver retractor, which is slipped into the anterior cul-de-sac and lifted superiorly to elevate the base of the bladder. This same traction results in a cephalad elevation of the intramural and lower segments of the ureter (Fig. 164).

With retractors in the 3-, 9-, and 12-o'clock positions, the cervix is now lifted superiorly to expose the posterior vaginal fornix. Traction in a posterior direc-

tion is applied to the cut edge of the vaginal mucosa, and countertraction is applied with the tenacula that are lifting the cervix superiorly. With Mayo scissors, the posterior cul-de-sac is exposed and the rectovaginal fascia and peritoneum are picked up and incised immediately adjacent to the posterior uterine wall (Fig. 165).

Occasionally, this can be a difficult dissection if an adhesive condition (usually endometriosis) is fixing the peritoneum of the posterior cul-de-sac firmly adjacent to the posterior wall of the uterus. Generally, if the dissection is continued superiorly, staying adjacent to the uterus, the cul-de-sac is entered in a higher position above the obliteration caused by the adhesive process. We prefer to use sharp dissection rather than finger fracturing or blunt dissection, which has the potential of tearing or perforating the rectal wall. Once the posterior cul-de-sac is entered, the incision is extended in both directions laterally to aid in the palpation and examination of the posterior cul-de-sac.

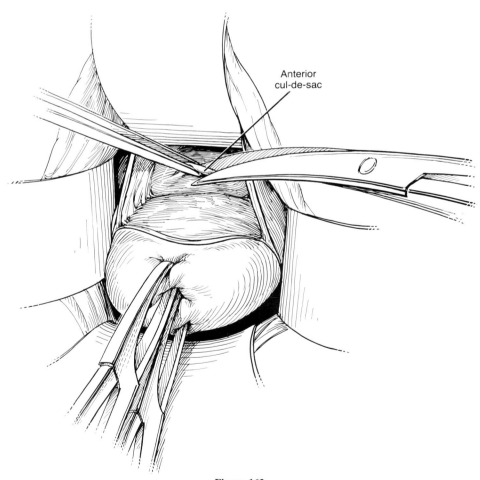

Anterior
cul-de-sac

Figure 162

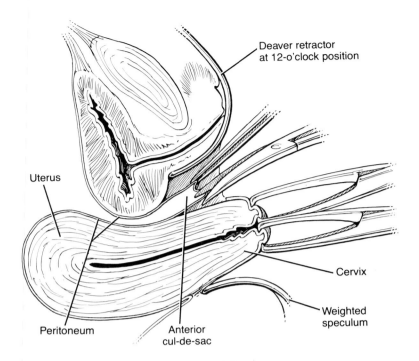

Deaver retractor
at 12-o'clock position

Uterus

Cervix

Peritoneum

Anterior
cul-de-sac

Weighted
speculum

Figure 163

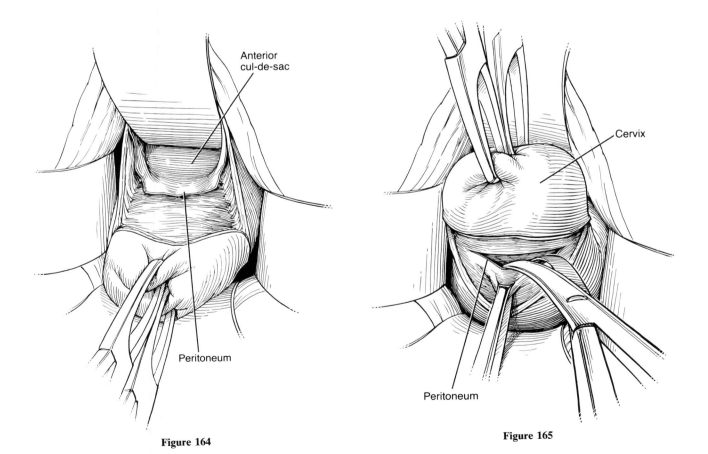

Anterior
cul-de-sac

Cervix

Peritoneum

Peritoneum

Figure 164

Figure 165

Traction is placed on the cervix, and it is pulled sharply to the patient's right; the previously incised vaginal mucosa is swept superiorly (with sharp and blunt dissection) with a gauzed finger to expose the underlying uterosacral and cardinal ligaments. A Heaney forceps is placed on the left uterosacral ligament as far lateral as feasible, with the curved tip directed toward the cervical canal (Fig. 166). This clamp occupies an increasingly cephalad position with each increasing degree of uterine procidentia. The ligament is divided, and a short remnant of tissue is left between the scissors and the forceps; the incision is continued around the tip of the forceps, and this will later accommodate the placement of a tie with a short pedicle.

With a needle (Mayo 6 caliber), a ligature of no. 1 delayed absorbable suture is passed through the tissues behind the Heaney forceps in the middle of the ligament, after which a single tie is placed on its inferior segment (Fig. 167A). This suture then is carried around the superior end of the pedicle and again tied with three knots (Fig. 167B). As the first tie is placed, the forceps is slowly opened to permit tightening of the tissues and yet prevent retraction of the vessels before the suture is in place (Fig. 167C). Once tied, the end of the suture is left long, and a straight forceps is tied to tag its distal ends. (Straight forceps identify uterosacral ligaments on both sides; curved forceps identify cardinal ligaments on both sides.) The purpose of tagging the ligament ties is

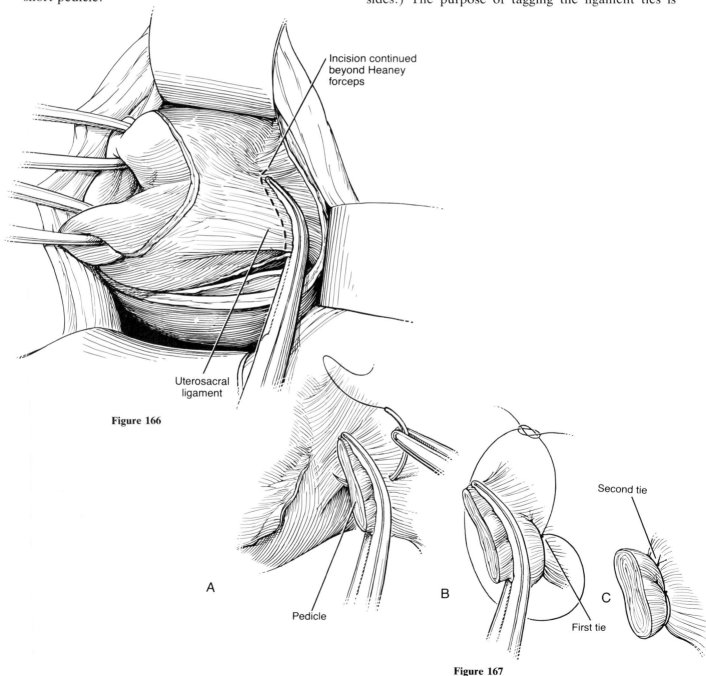

Incision continued
beyond Heaney
forceps

Uterosacral
ligament

Figure 166

Pedicle

A

B

First tie

Second tie

C

Figure 167

only for rapid identification of the pedicle and never for traction.

The surgeon's left index finger is inserted through the anterior cul-de-sac beneath the Deaver retractor, elevating the bladder and directed to the left lateral position to palpate the lower segment of the left ureter between the index finger and the surface of the Deaver retractor in the 3-o'clock position (Fig. 168). A characteristic pop can usually be heard when the ureter is snapped between the index finger and the retractor.

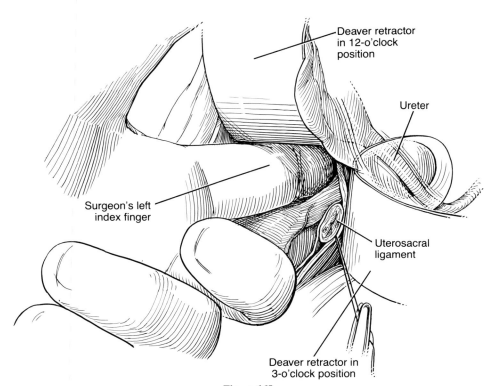

Figure 168

After the left ureter is identified, the Heaney forceps is placed on the lower portion of the cardinal ligament, again with the forceps pointed toward the cervical canal to direct it away from the superiorly (and laterally) located ureter (Fig. 169). The ligament is incised, suture-ligated, and tagged in a similar fashion to that of the uterosacral ligament, except that a curved forceps designates this as a first suture on the cardinal ligament.

The last clamp on the cardinal ligament incorporates the peritoneum of the posterior cul-de-sac with the peritoneum of the anterior cul-de-sac; the cut end of the uterine artery typically is located in the lower end of the jaws of the Heaney forceps (Fig. 170). This pedicle is cut and suture-ligated, and the distal ends of the tie are included in the curved forceps (the two pedicles represent the cardinal ligament). A similar procedure is done on the right side of the uterus, where the right uterosacral ligament is clamped, cut, and suture-ligated. The right ureter is palpated, this time with the surgeon's right index finger identifying the lower segment of the right ureter between the right index finger and the Deaver retractor placed in the 9- or 10-o'clock position. The cardinal ligament is again taken in two segments, each with separate ties, which are tagged with a single curved forceps. At this point, the uterus is held in place by the remaining portions of the broad ligament inferior to the round ligament and utero-ovarian vessels, but it is free enough such that the fundus of the uterus can be rotated and delivered through the posterior cul-de-sac into the vagina.

Initially, the right utero-ovarian pedicle is clamped. This step is accomplished with the surgeon's left hand being inserted behind the uterus and the Heaney forceps coming from above, pointed inferiorly and placed between the surgeon's fingers and the uterus (Fig. 171). The surgeon's fingers thus prevent the possibility of including the small bowel in this clamp.

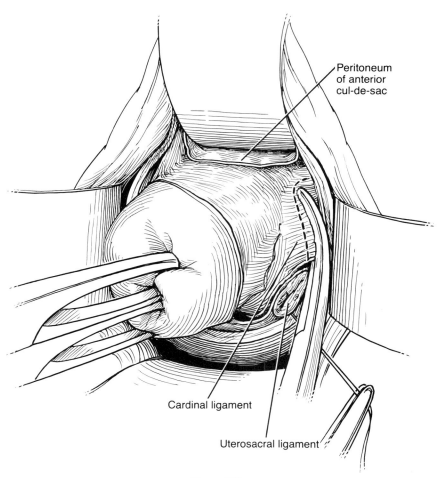

Peritoneum of anterior cul-de-sac

Cardinal ligament

Uterosacral ligament

Figure 169

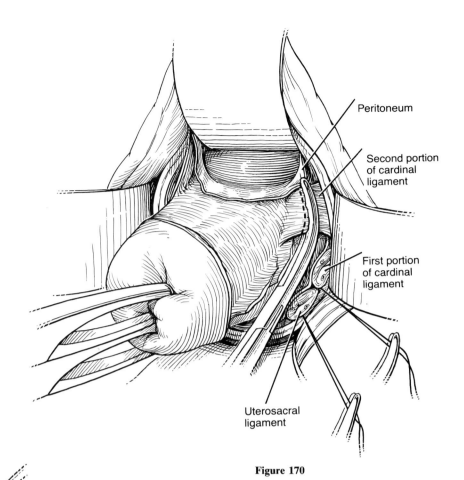

Peritoneum

Second portion
of cardinal
ligament

First portion
of cardinal
ligament

Uterosacral
ligament

Figure 170

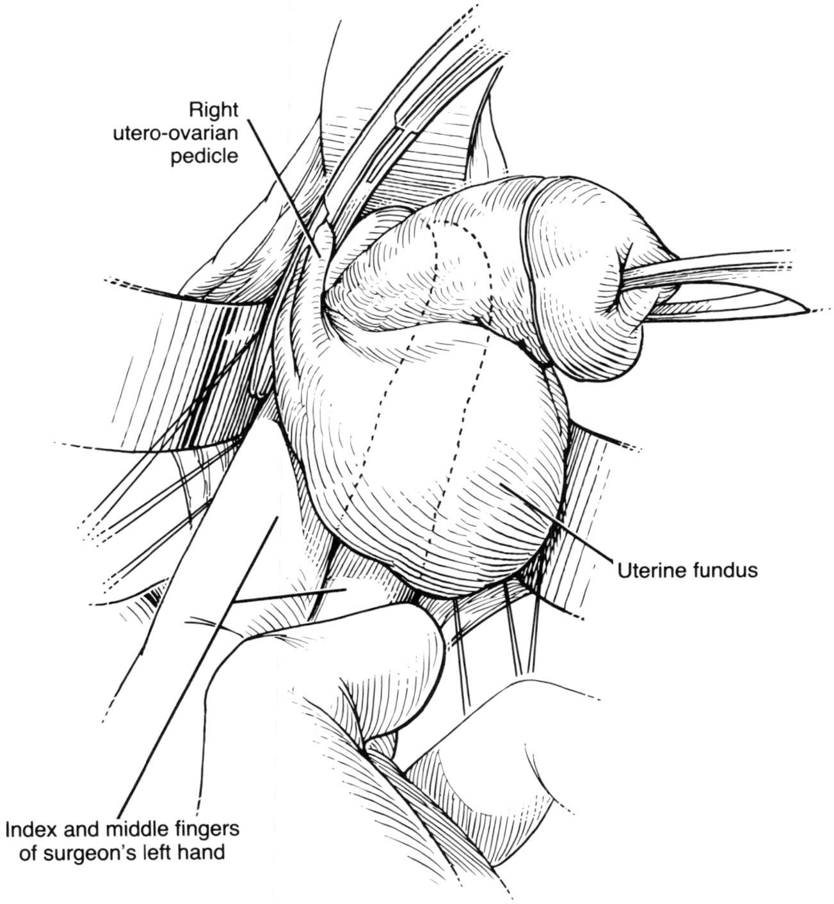

Right
utero-ovarian
pedicle

Uterine fundus

Index and middle fingers
of surgeon's left hand

Figure 171

When the right side of the uterus is freed, the fundus is rotated, and the Heaney forceps is placed on the left utero-ovarian pedicle from an inferior to a superior position, again with the surgeon's fingers behind the uterus to prevent injury to bowel that might be prolapsed in this position (Fig. 172). The Heaney clamp includes the tube and round ligament and any remaining portion of the broad ligament.

The uterus is then removed; removal permits direct visualization of the cut ends of the utero-ovarian pedicles, which then are suture-ligated. The distal ends of the tags are identified with straight forceps. Careful inspection is then done to ensure that there are no free bleeding vessels in the small spaces between each of the tied pedicles. Occasionally, bleeding from the posterior edge of the vaginal wall is sufficient to justify the placement of several interrupted, fine absorbable sutures. The tubes and ovaries are carefully inspected to ensure that they are normal.

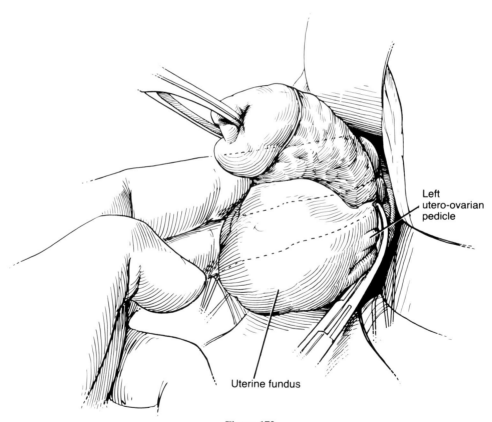

Left
utero-ovarian
pedicle

Uterine fundus

Figure 172

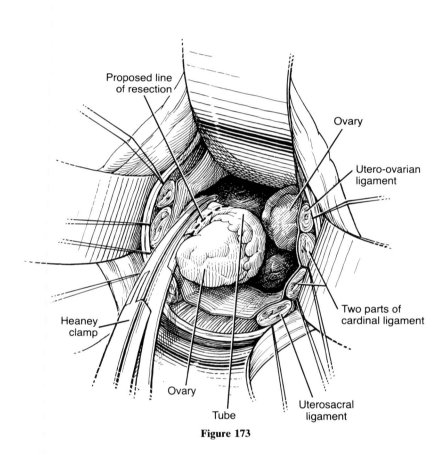

In the appropriate patient, a salpingo-oophorectomy can be accomplished at this time (Fig. 173). With Deaver retractors in the 9- and the 12-o'clock positions, the right tube and ovary are delivered into the field with Russian forceps. A Heaney clamp is placed proximal to the tube and ovary, incorporating the infundibulopelvic ligament. The clamp is placed so as to ensure that the entire tube and ovary are excised but that the ureter, which is just cephalad from the clamp, is not incorporated in the clamp or tie. After resection, the stump is suture-ligated with a 0 delayed absorbable suture and permitted to retract into the abdomen. The left tube and ovary are removed in a similar manner.

Proposed line of resection

Ovary

Utero-ovarian ligament

Heaney clamp

Two parts of cardinal ligament

Ovary

Tube

Uterosacral ligament

Figure 173

Although there are several equally acceptable techniques for hysterectomy, probably of greater significance are the steps taken for appropriate reconstruction of the pelvis. When complete hemostasis is obtained, the posterior cul-de-sac is carefully evaluated for the presence of a potential or true enterocele (Fig. 174). Usually there is some redundancy of the posterior cul-de-sac, for which we excise the peritoneal lining. The cut edge of the peritoneum is elevated with toothed forceps; with Mayo scissors the rectum is reflected posteriorly; and the sheet of peritoneum, the posterior cul-de-sac, and the sigmoid colon are resected flush with the longitudinal fibers of the rectosigmoid (Fig. 175). The anterior peritoneum beneath the base of the bladder may be treated in a similar fashion if the excess is sufficient to justify this procedure.

If there is a patulent posterior cul-de-sac, an internal McCall suture may be placed before the later placement of an external McCall suture. To place the internal McCall suture, the surgeon depresses the sigmoid colon down and to the patient's right with the left index and middle fingers. The monofilament 0 suture is placed deeply into the left pararectal fascia, after which the suture continues across the front of the sigmoid colon, where the surgeon depresses the sigmoid down and to the patient's left side for a similar deep placement of the suture in the right pararectal fascia (Fig. 176). This suture is tagged, after which the external McCall suture is placed.

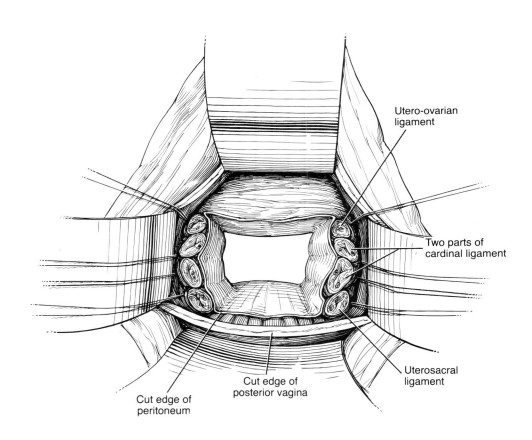

Utero-ovarian ligament

Two parts of cardinal ligament

Uterosacral ligament

Cut edge of posterior vagina

Cut edge of peritoneum

Figure 174

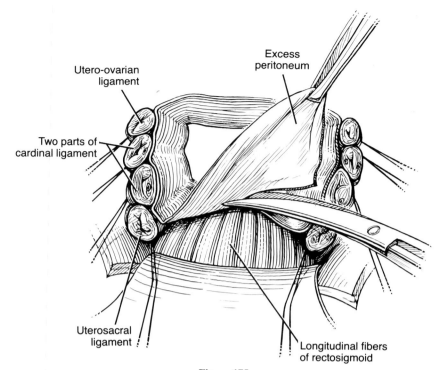

Utero-ovarian ligament

Excess peritoneum

Two parts of cardinal ligament

Uterosacral ligament

Longitudinal fibers of rectosigmoid

Figure 175

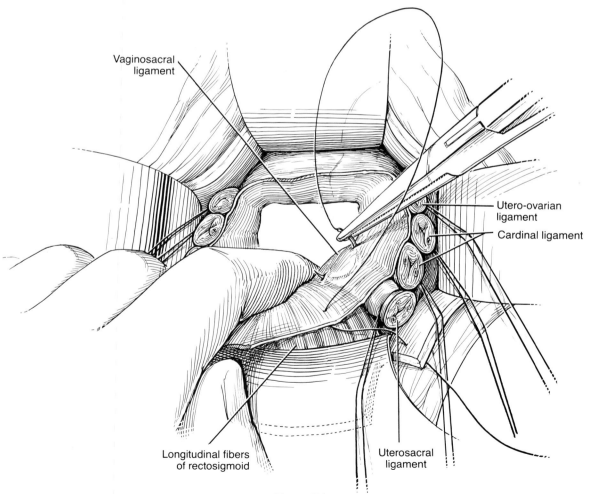

Vaginosacral ligament

Utero-ovarian ligament

Cardinal ligament

Longitudinal fibers of rectosigmoid

Uterosacral ligament

Figure 176

The external McCall suture begins with passage of a 0 delayed absorbable suture through the posterior vaginal wall and peritoneum to then incorporate the same pararectal fascia described for an internal McCall suture, but it is placed in a more cephalad position (Fig. 177). The suture is continued across the front of the sigmoid to the right pararectal fascia and brought out the vagina, where it is tagged to be tied at a later time. If the degree of redundancy does not warrant an internal McCall suture, a simple external McCall suture may be sufficient (Fig. 178).

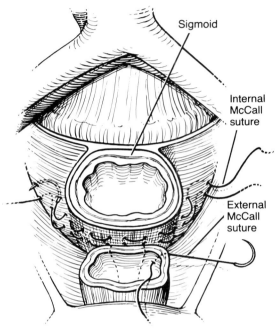

Figure 177

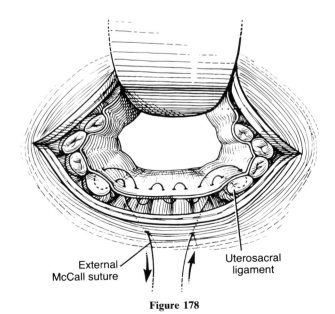

Figure 178

In all patients, a reperitonealizing suture is accomplished as follows. The anterior Deaver retractor is rocked forward to expose the anterior peritoneum, which is grasped with a broad Allis forceps or pickup forceps by the first assistant. The bladder may be gently separated from the peritoneum to give adequate clearance for the later reperitonealizing suture. The reperitonealizing suture passes through the peritoneum cephalad to the previously placed internal and external McCall sutures, picking up the peritoneum over the uterosacral and cardinal ligaments, and is passed lateral to the left utero-ovarian and round ligaments and then back through the anterior peritoneum (Fig. 179A). A straight clamp is placed on the distal ends of the utero-ovarian pedicle and pulled down by the first assistant while the surgeon

ties the first half of the pursestring suture, thus placing a second tie around the left utero-ovarian ligament. The pursestring suture is then continued from the 6-o'clock position clockwise above the McCall sutures on the right side in a similar fashion to that just completed on the left side (Fig. 179B). This suture exteriorizes the ligament stumps and permits the placement of a second tie on the right utero-ovarian ligament. The same needle is then passed through the right posterior vagina and a bare no. 6 Mayo needle is placed on the free end of the pursestring suture and brought out the left posterior vagina. The ends of the pursestring sutures are then tagged with a straight clamp and left hanging in a straight downward position.

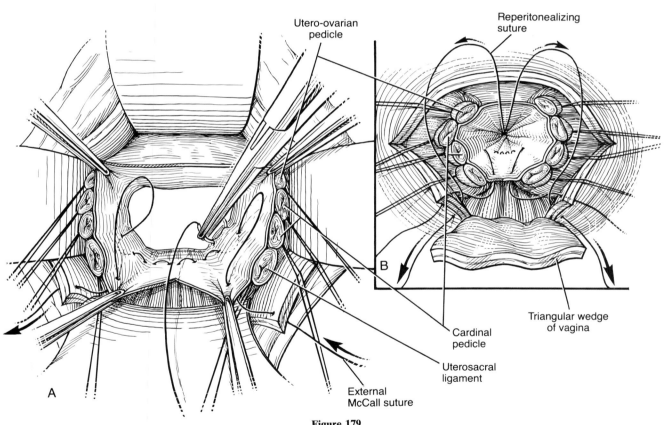

Figure 179

After perfect hemostasis is ensured, the vaginal vault is ready for closure. This is accomplished with the use of 2-0 delayed absorbable sutures placed as follows. At the left corner (patient's left) in the 3-o'clock position, a simple suture is placed starting through the posterior vaginal wall (proximal to the tie on the uterosacral ligament and distal to the ties on the cardinal and utero-ovarian ligaments) and coming out the anterior vaginal wall, where it is tied so that the edges of the vagina are approximated but not strangulated (Fig. 180*A*). Second and third more medially placed sutures incorporate the edges of the vagina, but usually the stumps of the pedicles are sufficiently lateral that they cannot be incorporated with this suture (Fig. 180*B*). The right side of the vaginal vault is closed in a similar fashion, again stick-tying the ligament stumps to the corners of the vaginal vault. The McCall sutures are now tied in the order in which they were placed (Fig. 181). Frequently, the high position of the McCall sutures results in a tenting-up of the posterior cul-de-sac as it pulls the posterior vagina to the level of the pararectal fascia (Fig. 182). If no additional repair is required, a small pack is placed in the vagina and a no. 16 Foley catheter is placed in the bladder.

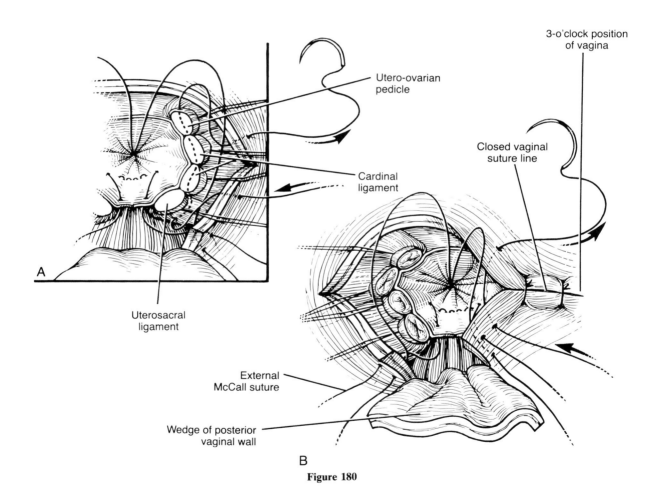

Utero-ovarian pedicle

Cardinal ligament

3-o'clock position of vagina

Closed vaginal suture line

Uterosacral ligament

External McCall suture

Wedge of posterior vaginal wall

A

B

Figure 180

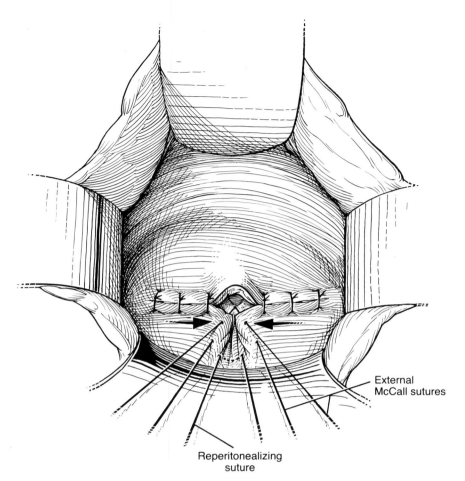

External
McCall sutures

Reperitonealizing
suture

Figure 181

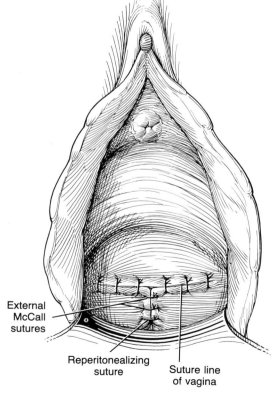

External
McCall
sutures

Reperitonealizing
suture

Suture line
of vagina

Figure 182

During the attempt to enter the anterior cul-de-sac, one may be a layer too far anterior and, as a result, enter the bladder. We purposely do not place a catheter in the bladder, nor do we empty the bladder preoperatively. As a result, if the bladder is entered, one encounters a gush of clear fluid, signaling the possibility of having entered the bladder. Infrequently, the amount of peritoneal fluid is sufficient to gush forth when the peritoneal cavity is entered, but generally its quantity is not comparable to that if the bladder is entered. Also, fat or bowel may be identified to establish the entrance as the peritoneal cavity. If the bladder is entered, there are two choices regarding its management. Because the cystotomy is readily available and easily exposed, one may want to close the cystotomy at this time. The disadvantage of immediate closure is that in the process of performing the forthcoming hysterectomy, the previously accomplished closure of the cystotomy can be disrupted (from pressure applied with the retractors or tension applied to the uterus). A preferred approach to closure of the cystotomy is to leave it undisturbed and proceed with dissection of the anterior vesicouterine space in a cephalad direction one layer closer

to the uterus to enter the anterior cul-de-sac. The hysterectomy is then accomplished in the customary fashion and the appropriate McCall sutures are placed. At this point, Allis forceps are placed on the edges of the bladder to provide traction and exposure of the cystotomy.

Closure is accomplished with either a running or an interrupted 3-0 delayed absorbable suture placed within the muscularis of the bladder in an extramucosal position (Fig. 183A). The closure extends one suture beyond the cystotomy in each direction. This initial layer is inverted with a second layer of the same suture, and again the closure extends lateral to the most lateral sutures of the original suture line, in either a running or an interrupted fashion in an extramucosal position (Fig. 183B). The peritoneum is pulled from the back of the bladder and covers the two-layered closure just accomplished (Fig. 183C). Then the pelvis is reperitonealized (as described earlier), the ligament stumps are suture-ligated to the corners of the vagina, and the vaginal suture line is closed. The catheter is left in for approximately 5 days instead of being removed the next morning.

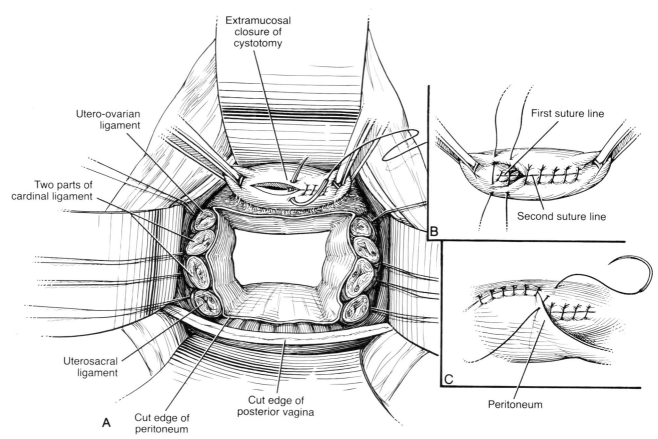

Figure 183

Vaginal Hysterectomy for Uterine Procidentia with Associated Cystocele, Enterocele, and Rectocele

Uterine prolapse occurs more frequently in the multiparous woman as a result of stretching, attenuation, or actual splitting of the endopelvic fascia and its condensations, the uterosacral and cardinal ligaments. The same stretching or lacerations of the muscles of the levator plate and perineal body further enhance descensus of the uterus. There are inherited differences in the quality and quantity of the supporting structures (endopelvic fascia and its condensations—the cardinal and uterosacral ligaments—and levator muscles), the shape of the bony pelvis, and the position of the uterus and its alignment in the axis of the vagina that may enhance pelvic relaxation. Local conditions such as obesity, chronic lung disease, and neurologic defects involving the pelvic floor musculature are additional factors affecting loss of pelvic support. Some degree of uterine descensus can be demonstrated in virtually all parous women; however, the condition may not become symptomatic until after the menopause, when the fascial and muscular supports become further attenuated by the progressive involutional changes.

Uterine prolapse invariably is associated with a potential or actual enterocele, which usually progresses in size with the degree of uterine descensus. Enterocele is a herniation of the pouch of Douglas into the rectovaginal septum that presents as a bulging mass in the posterior fornix and upper portion of the vaginal wall. Surgical correction consists of excision and a high ligation of the enterocele sac and approximation of the uterosacral (and vaginal sacral) ligaments and endopelvic (pararectal) fascia anterior to the rectum. Descent of the anterior vaginal wall (posterior wall of the bladder) is a result of the same factors responsible for descensus of the uterus. The resultant sagging support of the bladder and urethra (and thus changes in the angular relationships of the urethra and bladder neck) leads to urinary incontinence, or if there is sufficient relaxation, the urethra may be kinked and various degrees of urinary retention may result. When the cystocele is large and results in the potential for retained urine, or if the changes associated with urinary stress incontinence occur, operative repair is then required. A cystocele represents one component of the composite of pelvic relaxation; it specifically involves the attenuation, splitting, or simple sagging of the cervicopubic fascia supporting the bladder and urethra. Vaginal repair of the anterior vaginal wall, properly accomplished, results in effective correction of the symptoms and is associated with an excellent prognosis for satisfactory long-term results.

Although the degree of pelvic relaxation varies, Figure 184 is representative of true uterine procidentia. A weighted speculum is placed in the vagina in the 6-o'clock position. The second assistant, on the surgeon's left, provides exposure with Deaver retractors in the 9- and the 12-o'clock positions. The first assistant, on the surgeon's right, holds the Deaver retractor in the 3-o'clock position. Vulsellum tenacula are placed on the anterior and posterior lips of the cervix, and care is taken to include a greater portion of the endocervix and a lesser portion of the portio vaginalis in the clamp. The surgeon grasps the tenacula, applying traction with the left hand to pull the cervix down and, in this case, completely out of the vagina (Fig. 185). The superior extent of the future corner of the vagina is established at the 9-o'clock position, and this incision thus determines the future depth of the vagina. The incision is carried down through the cervicopubic fascia (from the 9- to the 12- to the 3-o'clock position—anterior incision—and, similarly, from the 3- to the 6- to the 9-o'clock position—posterior uterine incision), which can be seen to strip away from the anterior aspects of the cervix. The first assistant then takes the tenacula in the left hand and maintains firm, downward traction while the surgeon uses the tooth forceps to pick up the anterior vaginal wall and, with curved Mayo scissors, dissects free the anterior vaginal wall and bladder from the anterior aspect of the cervix, being careful to keep the point of the curved scissors toward the cervix.

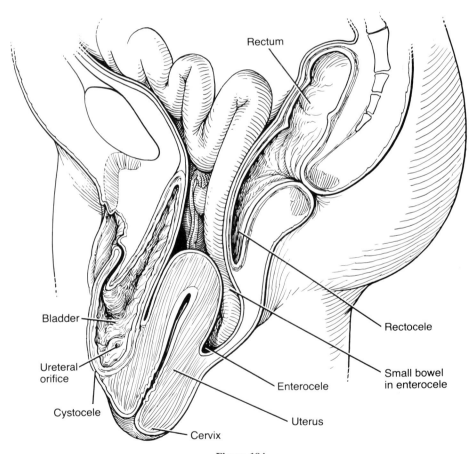

Rectum

Bladder

Ureteral orifice

Cystocele

Cervix

Enterocele

Uterus

Rectocele

Small bowel in enterocele

Figure 184

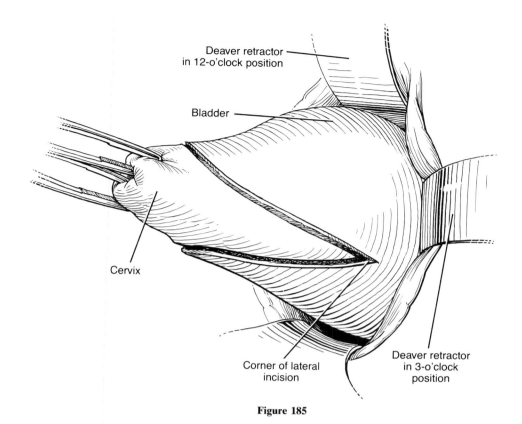

Deaver retractor in 12-o'clock position

Bladder

Cervix

Corner of lateral incision

Deaver retractor in 3-o'clock position

Figure 185

As the anterior vaginal wall and the underlying bladder are being separated from the anterior surface of the uterus, the second assistant moves the Deaver retractor from the 12-o'clock position under the anterior vaginal wall and bladder, placing these structures on tension and thus exposing the white fold of the peritoneum (Fig. 186). The surgeon then incises the fold of peritoneum transversely with a curved scissors. The tips of the scissors are inserted into the peritoneal defect and spread. (A Russian forceps can be inserted through this opening and the fundus pushed down in order to detect the epiploic tags or bowel and so ensure that the peritoneal cavity has been entered. If there was urine in the bladder, a gush of fluid would obviously be seen were the bladder to be entered.) Having entered the anterior cul-de-sac, the second assistant then inserts the anterior Deaver retractor (12-o'clock position) inside the peritoneal cavity.

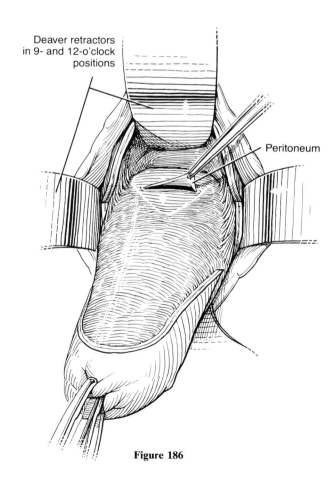

Deaver retractors in 9- and 12-o'clock positions

Peritoneum

Figure 186

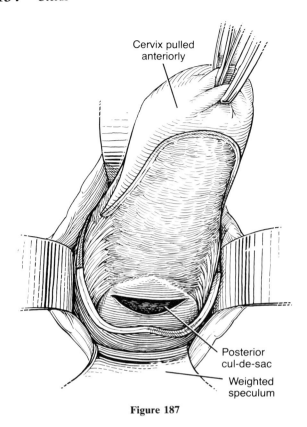

Cervix pulled
anteriorly

Posterior
cul-de-sac

Weighted
speculum

Figure 187

The first assistant then pulls the tenacula in the cephalad position toward the symphysis pubis, thus exposing the posterior vaginal wall. The surgeon applies countertraction to the cut edge of the vagina (with toothed forceps) and, with curved scissors, separates the posterior vaginal wall from the back of the uterus and enters the posterior cul-de-sac (Fig. 187). The posterior cul-de-sac is examined for any adhesions or bowel. The second assistant now removes the Deaver retractor from the 9-o'clock position, grasps the tenacula, and retracts them to the patient's right, thus placing the left uterosacral and cardinal ligaments on tension. The lateral vaginal wall is further (bluntly) mobilized with the gauzed index finger of the surgeon's right hand, and the upper aspects of the attenuated uterosacral-cardinal ligament complex are thus exposed.

A Heaney forceps grasps the uterosacral ligament far superior (6 to 9 cm) from the incision on the anterior vaginal wall and thus captures the most substantial supportive tissues available in this ligament (Fig. 188). The ligament is cut and suture-ligated in a fashion similar to that used for a straight vaginal hysterectomy. With a no. 6 Mayo needle, a ligature of no. 1 delayed absorbable suture is passed through the tissue behind the Heaney forceps in the middle of the ligament, after which a single tie is placed on its inferior segment. This suture is carried around the superior end of the pedicle and tied with three knots (Fig. 189).

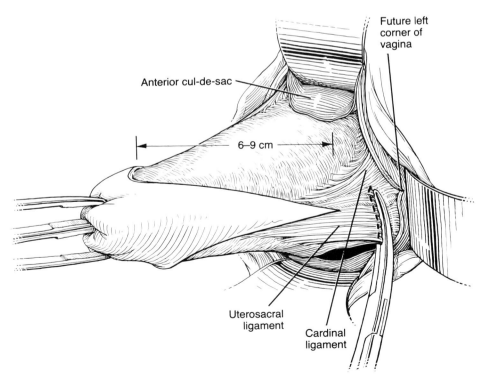

Future left
corner of
vagina

Anterior cul-de-sac

6–9 cm

Uterosacral
ligament

Cardinal
ligament

Figure 188

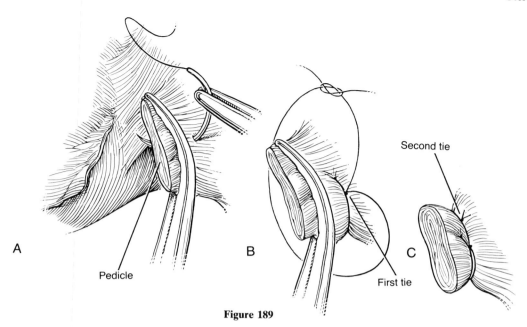

A

Pedicle

B

Second tie

C

First tie

Figure 189

Because of the extreme degree of prolapse, it is imperative to identify the ureter, which frequently is outside the vagina just cephalad to the uterosacral ligament tie. To identify the ureter, the surgeon inserts the left index finger in the anterior cul-de-sac and palpates the exact location of the left ureter between the index finger and the Deaver retractor in the 3-o'clock position (Fig. 190A). If there is any question, the index finger can be kept in the anterior cul-de-sac (against the ureter) during placement of the Heaney forceps to be absolutely sure that clamping this tissue does not compromise the ureter (Fig. 190B).

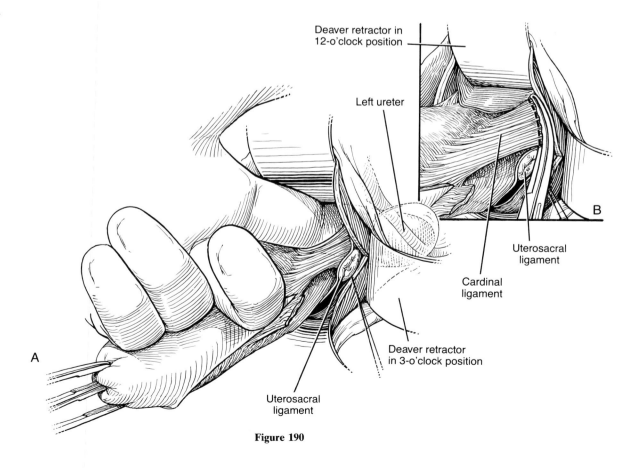

Deaver retractor in 12-o'clock position

Left ureter

Uterosacral ligament

Cardinal ligament

Deaver retractor in 3-o'clock position

Uterosacral ligament

A

B

Figure 190

With Mayo scissors, the cardinal ligament pedicle is cut distal to the clamp, and an adequate cuff must be left and extended about the tip of the clamp to permit secure placement of the ligature. This is tagged with a curved forceps, which is placed on the patient's left side. The remainder of the cardinal ligament and its enclosed uterine artery are clamped and tied in the same fashion, including a portion of the anterior and posterior peritoneum (Fig. 191). This tagged suture is placed in the same curved forceps as the original cardinal ligament pedicle. (The pedicle is tagged to assist in rapid identification, and at no time is traction applied to the tie.)

The Deaver retractor in the 3-o'clock position is now passed from the first assistant to the second assistant and placed in the 9-o'clock position. The tenacula are grasped by the first assistant, and the cervix and uterus are pulled to the patient's left. The right uterosacral and cardinal ligaments are dealt with in the same way as those on the patient's left side. At this point, it is important to emphasize that when tying a ligament stump, the surgeon must be careful to tie the knots far enough back on the stump to include all of the vessels and not allow any of them to slip out of the grasp of the knot. Each pedicle should be immediately adjacent to the next pedicle, such that there would not be a space between them sufficient to allow postoperative bleeding. The surgeon now delivers the fundus through the posterior cul-de-sac by means of anterior traction on the tenacula. Occasionally, it may be necessary to move one of the tenacula from the cervix back onto the fundus in order to deliver the fundus. A Heaney clamp is placed on the right utero-ovarian and round ligaments, and, with Mayo scissors, the surgeon divides these ligaments medial to the clamp (Fig. 192). The left utero-ovarian and round ligaments are dealt with in the same manner (Fig. 193), and the specimen is sent for immediate frozen-section histologic study. The utero-ovarian and round ligaments are then suture-ligated and tagged with straight forceps, which are placed on the abdomen of the patient. With all ligatures visible, hemostasis can be assessed and the tubes and ovaries examined.

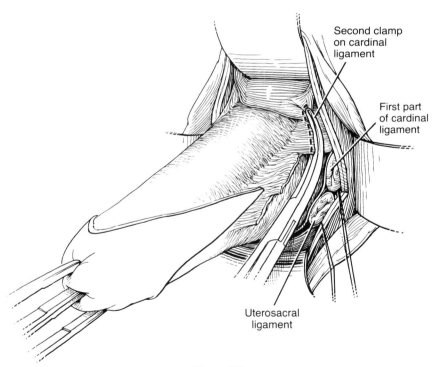

Second clamp
on cardinal
ligament

First part
of cardinal
ligament

Uterosacral
ligament

Figure 191

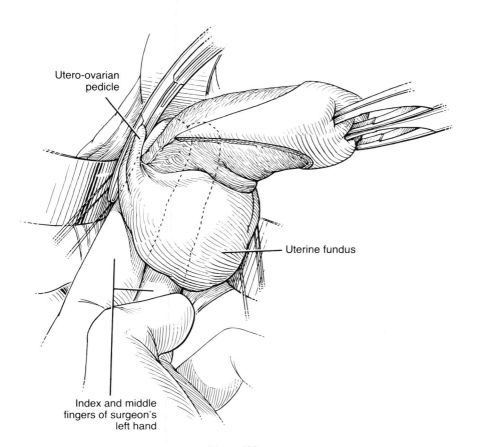

Utero-ovarian
pedicle

Uterine fundus

Index and middle
fingers of surgeon's
left hand

Figure 192

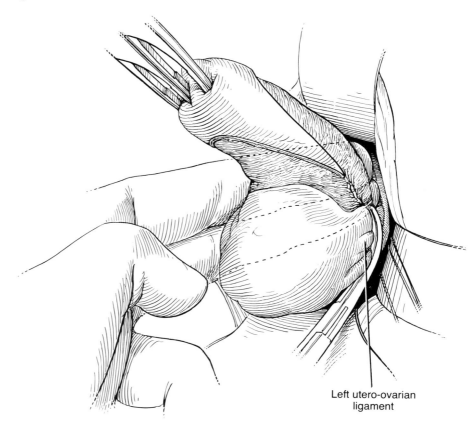

Left utero-ovarian
ligament

Figure 193

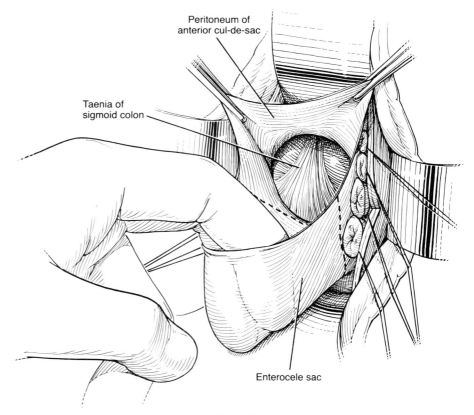

Peritoneum of
anterior cul-de-sac

Taenia of
sigmoid colon

Enterocele sac

Figure 194

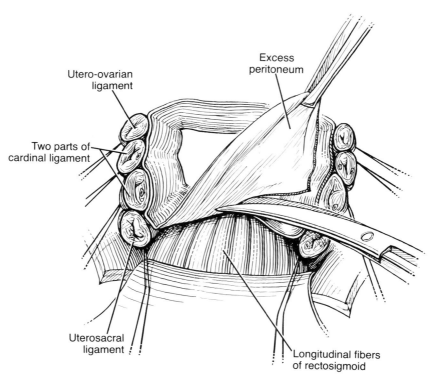

Utero-ovarian
ligament

Excess
peritoneum

Two parts of
cardinal ligament

Uterosacral
ligament

Longitudinal fibers
of rectosigmoid

Figure 195

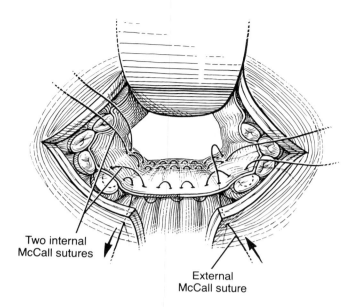

Two internal
McCall sutures

External
McCall suture

Figure 196

The degree of enterocele present varies, but there always is some enterocele present with true procidentia (Fig. 194). A small abdominal pack is placed through the incision, and the table is altered to a slight Trendelenburg position to prevent the intestines from prolapsing into the operative field. An Allis forceps may be placed on the peritoneum of the posterior cul-de-sac, and, with Mayo scissors, the rectum and lower sigmoid are separated from the peritoneum, the excess of which is excised (Fig. 195). At this point, the redundancy of the posterior vagina is assessed, and the appropriate-sized wedge of posterior vagina is reflected and placed under the tongue of the weighted speculum. Again, depending on the size of the enterocele, one to three internal McCall sutures (Fig. 196) and one or two external McCall sutures followed by a final reperitonealizing suture are placed (in the order given), each in an increasingly cephalad position within the pelvis (Fig. 197). A

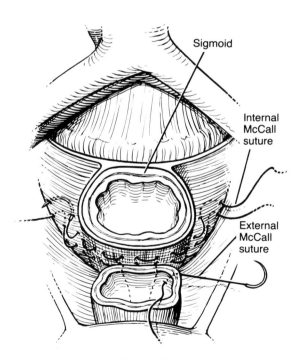

Sigmoid

Internal
McCall
suture

External
McCall
suture

Figure 197

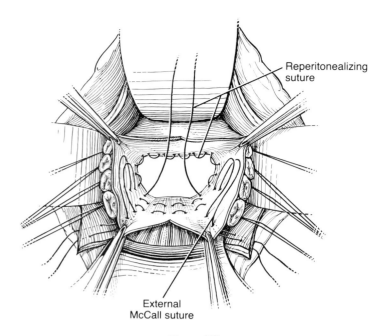

Reperitonealizing suture

External McCall suture

Figure 198

reperitonealizing suture is placed in the most cephalad or superior level (Fig. 198). The technique of placement of the internal and external McCall and reperitonealizing sutures is the same as that described for correction of the enterocele for posthysterectomy vaginal vault prolapse (see page 85).

The vaginal vault closure is accomplished with 2-0 delayed absorbable suture, as follows. At the left vaginal corner, a simple suture is placed starting through the posterior vaginal wall and passing through and proximal to the tie of the uterosacral ligament but distal to the tie on the two portions of

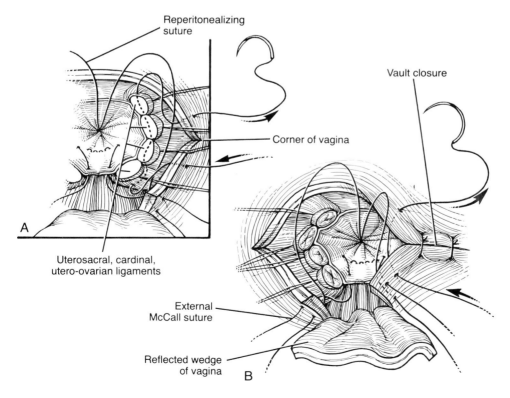

Reperitonealizing suture

Corner of vagina

Uterosacral, cardinal, utero-ovarian ligaments

External McCall suture

Reflected wedge of vagina

Vault closure

A

B

Figure 199

the cardinal ligament and the utero-ovarian pedicle, and then it is continued through the anterior vaginal wall. This is tied and cut along with the previously tagged ligament stump ties on the left side (Fig. 199*A*). A second stitch is placed medial to the original suture, thus incorporating the very distal ends of the ligament stumps and the vaginal wall. Usually, a third suture is placed in the same fashion, but it is too far medial to include any portion of the vaginal stumps (Fig. 199*B*). The right side of the vaginal vault is closed in the same fashion, again stick-tying the ligament stumps to the corners of the vagina. Hemostasis is carefully evaluated as the procedure is accomplished, and while the edges of the vagina are approximated, care is taken that undue tension is not placed on the suture, which could potentially necrose the edge of the vagina. At this point, some surgeons prefer to tie the McCall sutures in the order in which they were placed. As each subsequent McCall suture

is placed, a lower level of the cut edge of the vagina is approximated with a higher level of the pararectal fascia. We prefer to leave the McCall and reperitonealizing sutures tagged, thus avoiding elevation of the posterior vagina, which tends to pull the anterior vaginal wall superiorly (and makes the dissection for the modified Kennedy anterior colporrhaphy more difficult).

The anterior colporrhaphy is accomplished in the following manner. Straight clamps are placed on the corners of the anterior vaginal wall and medial border of the vault closure, and a third clamp is placed just below the external urethral meatus (Fig. 200). Proper traction by an assistant places the vaginal wall under tension in a triangular fashion, thus permitting the surgeon, with pickup forceps in the left hand, to proceed in the midline to separate the vaginal wall carefully from the underlying cervicopubic fascia cov-

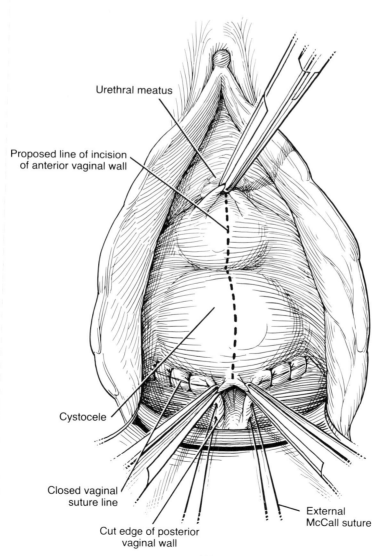

Urethral meatus

Proposed line of incision
of anterior vaginal wall

Cystocele

Closed vaginal
suture line

Cut edge of posterior
vaginal wall

External
McCall suture

Figure 200

ering the bladder and urethra. The tips of the scissors are immediately adjacent to the undersurface of the anterior vaginal wall, and the points of the scissors are directed away from the bladder (Fig. 201). This dissection is best accomplished with slight spreading of the tips of the scissors to aid in separation of the vaginal mucosa from the cervicopubic fascia. As each segment (2 to 3 cm) is freed, the vaginal wall is incised in the midline; this approach provides access for the continued separation of the anterior vaginal wall from the underlying cervicopubic fascia (Fig. 202).

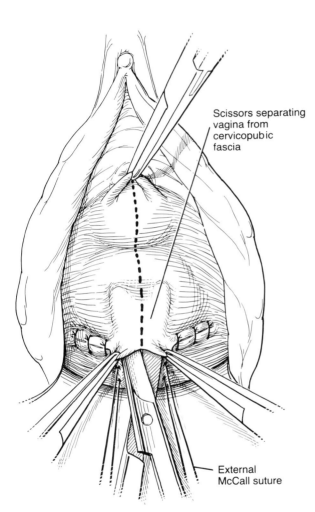

Scissors separating vagina from cervicopubic fascia

External McCall suture

Figure 201

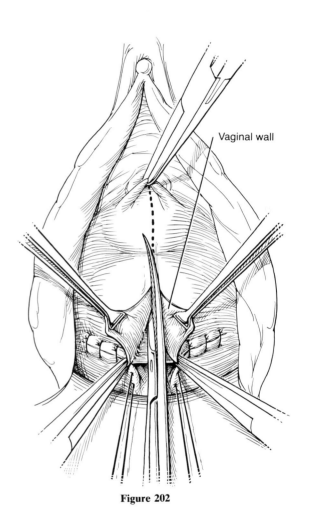

Vaginal wall

Figure 202

Dissection and incision of the anterior vaginal wall are continued all the way to the straight forceps fixed just short of the external urethral meatus. Two Allis forceps are placed on each side of the cut edge of the vaginal wall, and the previously placed straight Kocher clamp is repositioned on the tip of the anterior vaginal wall in the medial position. As the assistant applies spreading traction on the clamps on the anterior vaginal wall, the surgeon, with toothed forceps in the left hand, applies countertraction on the bladder and, using Mayo scissors, sharply dissects the bladder with its cervicopubic fascia from the inferior surface of the vagina (Fig. 203A). This dissection is continued laterally and superiorly adjacent to the left descending pubic ramus (Fig. 203B). The anterior vaginal wall is more intimately attached to the endopelvic fascia at the level of the bladder neck and urethra. With appropriate traction and countertraction, sharp dissection permits mobilization in the same plane laterally to ensure adequate mobility for later plication. Adequate mobilization is very important to ensure the surgeon the freedom to develop adequate plication of the bladder neck and urethra and so provide the proper angular relationships between the urethra and base of the bladder to result in urinary control. Adherence to the basic principles of traction and countertraction helps the surgeon avoid buttonholing of the vaginal wall and yet ensures that the fascial capsule of the bladder remains attached to the bladder.

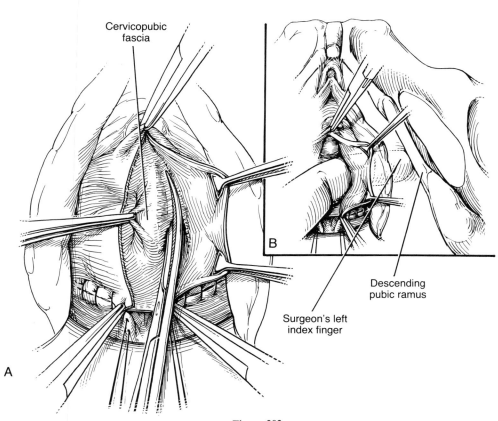

Figure 203

A similar dissection is repeated on the right side, where the surgeon holds the Allis forceps in the left hand and may place the fingers on the outside of the vaginal wall; the assistant applies traction on the bladder to facilitate sharp, accurate, and wide dissection (Fig. 204).

Once the bladder neck and urethra are fully mobilized laterally to the pubic ramus, the imbricating sutures can be placed. We prefer to use interrupted 2-0 monofilament delayed absorbable sutures in the initial layer. The first suture is placed deeply, parallel and adjacent to the external urethral meatus on each side, sufficiently cephalad to incorporate the inferior as-

pects of the base of the posterior pubourethral ligament (Fig. 205). The sutures are tied, and each suture is appropriately placed (each succeeding suture is slightly more lateral than the previously placed suture) in lateral positions such that excellent support is obtained beneath the urethra, bladder neck, and base of the bladder (Fig. 206A). Additional sutures may be placed in the area of the proximal urethra and bladder neck; they further plicate the supporting tissues in the most critical area for urinary control (Fig. 206B). The fascial sutures result in plication of the cervicopubic fascia and also assist in controlling hemostasis.

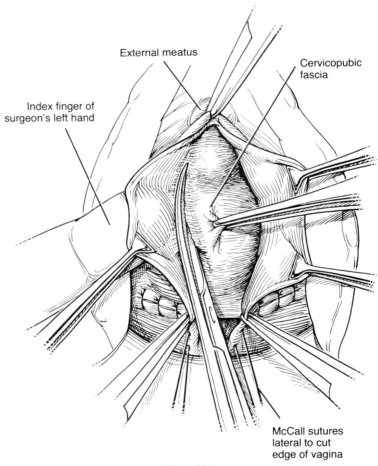

External meatus

Cervicopubic fascia

Index finger of surgeon's left hand

McCall sutures lateral to cut edge of vagina

Figure 204

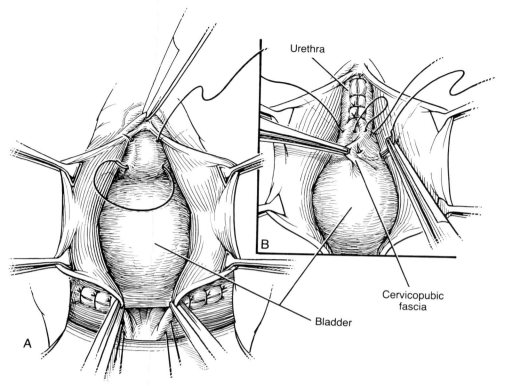

Urethra

Cervicopubic
fascia

Bladder

B

A

Figure 205

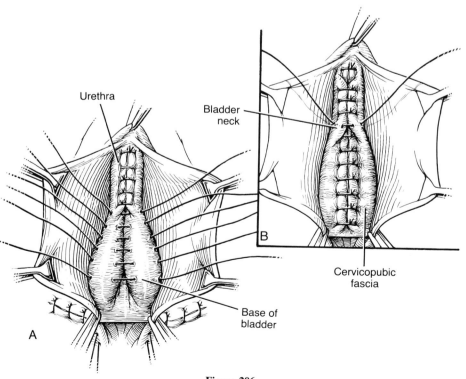

Urethra

Bladder
neck

Base of
bladder

Cervicopubic
fascia

B

A

Figure 206

The Allis forceps are then removed from the edges of the vaginal wall. The redundant vaginal wall is carefully resected with scissors (we do not apply traction on the vaginal wall), and care is taken to ensure that the resultant suture line can be closed free of tension (Fig. 207*A*). A similar resection is done on the right wall of the vagina such that the two vaginal edges fall into perfect approximation in the midline (Fig. 207*B*).

The vaginal edges are then approximated with interrupted 3-0 delayed absorbable sutures. As each edge of the vaginal wall is approximated, a small portion of the underlying cervicopubic fascia is incorporated to pull the vaginal wall to the level of the cervicopubic fascia and avoid potential dead space (Fig. 208). Care should be taken that the sutures do not perforate the wall of the urethra or bladder and that excessive tension is not placed on the vaginal wall, which could lead to slough of the approximated edges. Once the anterior vaginal wall is completed, we prefer to tie the previously placed McCall sutures, which further elevate the apex of the vagina superiorly and back toward the hollow of the sacrum (Fig. 209).

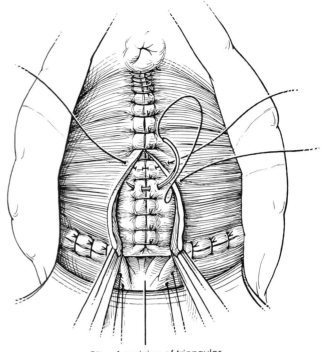

Site of excision of triangular
wedge of posterior vagina

Figure 208

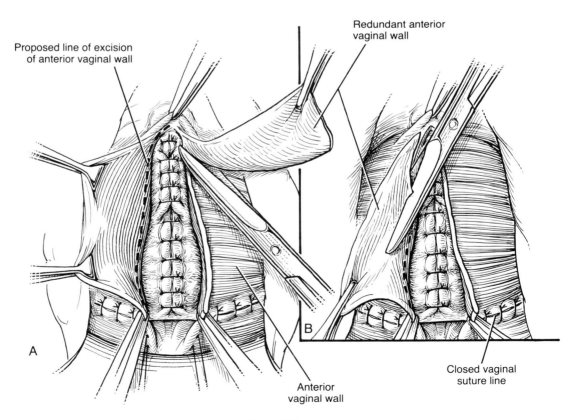

Proposed line of excision
of anterior vaginal wall

Redundant anterior
vaginal wall

Anterior
vaginal wall

Closed vaginal
suture line

Figure 207

A posterior colpoperineorrhaphy can now be completed. Two vulsellum tenacula are placed on the right and left perineum, approximately where the marks remain from the just-removed weighted speculum (Fig. 210). While assistants maintain traction on the tenacula, a knife is used to make a V-shaped incision between the tenacula (the shape of the incision is tailored to the size of the patient's perineal body). Using scissors with toothed forceps for traction, the surgeon dissects the posterior vaginal wall free from the anterior rectal wall, removing the appropriate strip of posterior vagina and its underlying fascia, which is flush with the anterior wall of the rectum (Fig. 211). With appropriate traction on the strip of vagina and with use of the scissors, the rectum is reflected off the posterior vaginal wall of the vagina.

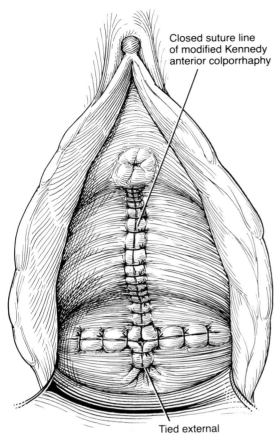

Closed suture line of modified Kennedy anterior colporrhaphy

Tied external McCall sutures

Figure 209

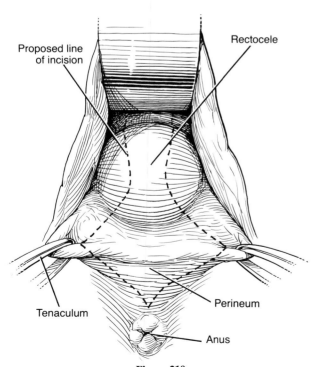

Proposed line of incision

Rectocele

Tenaculum

Perineum

Anus

Figure 210

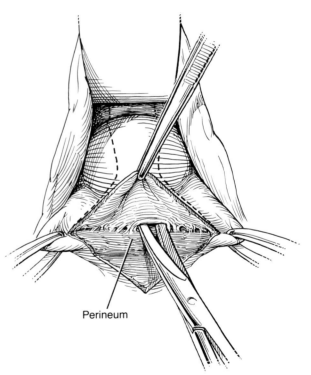

Perineum

Figure 211

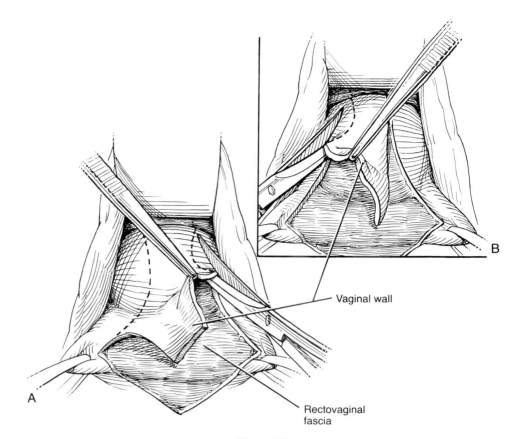

Vaginal wall

Rectovaginal
fascia

Figure 212

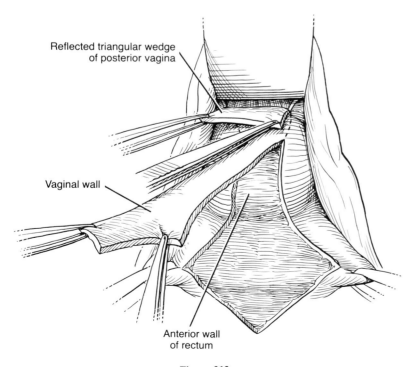

Reflected triangular wedge
of posterior vagina

Vaginal wall

Anterior wall
of rectum

Figure 213

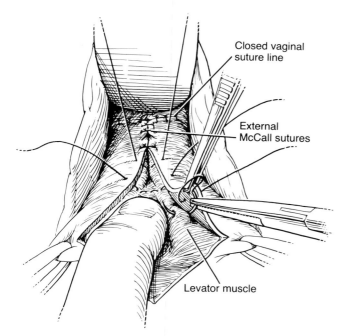

Closed vaginal
suture line

External
McCall sutures

Levator muscle

Figure 214

The surgeon, using scissors, cuts first on one side and then the other, being careful to stay free of the rectum and to maintain a symmetric resection of the redundant posterior vaginal wall (Fig. 212). The width of the strip of vagina removed is determined by the degree of relaxation of the posterior vaginal wall and the need to preserve a functional vagina.

The vaginal incisions are continued in a superior direction until they meet the reflected upper triangular wedge of posterior vagina that was initially placed under the weighted speculum (Fig. 213). With 3-0 delayed absorbable suture, the edges of the vaginal wall and the underlying rectovaginal fascia are closed with a single layer of interrupted suture (Fig. 214). As each suture is tied in the midline, the diameter of the vagina is evaluated to be sure that there is adequate room for vaginal function. At the appropriate level, the medial border of the underlying levator muscle is approximated as a separate layer, after which the overlying vaginal mucosa is closed with interrupted sutures (Fig. 215). Again, the aperture of the vaginal canal is evaluated to ensure that appropriate support has been developed without adversely compromising the vaginal diameter. The pro-

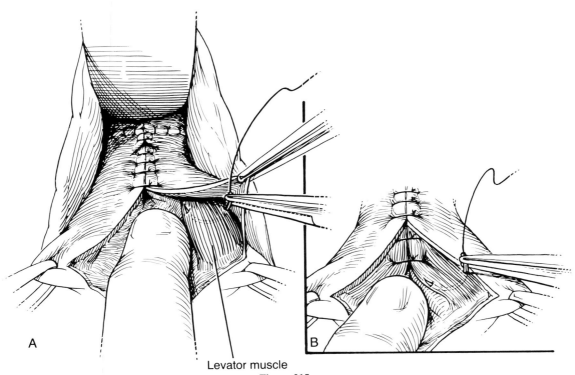

A

B

Levator muscle
Figure 215

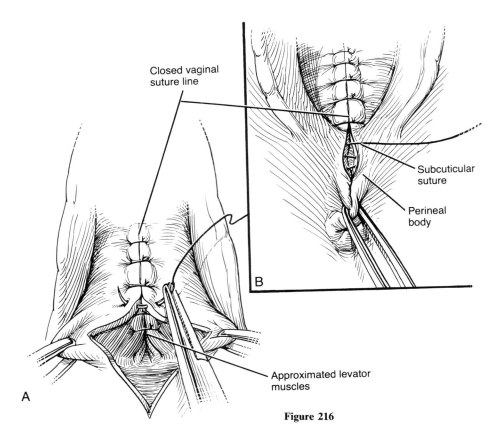

Figure 216

cedure is continued inferiorly with increasingly larger portions of the levator muscle approximated as the introitus is approached (Fig. 216*A*). The perineorrhaphy is completed by approximation of the perineal muscle and subcuticular closure of the skin (Fig. 216*B*). At completion, it is apparent that the apex of the vagina is well supported and that the patulent diameter of the vagina is corrected with excellent support all the way to the introitus.

The suture lines are carefully inspected to ensure that complete hemostasis has been obtained. The transverse suture line at the very apex of the vagina is far superior and pulled posterior toward the hollow of the sacrum. The anterior suture line demonstrates the urethra and bladder neck area tucked up under the symphysis pubis, with a gentle curve representing the base of the bladder. The apex of the posterior suture line is noted to point directly posterior toward the hollow of the sacrum with a gradual elevation over the area of the lower portion of the levators; this positioning results in a vagina of normal depth and diameter such that in the standing position the upper half to two thirds of the vagina is parallel to the floor (Fig. 217). A small pack is placed in the vagina and a no. 16 Foley catheter is placed in the bladder.

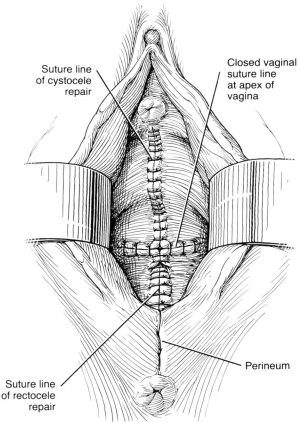

Figure 217

Difficult Vaginal Hysterectomy

Narrow Vagina—Schuchardt Incision

Occasionally in the nulliparous patient requiring a vaginal hysterectomy, exposure to the upper vagina and cervix can be compromised. To facilitate exposure and vaginal hysterectomy, an episiotomy-like incision (Schuchardt incision) can greatly enhance the safety of the procedure. The incision is initially made like that of a mediolateral episiotomy, extending through the perineal muscles laterally to the external anal sphincter and continuing posteriorly (the extent of the incision is determined by the individual need) around the anus, laying open the entire lower half of the vagina (Fig. 218). Individual bleeders should be identified and appropriately ligated. Appropriate traction on the cervix with Deaver retractors holding the vaginal wall superiorly and laterally facilitates visibility and the safety of the procedure.

We proceed with vaginal hysterectomy, using the technique just described. On occasion, because of some compromise in the exposure, it may be initially difficult to enter the anterior cul-de-sac. In such cases, one does not persist but, rather, enters the posterior cul-de-sac, where the uterosacral ligaments are clamped, cut, and suture-ligated bilaterally. With this maneuver, there is generally additional descent of the uterus; this facilitates visibility of the anterior cul-de-sac, which then can be safely entered. Once this is entered, the ureter is identified before placement of the cardinal ligament clamp. In the overwhelming majority of patients, the ureter is far superior and most unlikely to be injured. In some cases (because of the relatively high location of the ureter and the limited room of the anterior cul-de-sac), the ureter cannot be palpated, and then the cardinal ligament should be carefully examined in the area where the clamp is to be placed to obtain a "negative feel" (failure to palpate the ureter), which is further assurance that the clamp can be placed safely. The hysterectomy then proceeds in the fashion already described.

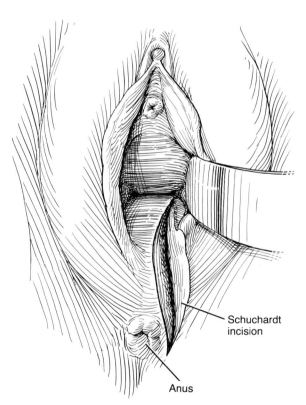

Schuchardt
incision

Anus

Figure 218

Previous Abdominal Suspension

Occasionally, a patient who has undergone uterine suspension later experiences the symptoms and has the physical findings of uterine prolapse (Fig. 219). In review of this group of patients, we have, with proper selection, been able to accomplish a vaginal hysterectomy with no increase in complications or morbidity. Sometimes the elongated uterus is difficult to deliver because of the fixation to the abdominal wall; rarely, an abdominal incision is required to free it from the anterior abdominal wall, which cannot be reached safely by the vaginal approach. For patients in whom an abdominal incision has been necessary to free a fixed uterus, we have always found a complicating condition that justified altering our planned approach. This is infrequent, and in the overwhelming majority of patients, we have been able to proceed with vaginal hysterectomy in the manner already described.

Uterine Enlargement Requiring Morcellation

Not infrequently, the size of the uterus to be removed is often taken as a major factor in deciding between an abdominal or vaginal approach to hysterectomy. However, large size, per se, is not a contraindication to vaginal hysterectomy; degree of mobility is also a factor. However, certain precautions should be taken to avoid complications. We always do a preliminary dilatation and curettage. Frozen sections are obtained, and a tissue diagnosis is immediately available to exclude endometrial malignancy. As in a regular vaginal hysterectomy, the anterior and posterior cul-de-sacs are entered. The uterosacral and cardinal ligaments are clamped, cut, and suture-ligated. With this degree of hemostasis, morcellation can be initiated; this is begun with a knife in the midline, and the cervix and lower uterine walls are divided (Figs.

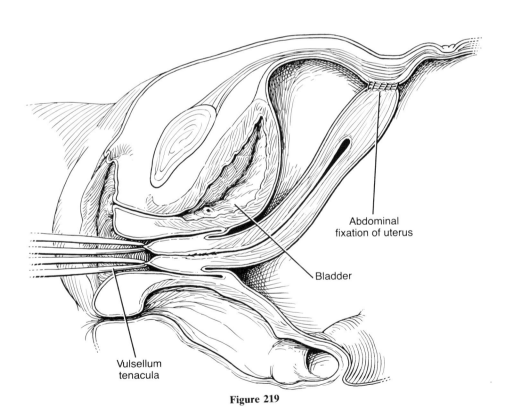

Abdominal fixation of uterus

Bladder

Vulsellum tenacula

Figure 219

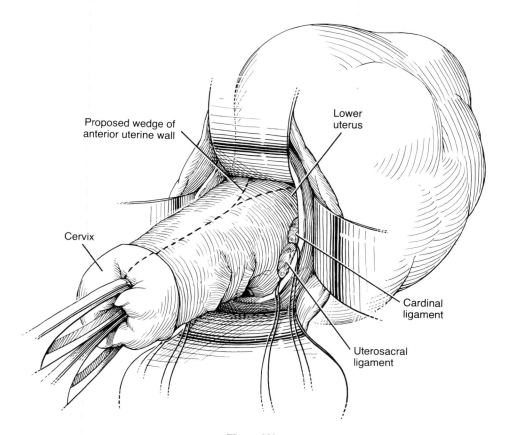

Proposed wedge of
anterior uterine wall

Lower
uterus

Cervix

Cardinal
ligament

Uterosacral
ligament

Figure 220

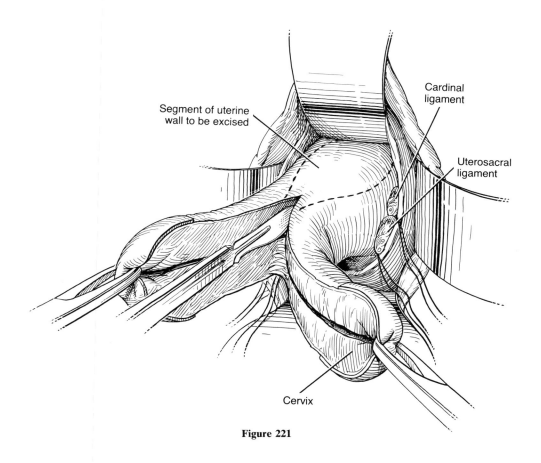

Segment of uterine
wall to be excised

Cardinal
ligament

Uterosacral
ligament

Cervix

Figure 221

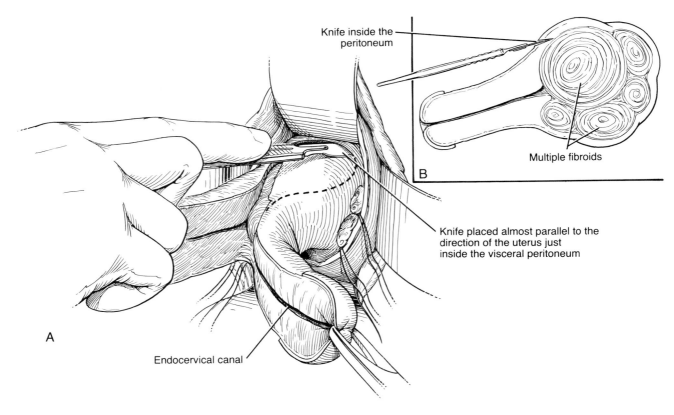

Knife inside the peritoneum

B

Multiple fibroids

Knife placed almost parallel to the direction of the uterus just inside the visceral peritoneum

A

Endocervical canal

Figure 222

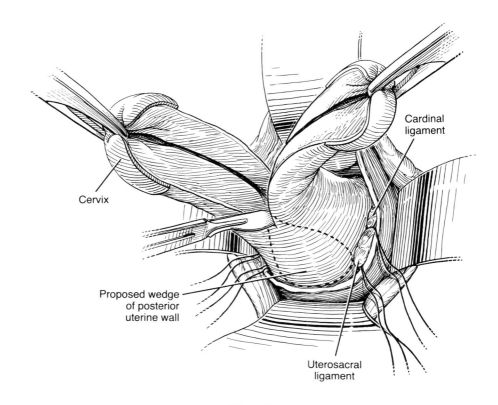

Cervix

Cardinal ligament

Proposed wedge of posterior uterine wall

Uterosacral ligament

Figure 223

220 and 221). A Deaver retractor is used to elevate the anterior vaginal wall, and, with a knife kept deep to the visceral peritoneum, a sizable portion of the anterior uterine wall is excised (Fig. 222). The uterus is then pulled anteriorly, and a similar segment of the posterior uterine wall is exposed; this is excised in the same fashion (Fig. 223). This procedure is continued in a superior direction, and the anterior and then the posterior vaginal walls are excised in a stepwise fashion; this approach thus reduces the diameter of the fundus of the uterus, permitting it to descend further into the vagina. The cutting on the uterus should never be higher than good exposure permits.

Frequently, one or several sizable fibroids are encountered within the wall of the uterus; these can be grasped directly with the third vulsellum tenaculum and sharply excised (Fig. 224). As the bulk of the uterine fundus is reduced, it can then be delivered out of the vagina. The surgeon then inserts the index

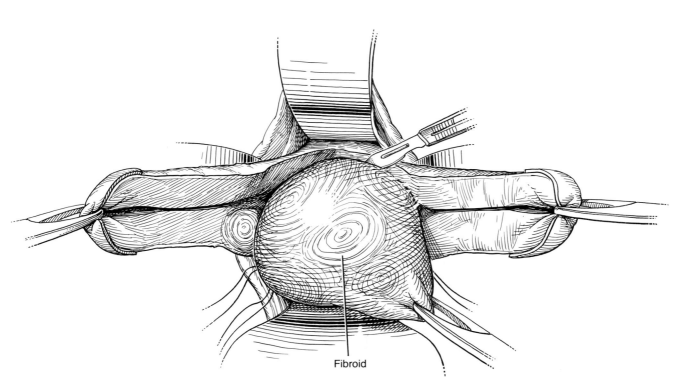

Fibroid

Figure 224

finger behind the uterine fundus to permit safe placement of the Heaney forceps on the utero-ovarian pedicle (tube, round and ovarian ligaments), which is divided to permit removal of the uterus (Fig. 225).

Cervical Elongation

If there has been significant injury or attenuation of the endopelvic fascia and its condensations (uterosacral and cardinal ligaments), increases in intra-abdominal pressure gradually lead to uterine prolapse in addition to cystocele, rectocele, and enterocele. If,

however, the integrity of the endopelvic fascia and its condensations has been maintained, the incompetency of the genital hiatus and levator muscles may be associated with only cervical elongation.

With cervical elongation, a thorough vaginal evaluation discloses that the anterior, posterior, and lateral vaginal fornices are in their customary high level and will descend minimally with straining (Fig. 226). The anterior and upper posterior vaginal walls are well supported with essentially no cystocele, enterocele, or rectocele.

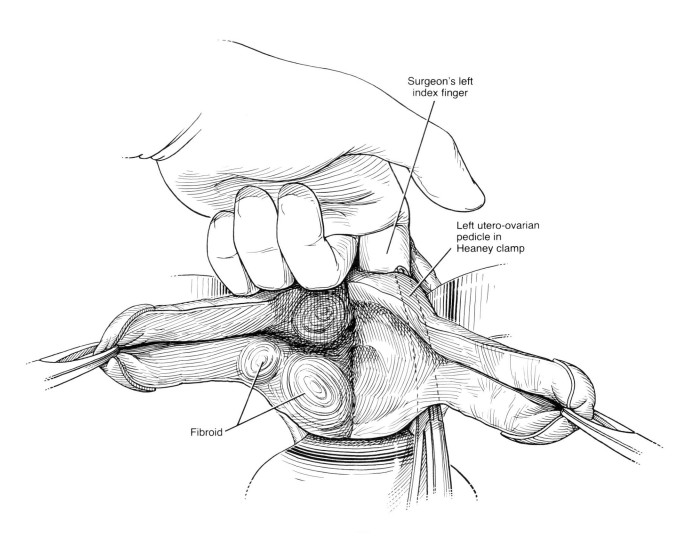

Surgeon's left index finger

Left utero-ovarian pedicle in Heaney clamp

Fibroid

Figure 225

With straining, the fundus of the uterus remains in a relatively high position at the apex of the vagina. However, the elongation of the cervix results in its presentation at the introitus or protrusion from the vagina. Because of the descensus and protrusion of the cervix, the patient may experience pelvic pressure or feel as though she is sitting on a ball. A vaginal hysterectomy is preferable and is indicated, and it can be accomplished safely. The important technical aspect of the operation is to recognize that the cul-de-sacs are in a high position in the pelvis (Fig.

226*B*). The incision about the cervix is made in the customary fashion. With the incision placed close to the uterus, the anterior vaginal wall and posterior surface of the bladder are dissected off the anterior surface of the uterus until the peritoneum is identified and entered. (The distance to the anterior cul-de-sac may represent 80% of the total length of the uterus.) A similar dissection is done posteriorly, after which the uterus is removed in the manner already described.

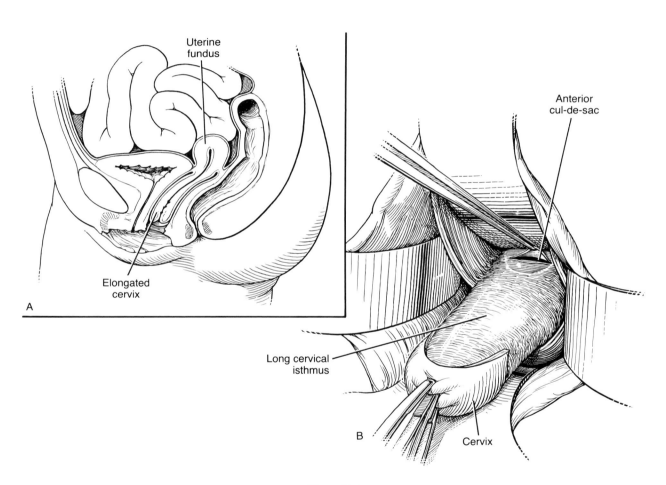

Figure 226

Total Abdominal Hysterectomy: Simple

Although total abdominal hysterectomy, properly performed, is safe and effective, a distressing number of patients sustain injuries to the bowel or urinary tract during the operation. Most injuries tend to occur not during operations complicated by large uterine fibroids, malignancy, or extensive pelvic inflammatory disease but during what should be simple hysterectomies for persistent menorrhagia, carcinoma in situ, or minimal endometriosis, when the uterus is anatomically normal and there is little, if any, alteration in the normal position of the bowel or urinary tract.

A definite, planned approach avoids useless, time-consuming, extra motion and permits the operation to be done safely and with dispatch. Certainly, because of a particular disease process, the operation may need to be altered extemporaneously, but the focus is always to return to the originally planned procedure.

The surgeon must have good lighting and excellent exposure through an adequate incision to perform an abdominal hysterectomy safely (regardless of the technique). An inadequate incision leads to inadequate exposure and dissection, and it may promote relatively blind clamping and oversewing, which are frequently responsible for the unrecognized injuries that account for genitourinary and intestinal fistulas after hysterectomy. We prefer a long midline incision that can be extended sufficiently to ensure a free field of operation.

In all pelvic operations, the first steps should be a general exploration of the contents of the abdominal cavity, mobilization of any adhesions, and an accurate assessment of the pelvic disease.

Sharp dissection should be used throughout the operation. The common practice of pulling or scooping out adnexa or fixed pelvic masses to begin a hysterectomy is to be deplored. Clean, sharp dissection averts injury to the adjacent structures such as the ureter, bladder, and rectum. It also promotes recognition of any such injuries and permits immediate repair, thus preventing the formation of a fistula.

Essential to any anatomic surgical dissection are proper traction and countertraction on the tissues to permit accurate definition of the correct tissue planes and to facilitate prompt identification of the important anatomic structures. We use a self-retaining retractor of the Balfour type, 30° of Trendelenburg position, and a large laparotomy pack inserted above the pelvic brim to keep the bowel out of the operative field. One or two retractors of the Harrington type may be helpful to keep the bladder, perivesical fat, or a redundant rectosigmoid out of the operative field— particularly if the pelvis is deep or if the patient is very obese.

Vital structures should be identified and cleanly mobilized by sharp dissection before any clamps are placed or pedicles transected. The ureters should be identified and mobilized from contiguous structures, as required in the individual operation. Freeing the bladder anteriorly and the rectum posteriorly prevents their inclusion during closure of the vagina and thus minimizes potential formation of a bladder fistula. The bladder and rectum should be sharply dissected to a point at least 1 cm beyond the site of the planned vaginal transection.

Although a contaminated organ (the vagina) is entered during the operation, the risk of postoperative infectious complications should be relatively low. Potential infection is minimized by adequate cleansing of the vagina; careful handling of the tissues; relatively nontraumatic, sharp dissection; use of low-reactive, fine absorbable suture material; avoidance of mass ligatures; and meticulous hemostasis.

In the operation described here, excellent support is given to the vaginal vault by securing the uterosacral-cardinal ligament complex to the lateral vaginal angles.

Adherence to these basic principles allows the surgeon to improvise the surgical dissection necessary for the specific condition and to accomplish the operation satisfactorily with minimal risk of morbidity or mortality.

The patient is placed in a deep Trendelenburg position (30°) and held in place with ankle straps (Fig. 227). A lower midline incision curving around the umbilicus permits accurate exploration of the upper and lower abdomen before proceeding with operation (Fig. 228). Straight Kocher forceps are placed across

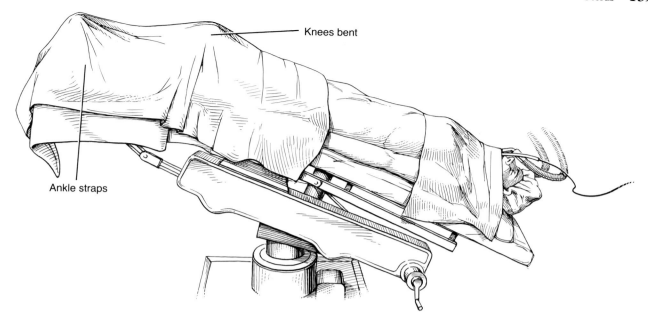

Figure 227

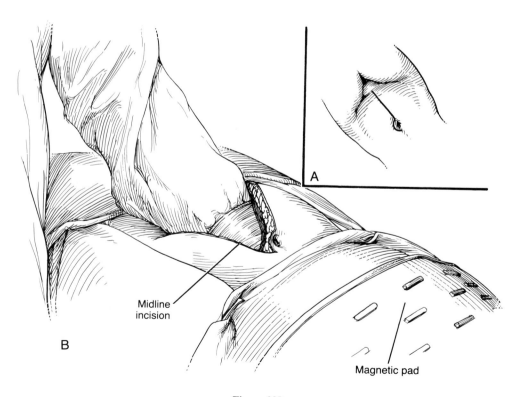

Figure 228

the cornual portion of the uterus so that they include the round ligament, the tubes, and the utero-ovarian vessels. In addition to preventing back bleeding later in the operation, continuous traction of these instruments expedites the entire dissection. The uterus is pulled vigorously up and to the left by the assistant (Fig. 229A). The round ligament on the right side is clamped (it will be cut) so that the underlying avascular space and the broad ligament are incised parallel to the tubes and ovarian vessels; the entire anterior leaf of the broad ligament is thus opened into the avascular area that exists below the tubo-ovarian vessels, above and medial to the internal iliac artery, and lateral to the ureter and uterine artery (Fig. 229B). The surgeon inserts the index finger of the left hand into the loose areolar tissue of the broad ligament and, with a Russian forceps, identifies the ureter. This dissection, when gently accomplished, does not carry any risk of damage to major vessels; the more vulnerable major veins (internal, external, and common iliac) are deep to the easily identifiable arteries. The leftward traction on the uterus and the

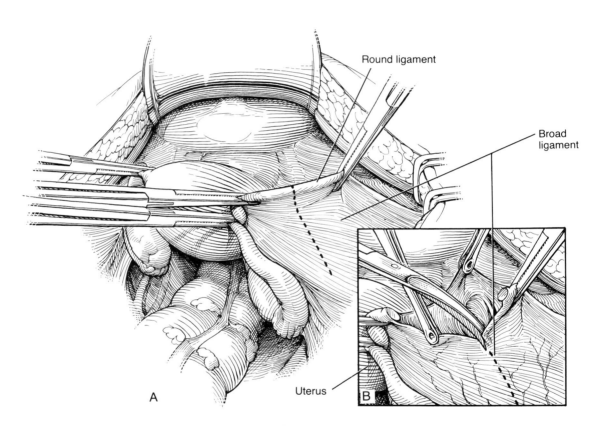

Figure 229

exposure of the internal iliac artery displace the posterior leaf of the broad ligament medially along with the ureter, which remains securely attached to the peritoneum. With abdominal hysterectomy, the ureter is often injured at the pelvic brim. To avoid injury to the ureter, it should be identified before the ovarian vessels and ovarian ligament are clamped, cut, or ligated. In thin patients, the ureter can be seen shining through the peritoneum just medial to the ovarian vessels; in obese patients, the posterior medial peritoneal leaf of the broad ligament can be grasped between the thumb and forefinger, and the ureter can be readily identified by the characteristic snap. Maintaining firm uterine traction anteriorly and to the left, the surgeon inserts an index finger through the opening of the posterior leaf of the broad ligament, just below the fallopian tube and utero-ovarian ligament; Figure 230 shows the position of the index finger when there is planned preservation of the ovary. Kocher clamps are placed across the fallopian tube and utero-ovarian ligament adjacent to the uterus.

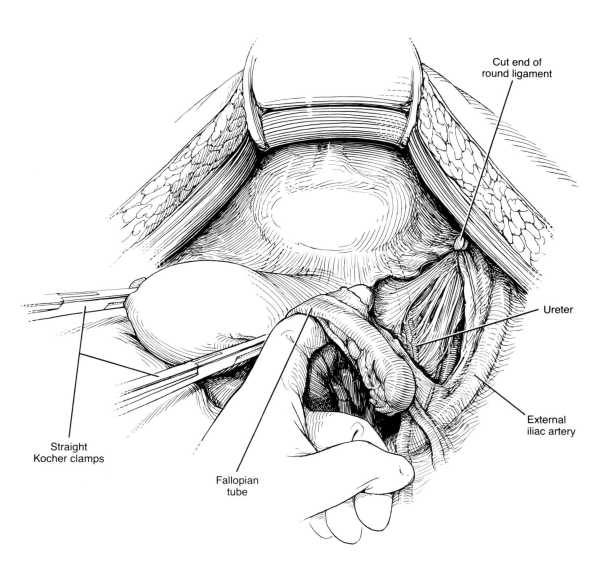

Figure 230

If the adnexa are to be removed, the ureter is identified along the medial leaf of the peritoneum. The index finger of the surgeon's left hand has perforated the peritoneum and elevates the blood supply for safe placement of the Kocher clamp (Fig. 231).

The same dissection is now repeated on the left side; the uterus is vigorously retracted to the patient's right side by the first assistant. The round ligament and ovarian vessels are ligated, and the ureter is exposed throughout its pelvic course down to the level of the uterine artery. Firm and constant cephalad traction

on the uterus is provided by the first assistant while upward countertraction is maintained on the peritoneum of the bladder with a pair of long Russian forceps (Fig. 232). This approach exposes the loose, white areolar tissue that exists between the bladder and the anterior portions of the cervix (Fig. 233). Incision of the vesicouterine peritoneal reflection proceeds from the left to the patient's right, joining the lateral openings previously made in the peritoneum of the anterior broad ligaments when the round ligament was divided.

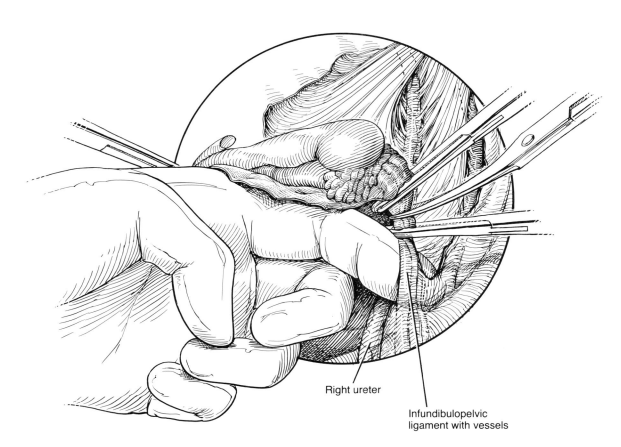

Right ureter

Infundibulopelvic
ligament with vessels

Figure 231

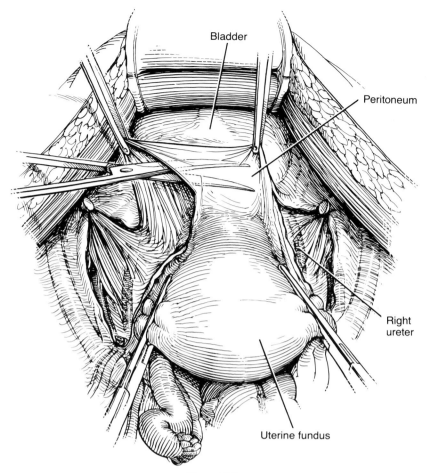

Bladder

Peritoneum

Right
ureter

Uterine fundus

Figure 232

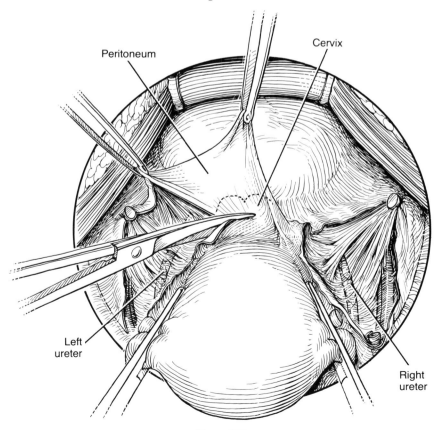

Peritoneum

Cervix

Left
ureter

Right
ureter

Figure 233

163

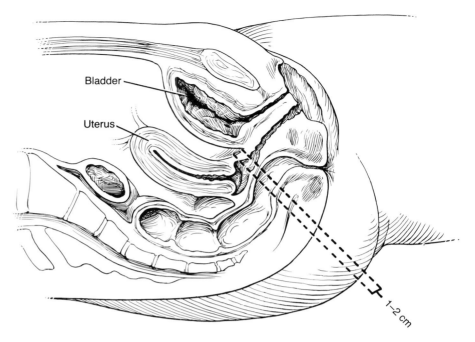

Bladder

Uterus

1–2 cm

Figure 234

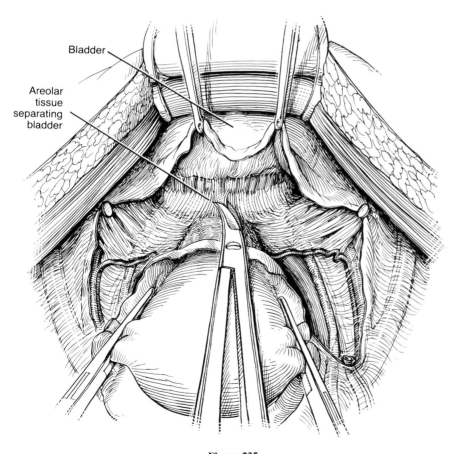

Bladder

Areolar
tissue
separating
bladder

Figure 235

With cephalad uterine traction and countertraction (toward the symphysis pubis) on the peritoneum of the bladder, a 1-cm area of loose areolar tissue can be noted between the relatively thin endopelvic fascia covering the bladder muscularis and the more dense, white fascia covering the anterior portion of the cervix. Sharp division of the central portion of this tissue with a pair of scissors allows entry into the proper avascular plane. Gentle spreading of the underlying tissue with the tips of the scissors and gentle snips allow the dissection to proceed down the midline, and the overlying bladder and underlying cervical and vaginal small vessels are avoided. Venous bleeding can be avoided by delaying far lateral dissection until the midline dissection progresses in the proper plane well down over the cervix onto the anterior vaginal wall. It must be emphasized that the bladder attachment curves upward on each side and lateral to the cervix, over lateral vaginal angles, and over the uterine vessels. The surgeon must expose 1 to 2 cm of the entire anterior vaginal wall below the level of the cervix or below the level of the planned vaginal transection (Fig. 234).

With the bladder elevated from the cervix and anterior vaginal wall, the surgeon can carefully proceed with sharp dissection of the areolar tissue, separating the bladder anteriorly from the lower uterine and cervical segments posteriorly (Fig. 235). The lateral view in Figure 236A shows the proper entry into the avascular cleavage plane between the bladder and the cervix.

The exact location of the cervix is best detected with a finger behind the uterus and a thumb compressing the area of the anterior portion of the cervix under the bladder. The lateral view in Figure 236B shows palpation and location of the cervix with the thumb and forefinger.

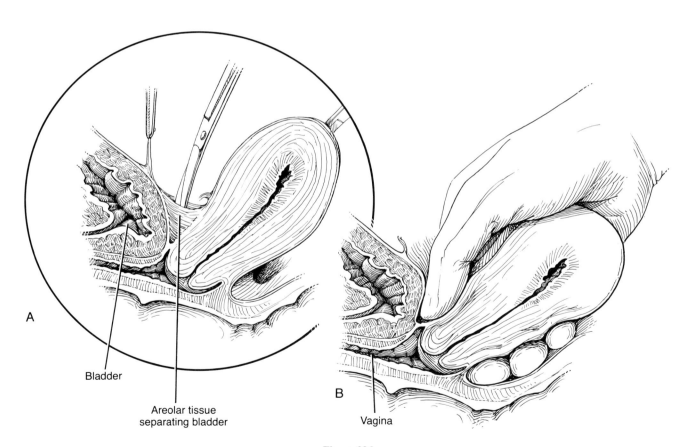

A

Bladder

Areolar tissue
separating bladder

B

Vagina

Figure 236

The lower 2 to 3 cm of ureter, as it passes under the exposed uterine artery and swings anteriorly and medially around the vaginal corner, can be "snapped" between the thumb and index finger (Fig. 237).

With strong traction maintained on the uterus, a Deaver retractor is placed anteriorly to maintain exposure by displacing the mobilized bladder away from the cervix on the upper portion of the vagina. With the uterus pulled first to the left and then to the right, a pair of Kocher forceps (a single forceps on each side) is placed well down on the right and then on the left side of the cervix and angled approximately 45° (Fig. 238). This clamp includes the uterine vessels, the superior portion of the cardinal ligaments, and the paracolpium immediately above the lateral vaginal fornix. The tips of the Kocher forceps slide off the side of the cervix as they are applied; thus, they engage the endopelvic fascia immediately above the lateral vaginal fornix.

When the uterine vessel–cardinal ligament complex is divided close to the cervix (medial to the Kocher clamp) and the tip is slightly undercut, a "fascial window" is opened; the anterior edge of this window is the cervicopubic fascia, which is subsequently developed and managed as a separate layer during the vaginal vault closure (Fig. 239). A similar procedure is done on the left side.

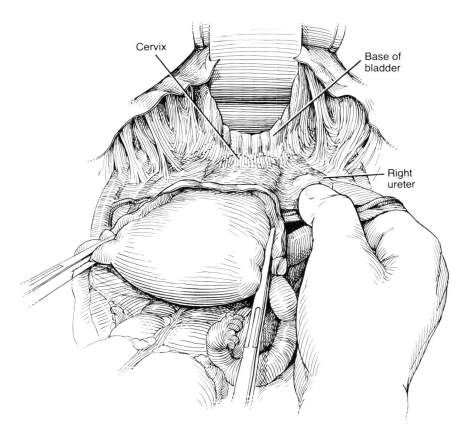

Cervix

Base of bladder

Right ureter

Figure 237

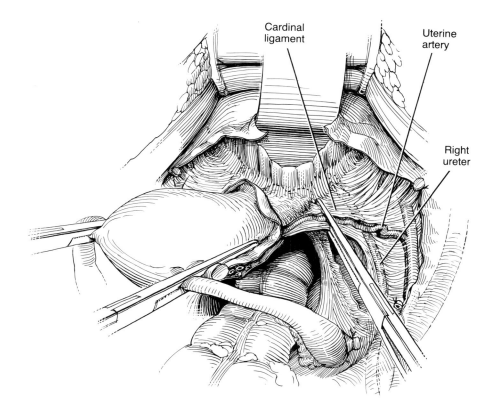

Cardinal
ligament

Uterine
artery

Right
ureter

Figure 238

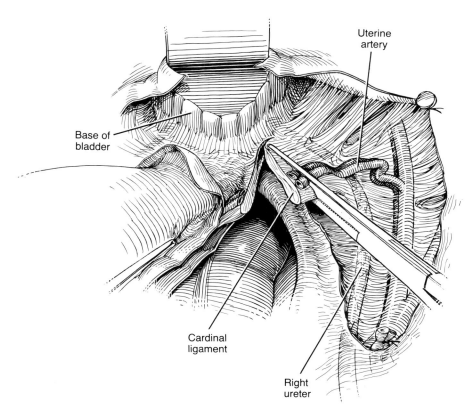

Uterine
artery

Base of
bladder

Cardinal
ligament

Right
ureter

Figure 239

With the uterine vessels and cardinal ligaments divided on each side, the uterosacral ligaments are made prominent by pulling the uterus up and anterior toward the symphysis pubis. When the uterosacral ligaments are cut at the proper place, close to the uterus, no important vessels are encountered, and the stump of the ligament is easily identified later (Fig. 240A). Thus, ligation of the uterosacral ligament is generally unnecessary at this time.

The cul-de-sac peritoneum is divided adjacent to the cervix; the proper degree of anterior traction on the uterus allows the rectum and uterosacral ligaments to slide inferiorly from the cervix and posterior vaginal fornix (Fig. 240B).

If the rectum is firmly attached to the cervix and the posterior vaginal fornix is obliterated, perhaps by endometriosis, the rectum can be readily mobilized

with firm anterior uterine traction up over the symphysis pubis while posterior countertraction is applied to the wall of the rectosigmoid with the sponge-covered fingers of the surgeon's left hand (Fig. 241). This maneuver facilitates sharp dissection of the proper plane just beneath the uterine peritoneum and underlying posterior cervicopubic fascia. Generally, when the dissection progresses below the level of scarring and fixation, the rectum is widely mobilized from the entire upper posterior vaginal walls. When the uterosacral ligaments have been divided, the uterus can be lifted to a higher level within the pelvis.

With cephalad traction, the cervicopubic fascia can now be incised transversely just above the level of the anterior vaginal fornix, connecting the two fascial windows joined on the lateral sides of the cervix. The cervicopubic fascia is dissected inferiorly from the anterior vaginal wall as a separate layer (Fig. 242).

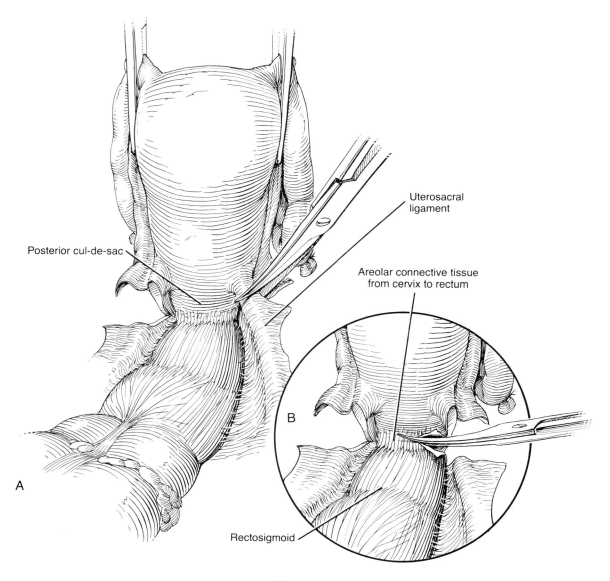

Figure 240

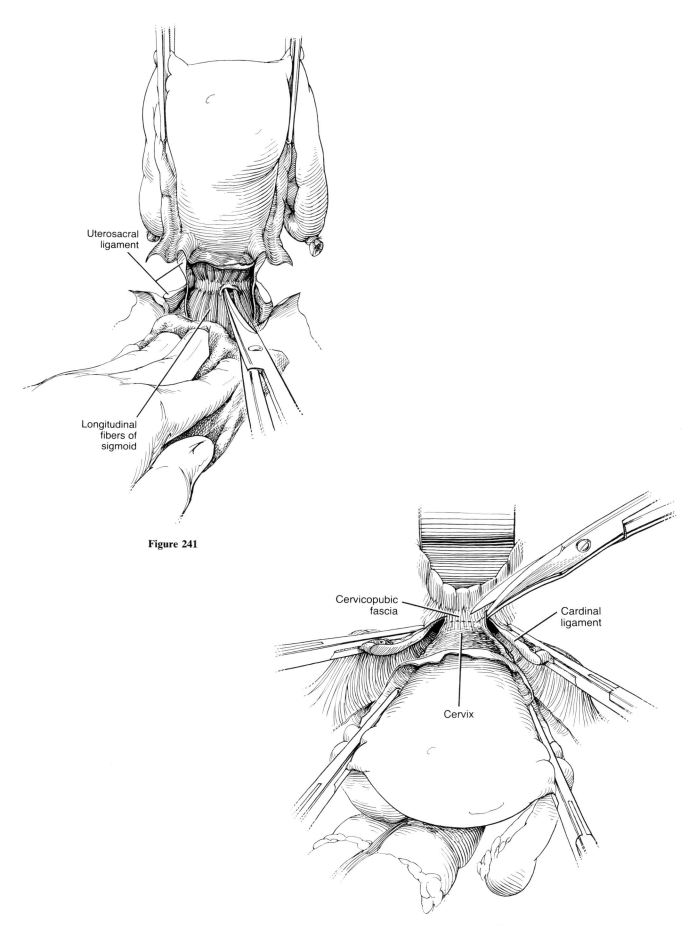

Uterosacral
ligament

Longitudinal
fibers of
sigmoid

Figure 241

Cervicopubic
fascia

Cardinal
ligament

Cervix

Figure 242

169

The uterus is retracted anteriorly and to the left, and the vagina is entered preferably posteriorly and laterally just above the stump of the right uterosacral ligament. The uterus can now be removed by circumcising the vagina as closely as possible to the cervix to avoid vaginal shortening (Fig. 243A). As the uterus is being removed, four vulsellum forceps are placed successively at the 3-, 12-, 9-, and 6-o'clock positions of the vaginal cuff as it is developed (Fig. 243B).

Traction by the first and second assistants on the four vulsellum forceps placed on the vaginal cuff serves to elevate and expose the entire circumference of the vaginal vault and so facilitate accurate closure of the vault while maintaining constant visualization of the bladder base and the rectum.

Closure of the vaginal vault provides satisfactory hemostasis, effected by a continuous suture of atrau-matic 3-0 polyglycolic acid material. Suturing is started with a right vaginal angle stitch, placed so that the small vaginal branch or branches of the uterine artery are ligated and, in addition, lateral supporting tissues from the base of the cardinal ligament are attached to the vaginal angle (Fig. 244A). The suture is continued toward the left, each bite placed submucosally so that the squamous edges are accurately approximated and inverted into the vagina. The suture does not enter the vagina and is not exposed to the contamination therein (Fig. 244B).

A generous portion of the left uterosacral ligament is included, following which the needle passes laterally to the vaginal fornix angle, through the lateral supporting tissues at the base of the cardinal ligament, and under the small vaginal vessels that can be noted. Anteriorly, the suture also includes the layer of cervicopubic fascia previously prepared (Fig. 245).

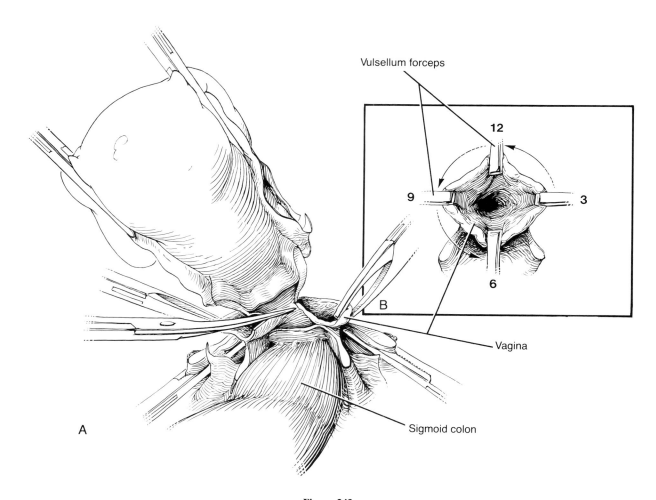

Figure 243

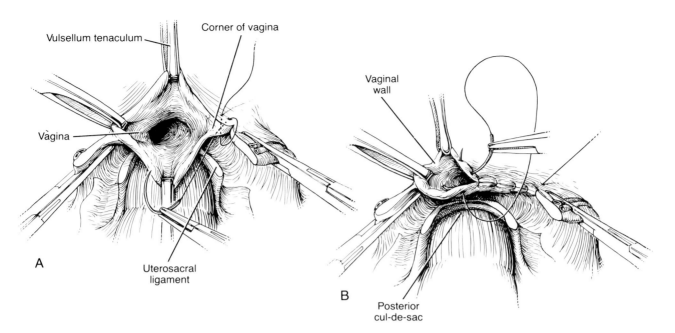

Vulsellum tenaculum

Corner of vagina

Vagina

Uterosacral ligament

A

Vaginal wall

Posterior cul-de-sac

B

Figure 244

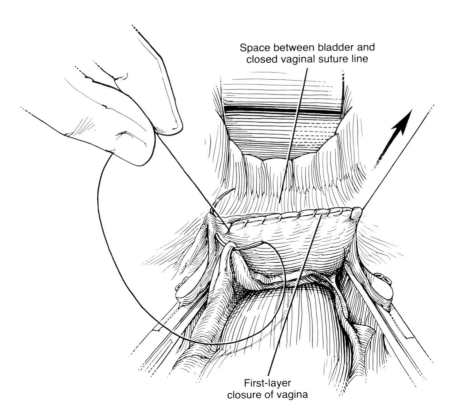

Space between bladder and closed vaginal suture line

First-layer closure of vagina

Figure 245

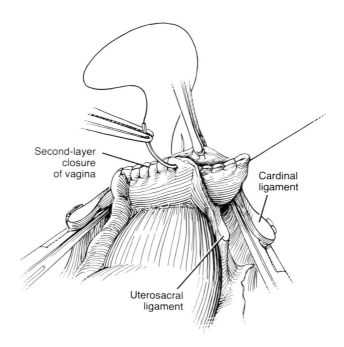

Second-layer
closure
of vagina

Cardinal
ligament

Uterosacral
ligament

Figure 246

The angle suture is securely locked in this position, and the suture is then returned across the vaginal vault, which includes the underlying endopelvic fascia posteriorly, small bites of the top of the previously closed vagina, and the cervicopubic fascia anteriorly (Fig. 246).

When the right vaginal corner is reached, a secure bite is obtained in the right uterosacral ligament, vaginal angle, and cervicopubic fascia anteriorly (Fig. 247). The suture is tied to the previously tagged suture and cut. A two-layer closure of the vaginal vault is accomplished with a single continuous suture that restores the continuity of the endopelvic fascia, the cervicopubic fascia anteriorly, the peritoneum (endopelvic fascia) and the uterosacral ligaments posteriorly, and the base of the cardinal ligament laterally.

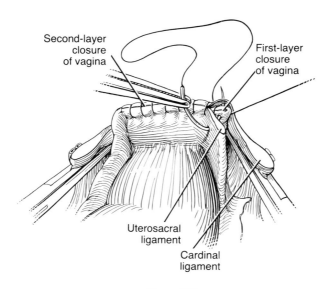

Second-layer
closure
of vagina

First-layer
closure
of vagina

Uterosacral
ligament

Cardinal
ligament

Figure 247

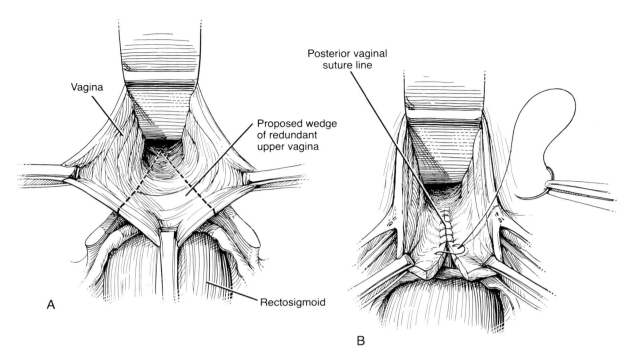

Figure 248

In patients with an unusually broad and copious upper vaginal vault associated with a wide, deep cul-de-sac (thus, potential candidates for development of a vault prolapse), a wide wedge of redundant vagina and cul-de-sac peritoneum is excised. Sharp and blunt dissection is used to mobilize and displace the rectum completely posteriorly to the level of the levator muscles. The width of the wedge depends on the width of the vaginal vault. A Deaver retractor is inserted through the vaginal vault to elevate the anterior vaginal wall and bladder and thus facilitate exposure and permit safe excision (and later repair) of the segment of posterior vaginal wall (Fig. 248A).

The defect is repaired with a continuous 2-0 locked polyglycolic acid suture placed within the vagina; each passage of the needle includes a full thickness of the vaginal wall and the rectovaginal fascia and picks up the lateral supporting tissues of the vagina adjacent to the levator fascia (Fig. 248B). This procedure increases the stability of the posterior vaginal wall, narrows the vaginal apex, and brings the lateral supporting tissues of the vagina and uterosacral ligaments toward the midline in front of the rectum.

After the vaginal vault is closed, the uterosacral ligaments can be approximated and the cul-de-sac obliterated with the use of additional interrupted no. 1 polyglycolic acid sutures (Fig. 249). Care needs to be taken not to incorporate the ureters, which are immediately underlying the peritoneum.

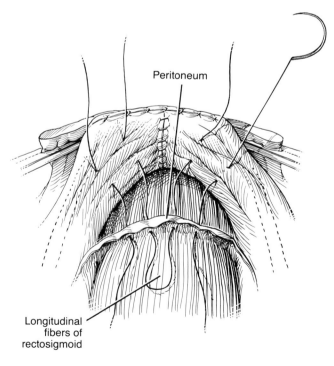

Figure 249

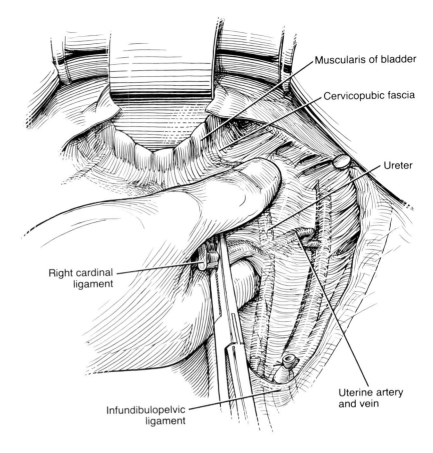

Figure 250

The previously placed Kocher clamp containing the upper portion of the cardinal ligament is now elevated toward the midline by the first assistant. The ureter is then palpated between the surgeon's index finger and thumb as it courses through the cardinal ligament toward the bladder. This maneuver provides a second check on the location of the ureter before the cardinal ligament is tied to the corner of the vault (Fig. 250).

The upper portion of the cardinal ligament containing the uterine artery is now attached securely to the vaginal angle and ligated. To accomplish this, the needle first enters the peritoneum, the right uterosacral ligament, and the right angle of the vagina just lateral to the suture used to close the vaginal vault (Fig. 251). This same procedure is accomplished on the opposite side. At this time, the pelvis should be completely inspected and meticulous hemostasis ensured.

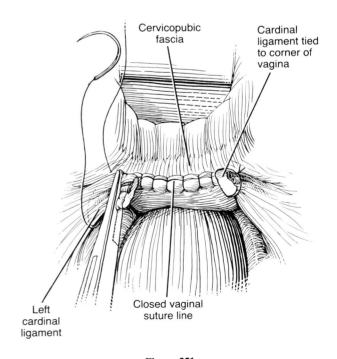

Figure 251

If the vaginal cuff or vaginal angles have been unusually "wet," the uterine artery can be additionally ligated lateral to the ureter at its origin from the internal iliac artery. This ligation requires only a few seconds because the area has been dissected and exposed initially. The ureter is identified and carried medially. The internal iliac artery is identified and followed inferiorly until the uterine artery is seen to branch in a medial direction. A forceps is placed underneath the uterine artery and vein, and a ligature

is carried through the space and tied. This should be accomplished bilaterally.

The pelvis is peritonealized with a continuous suture of 3-0 polyglycolic acid material. Suturing is started at the level of the right ovarian vessels in such a way that the vessels are again ligated, and the stump is extraperitonealized. Once more, care must be exercised during closing of the peritoneum to avoid the adjacent ureter (Fig. 252).

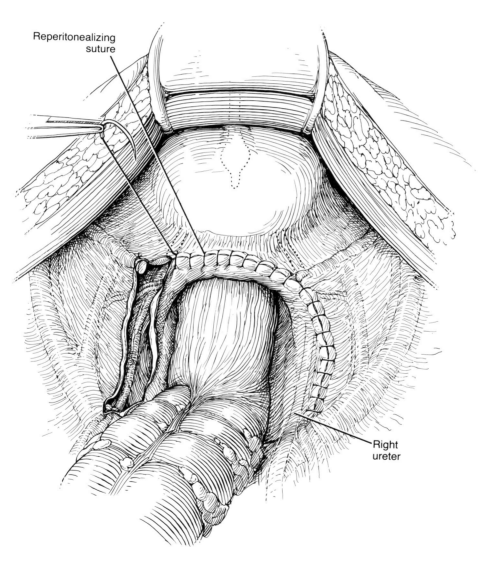

Figure 252

Endometrial Carcinoma

For patients with carcinoma of the endometrium who require a wide hysterectomy for adequate clearance, we vary the technique as follows.

The procedure for abdominal hysterectomy is followed to the point at which the lower parametrium and the tissues about the cervix are ready to be dissected. With traction pulling the uterus toward the patient's left side, the ureter is identified at the level where it crosses the common iliac artery. It is followed inferiorly to where it is crossed by the uterine vessels. A curved forceps is inserted under the uterine vessels as they cross the ureter; this maneuver exposes the underlying ureter (Fig. 253A). These vessels are then clamped lateral to the right ureter, and both ends are tied with 0 delayed absorbable suture (Fig. 253B). The ureter is then mobilized laterally, and a curved clamp is placed across the cardinal ligament medial to the ureter, 1 to 2 cm lateral to the cervix (Fig. 253C). This is cut and tied. The uterus is then pulled forward, and the uterosacral ligaments are cut. With the bladder mobilized sufficiently in an inferior direction, the vagina is entered, and the uterus is removed along with a small rim of vagina. The rest of the procedure is the same as that described for total abdominal hysterectomy.

We currently perform node sampling over the internal and obturator areas but do not do a formal node dissection for carcinoma of the endometrium.

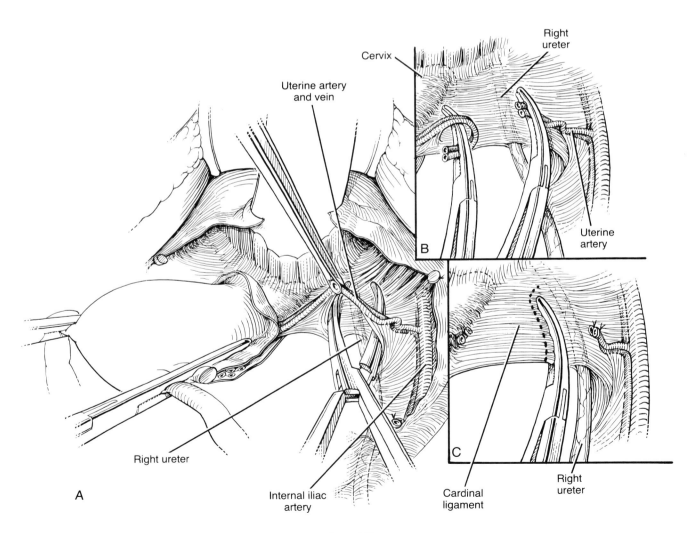

Figure 253

Myomectomy

Uterine myomas are the most commonly encountered tumors of the female genital tract, particularly during the childbearing years. Most of them remain asymptomatic and require nothing more than periodic evaluation. The most frequently reported indications for surgical extirpation of these tumors are pressure, menstrual abnormalities, rapid increase in size, infertility, and the inability to establish a definitive diagnosis. Although new medical therapies are being developed for their management, surgical treatment of myomas consists of either myomectomy or hysterectomy. The selection of abdominal myomectomy is predicated on the desire of the patient to retain or attempt to improve the possibility of future childbearing and on the inability to manage the myomas by curettage or posterior colpotomy. Except during pregnancy, abdominal myomectomy should be preceded by curettage to detect and possibly to remove submucous myomas and to exclude uterine malignant lesions. The patient and the surgeon should undertake operation with the understanding that it is impossible to tell with absolute certainty just what should be done until after the uterus is exposed. The myometrium has an abundant blood supply, especially in the young woman. To control excessive blood loss during myomectomy, we prefer to open the broad ligaments, identify the ureter, and place small rubber-shod, bulldog-type clamps on the uterine vessels adjacent to the uterus. Similar rubber-shod clamps are placed on the ovarian vessels, and again care is taken to avoid the ureters.

The decision about where the uterine incision is made is determined by the size, location, and number of leiomyomas present and by their proximity to the uterine vessels and fallopian tubes (Fig. 254). If possible, removal of all the leiomyomas should be accomplished through a single incision. The incision is carried down through the myometrium until it enters the surface of the underlying leiomyoma. The leiomyoma is then grasped with a single-tooth tenac-

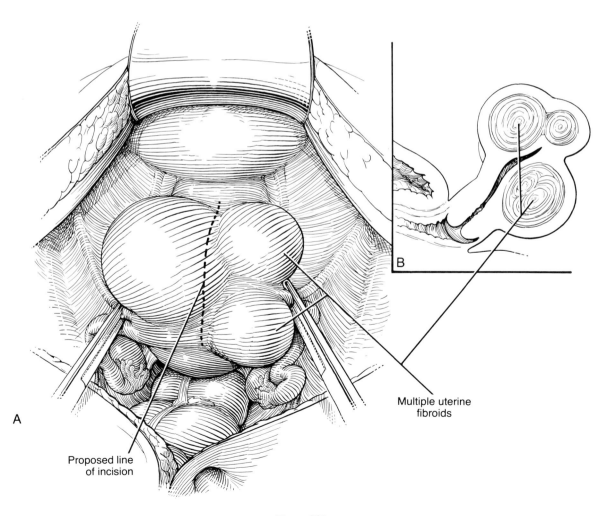

Proposed line of incision

Multiple uterine fibroids

Figure 254

ulum to apply appropriate traction. The plane of cleavage between the leiomyoma and the surrounding myometrium can usually be determined accurately, and this permits sharp dissection with scissors or, on occasion, blunt dissection with the finger enucleating the leiomyoma from its bed (Fig. 255). Any entry into the endometrial cavity should be noted and closed with fine extramucosal sutures. The defect in the myometrium is repaired with 2-0 delayed absorbable sutures, generally in two or three layers. The

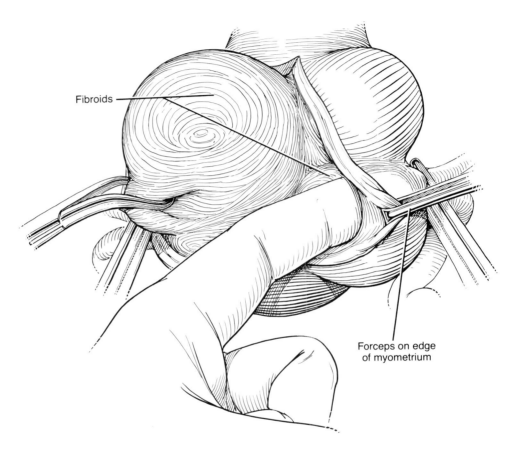

Figure 255

dead space is carefully closed, and hemostasis must be accomplished as each layer is closed (Fig. 256A). The serosa is closed with a subcuticular, subserosal 4-0 delayed absorbable suture (Fig. 256B).

The clamps previously placed on the uterine blood supply are removed, and the uterus is carefully inspected to ensure that complete hemostasis has been obtained.

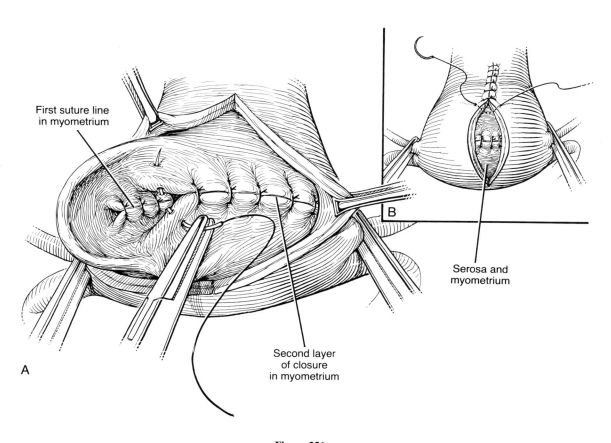

First suture line
in myometrium

Second layer
of closure
in myometrium

Serosa and
myometrium

A

B

Figure 256

Septate Uterus

Several different techniques are recommended for management of a septate uterus. We prefer to make a vertical incision between the horns of the uterus through the septum until the uterine cavity is entered (Fig. 257). Once the lower uterine cavity is entered, one blade of the Mayo scissors is inserted into the uterine cavity, and the other is kept on the outside of the cavity. An incision is made up the central portion of the left uterine horn, stopping approximately 1 cm medial to the isthmic portion of the fallopian tube (Fig. 258). A similar technique opens up the right uterine horn. No portion of the septum is removed; as it is incised, it becomes apparent that removal is unnecessary. Beginning at the inferior aspect on the anterior wall of the uterus, interrupted 3-0 delayed absorbable sutures are placed in an extramucosal fashion; this maneuver converts the uterus to a single cavity that is remarkably similar to a normal uterus in size and shape (Fig. 259). The myometrium is reapproximated in two or three layers, and care is taken that the sutures do not compromise the interstitial portion of the fallopian tubes. The technique is simple, conserving all of the myometrial tissue, and the result is a uterotubal junction that is in its normal lateral position.

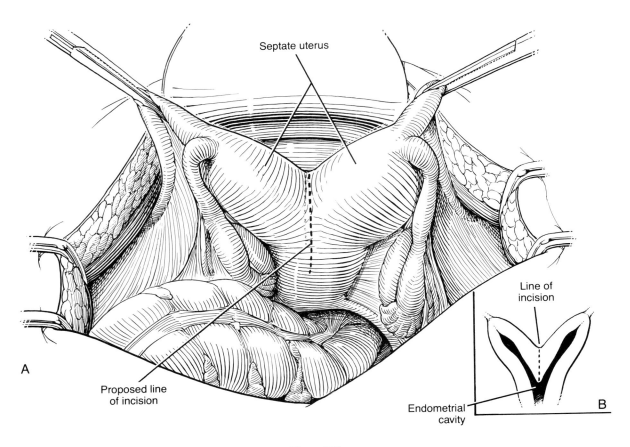

Figure 257

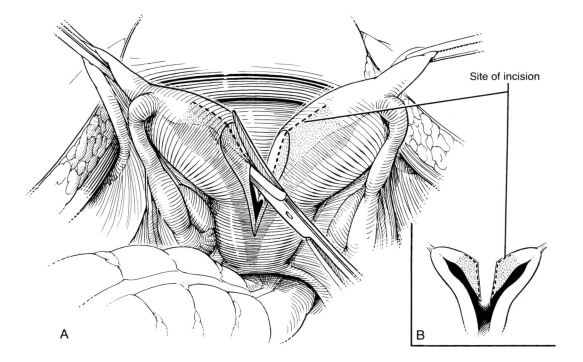

Figure 258

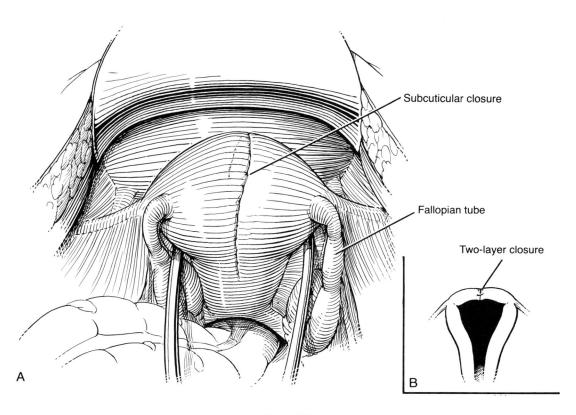

Figure 259

Radical Hysterectomy

Radical hysterectomy with pelvic lymph node dissection is an operation that is well suited for the management of International Federation of Gynecology and Obstetrics (FIGO) stages IA, IB, and IIA carcinoma of the cervix. Technical factors that are fundamental to ensure wide clearance of a centrally located lesion consist of early and accurate identification and development of the paravesical and pararectal spaces. These steps establish the tissue planes that define the remainder of the dissection, permit the dissection to be flush with the pelvic side walls and the roots of the sacral plexus, and minimize the chances of significant blood loss. The positions of the lower portions of the ureters make it impossible to achieve a complete en bloc resection of the central lesion. It is necessary to dissect the ureters and displace them cephalically and laterally out of the central mass of tissue, but this maneuver does not seem to have an adverse effect on the result of the operation. Certainly, if there is doubt regarding the proximity of the ureters, we resect the ureters superiorly to the suspicious area and reconstitute their anastomosis by ureteroneocystostomy. The endopelvic fascia encircling the vagina is circumferentially incised before the vagina is transected. Approximately 25% of the vagina is sacrificed with stage IB lesions, whereas the more extended partial vaginectomy with margins of clearance of 2 to 3 cm is performed with stage IIA lesions. Before closure of the vaginal vault, the resected borders of the vagina should be histologically examined by frozen section to ensure that there is adequate clearance of all disease.

Through a lower midline incision extending to the left side of the umbilicus, abdominal exploration is done to confirm that there is no extrapelvic spread of the cervical malignancy (Fig. 260A). The entire abdomen is carefully explored. Appropriate biopsy specimens (aortic nodes, liver, peritoneum) may be obtained as indicated. We prefer to use a Balfour retractor with the patient placed in a steep Trendelenburg position (30°).

With traction on the uterus being applied toward the patient's left side, the right round ligament is clamped and cut, and the broad ligament is incised parallel but lateral to the infundibulopelvic ligament; this incision widely opens the broad ligament (Fig. 260B and C). The ureter can be seen attached along the medial leaf of the peritoneum. By displacement of

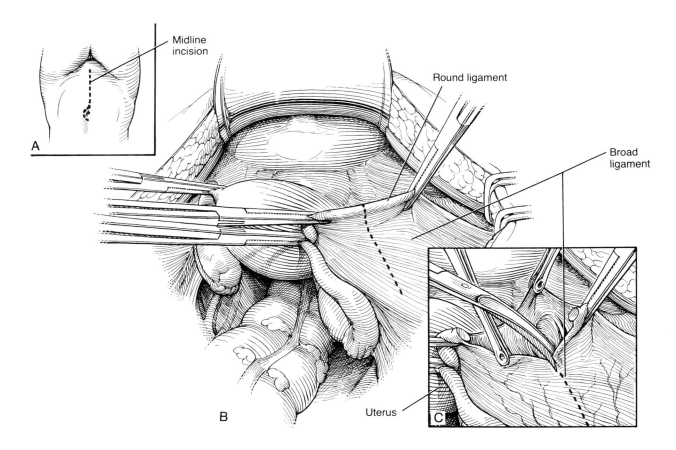

Figure 260

the peritoneum and attached ureter medially and of the anterior division of the internal iliac artery laterally with the surgeon's left index finger, the right posterior pararectal space is identified and dissected (with a Russian forceps) down to the base of the hollow of the sacrum. Care is taken not to disrupt the veins on the anterior surface of the sacrum (Fig. 261). Moving the left index finger anteriorly, the surgeon identifies the obliterated hypogastric vessels and mobilizes the vessels medially with the bladder. With Russian forceps, the anterior paravesical space is dissected and opened down to the superior surface of the levator fascia overlying the levator muscle. A wide Deaver retractor is inserted into the paravesical space, and traction is applied toward the patient's feet.

Thus, the steps described isolate the web of tissue that extends laterally from the cervix and the upper vagina toward the pelvic side wall. This includes the cardinal ligament complex, which contains the lower ureter medially and all of the vesical branches of the internal iliac vessels. The procedure also permits palpation of the paracervical and paravaginal tissues and lymph node areas to determine whether there is any extension of the malignancy that may require alteration of the planned technique.

A narrow Deaver retractor with traction superiorly and laterally elevates the abdominal wall and exposes the iliac fascia and external iliac vessels to the point at which they leave the abdominal cavity. The pelvic lymph node dissection is started at this point (the distal end of the iliac artery and vein). We prefer the use of long Russian thumb forceps and dissecting scissors or long, curved forceps to dissect all of the lymph node–bearing areolar fatty tissue cephalad and medially off the surface of the external iliac vessels (Fig. 261B). This dissection is continued superiorly above the bifurcation of the internal iliac vessels. This tissue is then displaced downward into the paravesical and obturator space. To dissect more superiorly, a wide Deaver retractor is inserted under the peritoneum and the ureter and lifted up and cephalad to expose the common iliac vessels up to the aortic bifurcation. In addition, the medial leaf of the peritoneum with the attached ureter is retracted toward the midline to expose this area. The lymph node–bearing areolar tissue is dissected downward from the common iliac artery in front of the vena cava and from the surface of the left common iliac vein, which courses from left to right just under and below the aortic bifurcation.

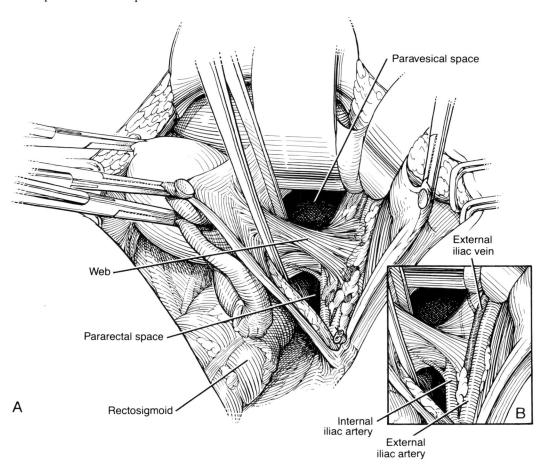

Paravesical space

External iliac vein

Web

Pararectal space

Rectosigmoid

Internal iliac artery

External iliac artery

A

B

Figure 261

The common and external iliac artery and vein are now displaced medially, and a Deaver retractor is used to retract the iliopsoas muscle laterally (Fig. 262). The obturator nerve and underlying lumbosacral trunk are seen lying on the pelvic brim as they emerge from beneath the iliopsoas muscle. The lymph node–bearing tissue is dissected downward and from the lateral surface of the external iliac vessels into the obturator fossa. The obturator nerve can be removed, without producing significant disability, if it is encased in metastatically involved lymph nodes, although removal is infrequently necessary.

With a vein retractor lifting the external iliac artery and vein laterally, the lymph node tissue along the anterior surface of the internal iliac vessel is teased inferiorly to bring together the lymph node–bearing tissue (including the obturator and external, common, and internal iliac lymph node–bearing tissue), which can be lifted out en bloc (Fig. 263). A frozen-section analysis of this tissue can be done during the time that a similar dissection is being done on the opposite side of the pelvis. In patients with positive pelvic nodes, the lymph node–bearing tissue is completely dissected up to the left renal vein (Fig. 264).

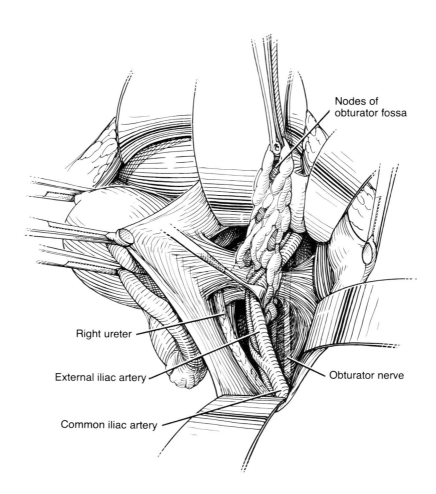

Nodes of obturator fossa

Right ureter

External iliac artery

Common iliac artery

Obturator nerve

Figure 262

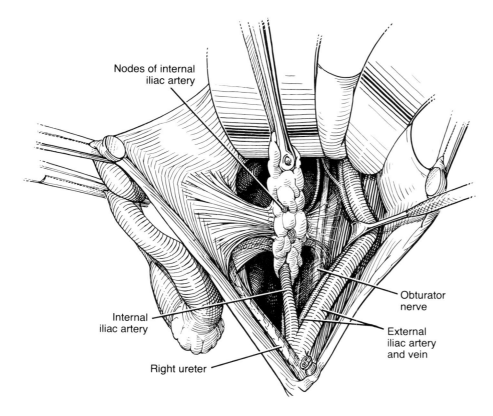

Nodes of internal
iliac artery

Internal
iliac artery

Right ureter

Obturator
nerve

External
iliac artery
and vein

Figure 263

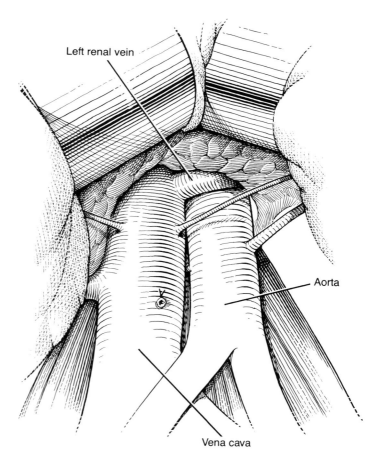

Left renal vein

Aorta

Vena cava

Figure 264

With the use of a right-angled forceps and by keeping it immediately adjacent to the lateral and inferior walls of the internal iliac artery, the iliac artery can be separated from the iliac vein in preparation for its being clamped, cut, and ligated with 0 delayed absorbable suture (Fig. 265A and B). If the surgeon wants to include the vein, the forceps is passed beneath the vessels and the vein is tied in a similar fashion (Fig. 265C).

With a wide Deaver retractor holding the bladder and the lower ureter medially and inferiorly and with traction on the uterine fundus toward the patient's left side, the surgeon palpates the potential window in the right broad ligament and perforates the tissue with the right index finger (Fig. 266). Once the window is developed, a long, curved Kelly clamp is placed flush with the lateral side wall, incorporating the web of the cardinal ligament (this contains the remaining visceral branches of the internal iliac artery).

The tissue is divided between the long, curved clamps and is suture-ligated on the pelvic side wall, flush with the sacral plexus (Fig. 267). Inaccurate accomplishment of this particular step may lead to troublesome venous bleeding, which can be controlled with adequate exposure and accurate clamping and suture ligation.

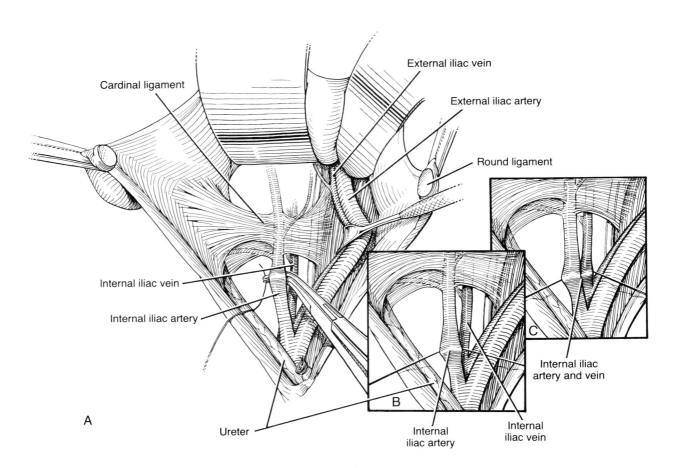

Figure 265

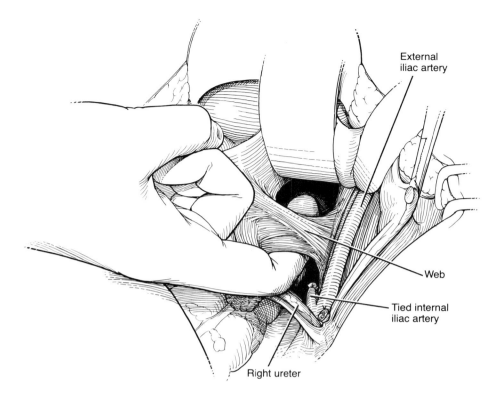

Figure 266

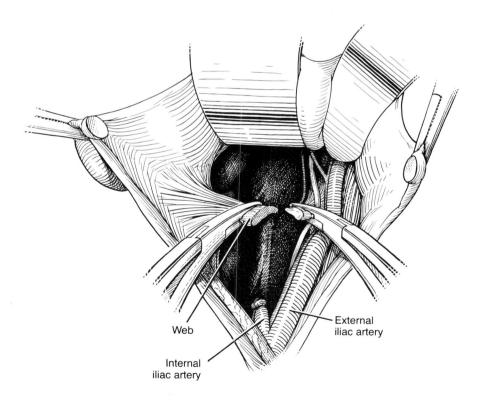

Figure 267

With vigorous anterior traction on the uterus and posterior countertraction on the rectosigmoid, the peritoneum behind the cervix is incised, and the rectum is dropped posteriorly from the back of the cervix and the upper vagina. If necessary, sharp dissection may be enhanced with countertraction on the rectosigmoid (Fig. 268A). The uterosacral ligaments can be clamped, cut, and ligated immediately adjacent to the anterolateral wall of the sigmoid colon. The rectum is easily mobilized with a sweeping action, using a sponge over the surgeon's index and middle fingers. If necessary, sharp dissection may be initiated. This results in the development of an arc of the lower uterosacral ligament (from the vagina to the sacrum), which swings laterally adjacent to the muscularis of the rectum to the front of the sacrum (Fig. 268B). If necessary, a narrow Harrington forceps can be inserted behind the posterior wall of the vagina and lifted anteriorly to aid in accurate placement of the curved Kelly clamp, which is placed across this tissue in a lateral posterior position to the rectal side wall, and the tissue is divided (Fig. 268C). This dissection allows additional upward mobility of the uterus and cervix, thus permitting a more accurate and atraumatic dissection of the ureters.

A

Figure 268

With vigorous cephalad traction on the uterus, the peritoneum overlying the bladder is transected to permit mobilization of the bladder from the anterior surface of the uterus, the cervix, and the anterior vaginal wall. This is accomplished in an avascular fashion with sharp dissection, dividing the layer of areolar tissue between the bladder and the uterus, cervix, and vagina. Demonstration of the proper plane is aided by sharp cephalad traction on the uterus and countertraction on the bladder and the peritoneum. Once the bladder is mobilized sufficiently in an inferior direction, it is held in place with a wide Deaver retractor. Proper traction on the uterus to the patient's left side and countertraction on the base of the bladder with a Deaver retractor permit accurate dissection of the lower 2 cm of the ureter to its entrance into the bladder (Fig. 269A). The tissue is divided between two clamps; the roof of the underlying ureter is thus freed (Fig. 269B).

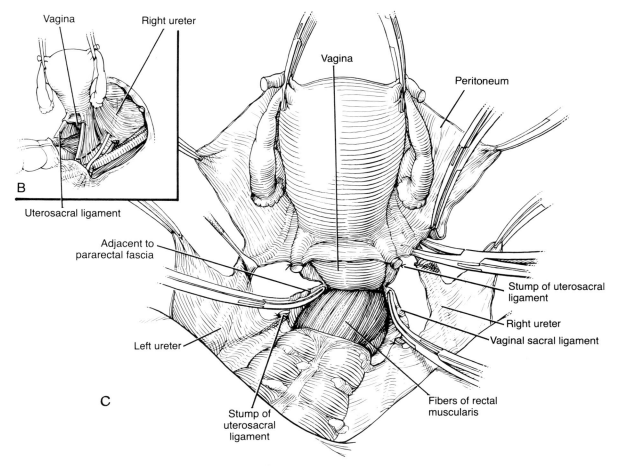

Figure 268 *Continued*

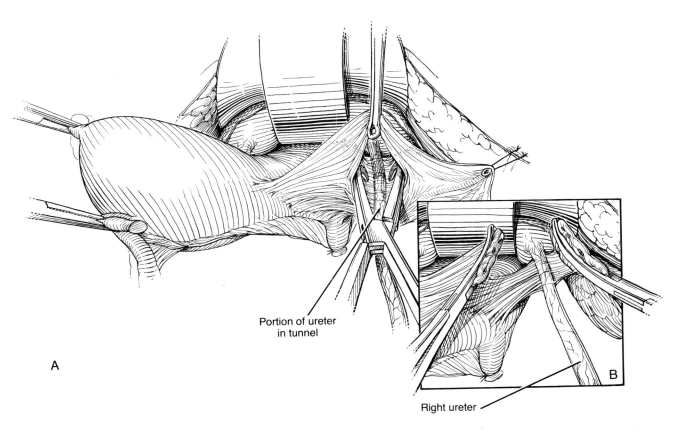

Figure 269

189

The previously placed lateral clamp of tissue originating from the superior surface of the ureter is now mobilized under the ureter and medially (Fig. 270*A*); this maneuver completely frees the lower 2 cm of the ureter (thus, the lower few centimeters of the blood supply of the ureter is totally dependent on an intact sheath and its enclosed blood supply) (Fig. 270*B*). The bladder has been dissected far inferiorly and laterally, the superior forceps is on the web of tissue, and the inferior forceps is on the tissue from over the superior surface of the ureter; thus, this positioning demonstrates the wide lateral clearance from the surface of the ureter.

The dissection has been completed. The uterus is pulled cephalad, and the bladder and ureters are displaced downward with a wide Deaver retractor. The paravaginal and paracervical tissues have been stretched laterally to show the wide central dissection (extending to the pelvic side wall) (Fig. 271). This is the essential and fundamental feature of this operation.

With the paravaginal clamps in place, the vagina is entered anteriorly and transected with scissors (Fig. 272*A*). Tenacula are placed in each vaginal corner to elevate the remaining portion of the vagina and to facilitate accurate vaginal closure. The right-angled clamp placed inferior to the ureter and including the low paravaginal tissue remains in place until the vagina is closed. We generally remove approximately a third of the vagina.

The vagina is closed with continuous 3-0 delayed absorbable suture placed in a subcuticular fashion that accurately approximates and inverts the anterior and the posterior squamous edges (Fig. 272*B*). This technique provides hemostasis for the vaginal edges and is continued back, left to right, approximating the cervicopubic fascia. The suture is then tied at the right vaginal angle to the previously tagged suture. The paravaginal tissues included in the right-angled forceps can now be suture-ligated to the sides of the vagina. This closure provides excellent hemostasis with good primary healing of the vaginal vault. The operative area is then vigorously irrigated with a large quantity of saline solution, and meticulous hemostasis is obtained with fine suture ligation or judicious use of cautery.

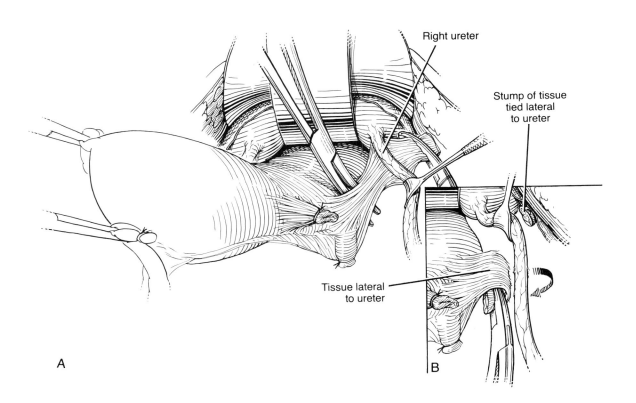

Right ureter

Stump of tissue tied lateral to ureter

Tissue lateral to ureter

A

B

Figure 270

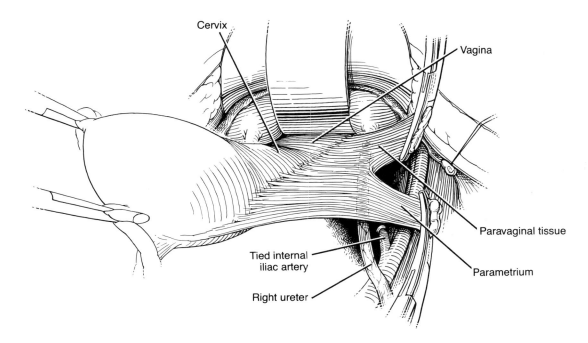

Figure 271

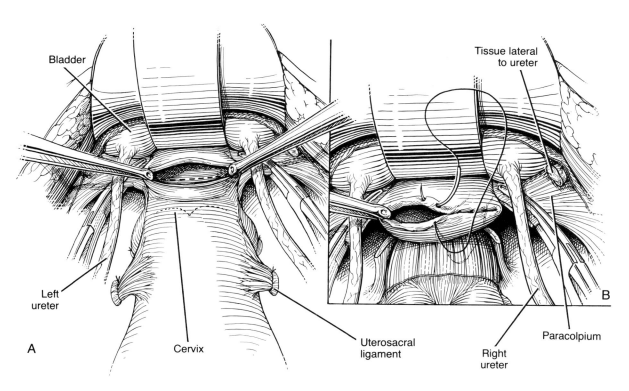

Figure 272

Careful inspection reveals ties on the internal iliac artery, lateral web, and round ligament on both side walls. Anteriorly, there are ties on the distal ends of the obliterated hypogastric vessels and a tie on the tissue lateral to the ureter adjacent to the bladder. The ureter skirts the pelvis like a telephone wire, free of support, from the pelvic brim until its entrance into the bladder, approximately 5 cm cephalad to the closed vagina (it may be farther, depending on the amount of vagina resected) and 10 cm above the sigmoid colon (Fig. 273).

To provide drainage of the retroperitoneal space, a large suction catheter is inserted on each side through a separate extraperitoneal stab wound lateral to the midline incision and is placed in the external iliac-obturator fossa.

The pelvis is reperitonealized in a transverse direction beginning in the area of the right infundibulopelvic ligament and proceeding in a continuous fashion toward the bladder and up to the left infundibulopelvic ligament; care is taken to avoid transfixing the drains previously placed in the obturator area. The previously closed vagina can be seen as it lies inferior to the peritoneal closure under the base of the bladder (Fig. 274A).

The abdominal incision is closed in layers, and the skin is closed with 4-0 subcuticular suture (Fig. 274B). The excised specimen consists of the uterus, the tubes, the ovaries, the entire broad ligament containing the parametrium and paracervical tissue, and the paracolpium with approximately 30% of the vagina (Fig. 275).

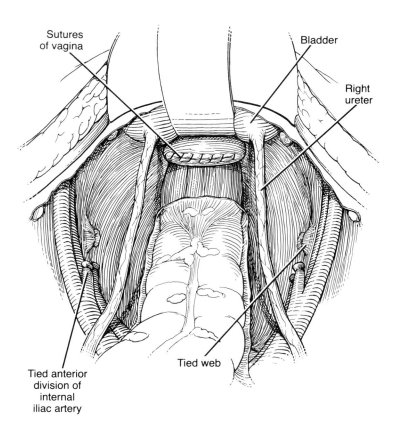

Figure 273

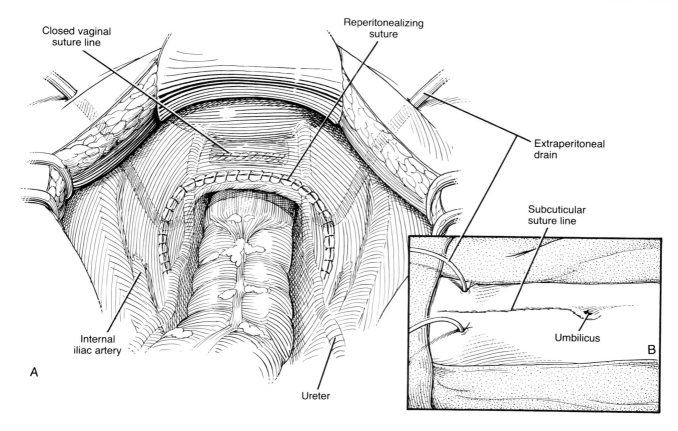

Closed vaginal suture line

Reperitonealizing suture

Extraperitoneal drain

Subcuticular suture line

Umbilicus

B

Internal iliac artery

A

Ureter

Figure 274

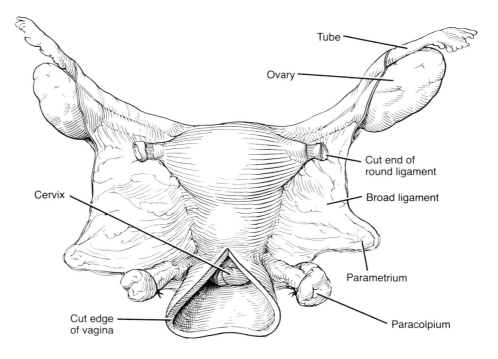

Tube

Ovary

Cut end of round ligament

Broad ligament

Cervix

Parametrium

Cut edge of vagina

Paracolpium

Figure 275

Radical Parametrectomy

Occasionally, a patient undergoes total abdominal or vaginal hysterectomy and the postoperative histologic study of the specimen reveals invasive carcinoma of the cervix. The patient should then have radical parametrectomy, upper vaginectomy with pelvic node dissection, or radiotherapy. The choice is based on what is preferable for the individual patient. Frequently, affected patients are young; for that reason, we have preferred immediate reoperation consisting of radical parametrectomy, upper vaginectomy, and node dissection. The morbidity associated with surgical staging and treatment of this condition is the same as or less than that associated with the Wertheim hysterectomy. In addition, this therapy avoids the effects of radiation therapy, which are detrimental to the function of the vagina, ovary, and gastrointestinal tract. The single disadvantage of operation in this circumstance is that the surgeon does not have the uterus with which to apply appropriate traction, which normally aids in surgical resection of the parametrium and paracolpium. In Figure 276, a vaginal hysterectomy had been performed previously, but an unsuspected invasive carcinoma of the cervix was found 3 days later in the specimen. Through a lower midline incision (Fig. 276A), the operation is begun with placement of a straight Kocher clamp on the round ligament (Fig. 277A) and with opening of the broad ligament (Fig. 277B). The ureter is identified, and the infundibulopelvic ligament is managed appropriately according to whether the ovary is to be preserved or resected.

The paravesical and pararectal spaces are developed in the same fashion as that accomplished with radical hysterectomy (Fig. 278). The node dissection is done

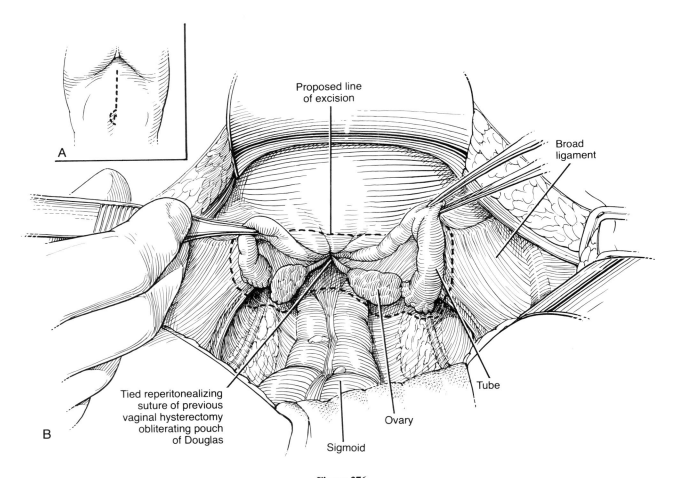

Proposed line of excision

Broad ligament

Tube

Ovary

Sigmoid

Tied reperitonealizing suture of previous vaginal hysterectomy obliterating pouch of Douglas

Figure 276

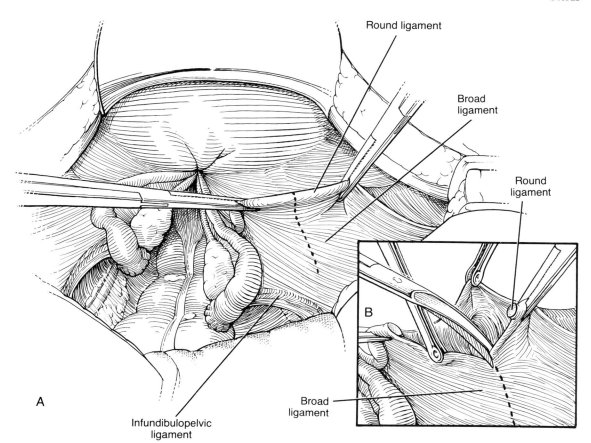

Round ligament

Broad
ligament

Round
ligament

B

Broad
ligament

A

Infundibulopelvic
ligament

Figure 277

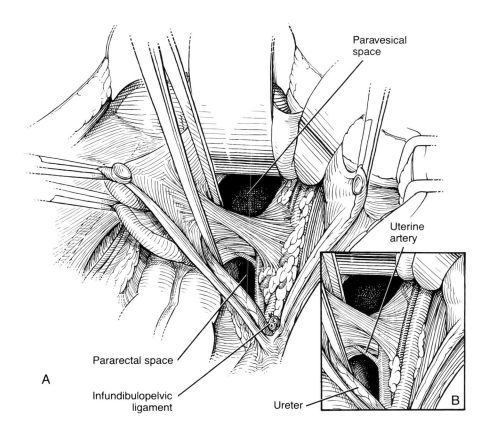

Paravesical
space

Uterine
artery

Pararectal space

A

Infundibulopelvic
ligament

Ureter

B

Figure 278

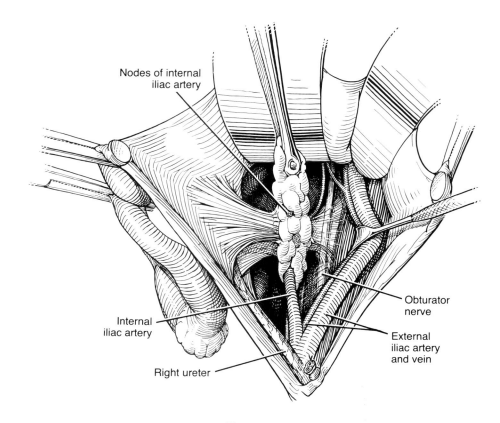

Nodes of internal
iliac artery

Obturator
nerve

External
iliac artery
and vein

Internal
iliac artery

Right ureter

Figure 279

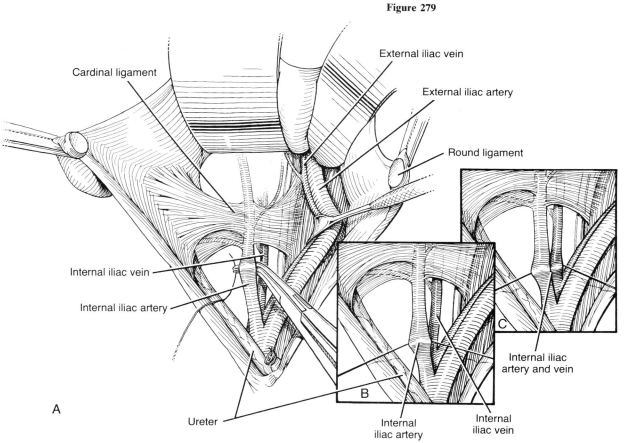

Cardinal ligament

External iliac vein

External iliac artery

Round ligament

Internal iliac vein

Internal iliac artery

A

Ureter

B

Internal
iliac artery

Internal
iliac vein

C

Internal iliac
artery and vein

Figure 280

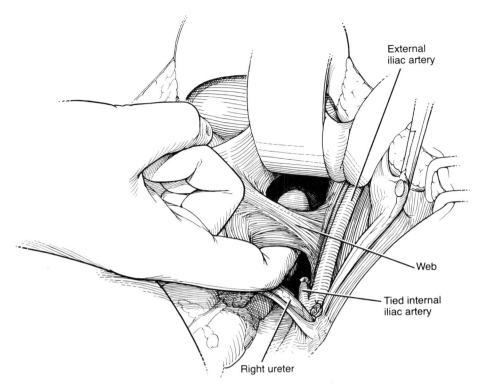

External
iliac artery

Web

Tied internal
iliac artery

Right ureter

Figure 281

over the external, internal, common iliac, and obturator areas (Fig. 279). The internal iliac vessels are
clamped, cut, and tied in the same manner as that in
radical hysterectomy (Fig. 280). The inferior portions
of the web are palpated, and a window is developed
through the loose areolar tissue beneath the cardinal
ligament by blunt passage of the index finger of the
surgeon's right hand (Fig. 281). This allows the placement of a long, curved clamp parallel and immediately adjacent to the pelvic side wall (Fig. 282). In
the nonirradiated patient, the web frequently can be
simply tied with a heavy, delayed absorbable suture.

To some degree, the postoperative bladder atonicity
and dysfunction are reflections of the degree of radicality with which this portion of the resection is
performed. Occasionally in the properly chosen patient, the surgeon may "slack off a little" to reduce
the radicality and thus reduce the potential for postoperative bladder dysfunction.

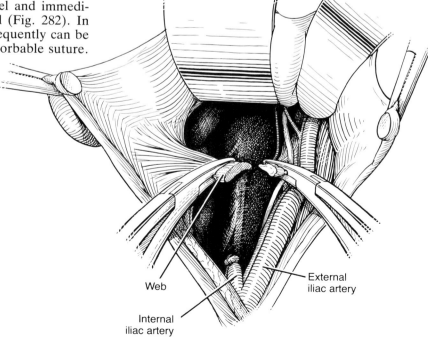

Web

Internal
iliac artery

External
iliac artery

Figure 282

With vigorous anterior traction on the Kocher clamps across the round ligaments and the proximal ends of the fallopian tube and ovarian pedicle and posterior countertraction on the rectosigmoid, the peritoneum behind the vagina is incised and the rectum is reflected posteriorly (Fig. 283). The uterosacral ligament can be clamped, cut, and suture-ligated immediately adjacent to the anterior lateral surface of the sigmoid colon, and the rectum is further mobilized with a sweeping action to develop an arc of the lower vaginosacral ligament adjacent to the muscularis of the rectum and in front of the sacrum (Fig. 284). The vaginal sacral ligaments are cut and suture-ligated with 0 delayed absorbable suture. The peritoneum over the back of the bladder is then incised, and the bladder is reflected far inferiorly (Fig. 285). With

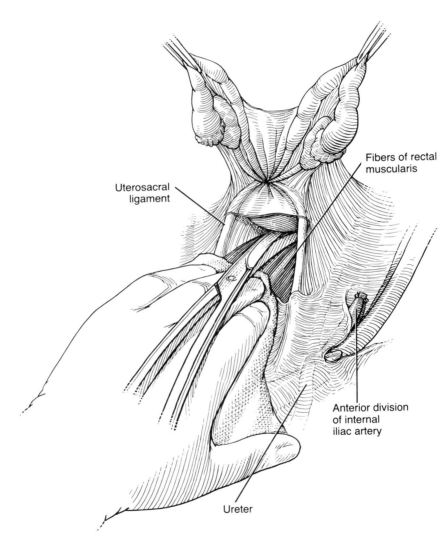

Figure 283

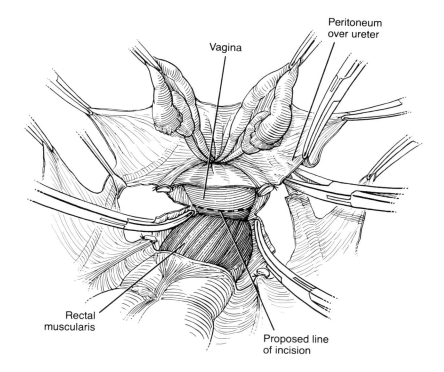

Vagina

Peritoneum over ureter

Rectal muscularis

Proposed line of incision

Figure 284

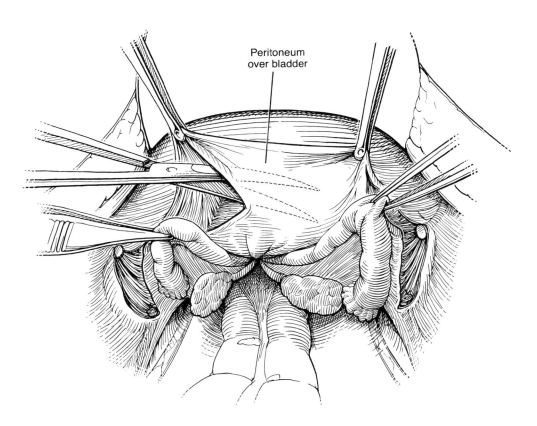

Peritoneum over bladder

Figure 285

traction on the specimen toward the patient's left side and countertraction with the wide Deaver retractor under the base of the bladder, the ureter is dissected out of its tunnel (Fig. 286A), and care is taken to avoid injury to the sheath and the longitudinal blood supply contained therein (Fig. 286B). The superior surface of the ureter is exposed all the way to its entrance into the bladder (Fig. 287A). The paracolpium is freed from the undersurface of the ureter, and the clamp on this tissue is brought beneath (and medial to) the ureter; the lower ureter is thus completely freed (Fig. 287B). A similar dissection is done on the left side.

A Harrington retractor is used to lift the bladder and the lower portion of the ureter superiorly, and countertraction is placed on the specimen superiorly and to the patient's left; this maneuver permits placement of a long, curved forceps perpendicular to the direction of the vagina and inferior to the ureter to include the paravaginal tissues (paracolpium), which are clamped and cut and will be ligated later (Fig. 288A). The vagina is entered at the 12-o'clock position; tenacula are placed on each vaginal corner, and the specimen is removed (Fig. 288B).

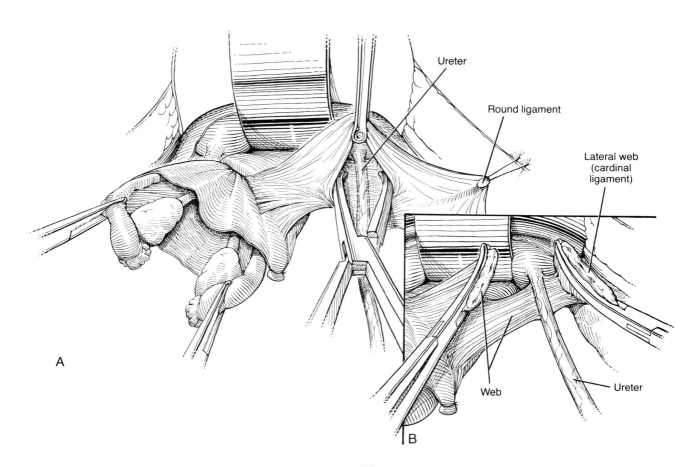

Figure 286

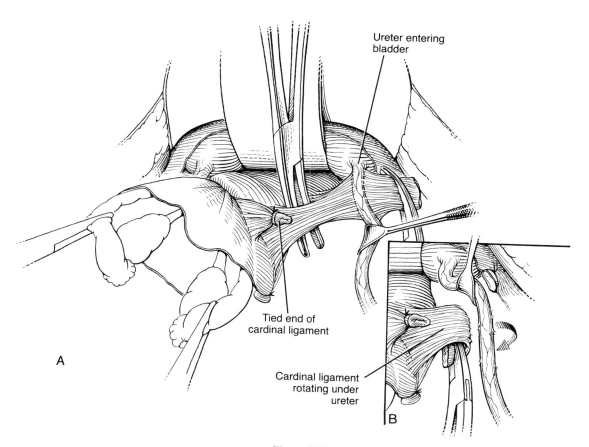

Ureter entering
bladder

Tied end of
cardinal ligament

Cardinal ligament
rotating under
ureter

A

B

Figure 287

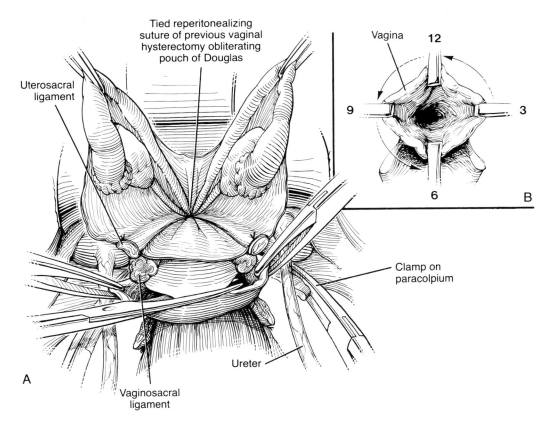

Tied reperitonealizing
suture of previous vaginal
hysterectomy obliterating
pouch of Douglas

Uterosacral
ligament

Vagina

12

9

3

6

B

Clamp on
paracolpium

Ureter

A

Vaginosacral
ligament

Figure 288

The vagina is closed with a 3-0 delayed absorbable suture placed in the subcuticular fascia; the vaginal edges are accurately approximated and inverted into the vagina (Fig. 289). A second layer of closure is accomplished with the same suture, approximating the cervicopubic fascia. The paravaginal tissues included in the clamps are now suture-ligated, as are the vaginosacral ligament tissues. The operative area is vigorously irrigated, suction catheters are placed and brought out separate stab wounds lateral to the midline incision, and the pelvis is reperitonealized (Fig. 290A). The abdominal incision is closed, and the suction catheters are connected to light suction (Fig. 290B). The excised specimen shown in Figure 291 includes both tubes and ovaries with parametrial and paracolpium tissues that reach the pelvic side walls and approximately 30% of the vagina.

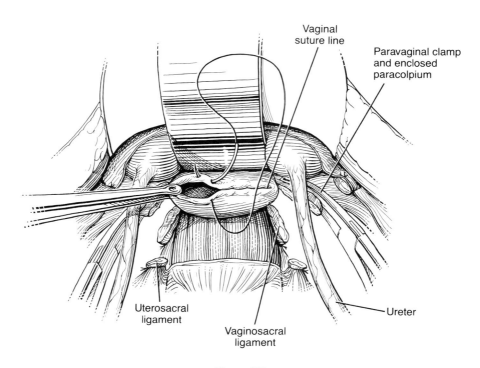

Figure 289

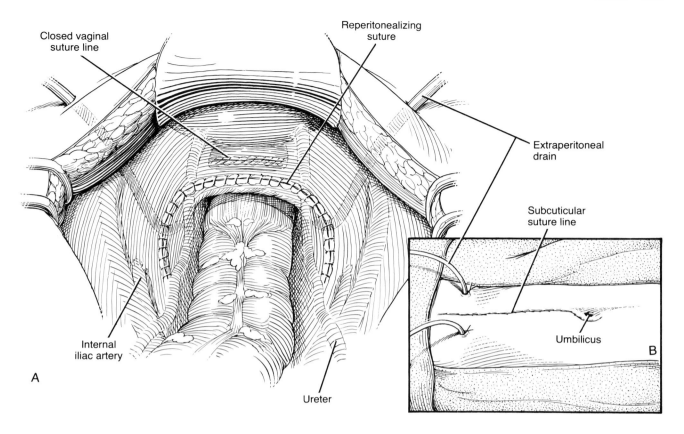

Closed vaginal suture line

Reperitonealizing suture

Extraperitoneal drain

Subcuticular suture line

Umbilicus

Internal iliac artery

Ureter

A

B

Figure 290

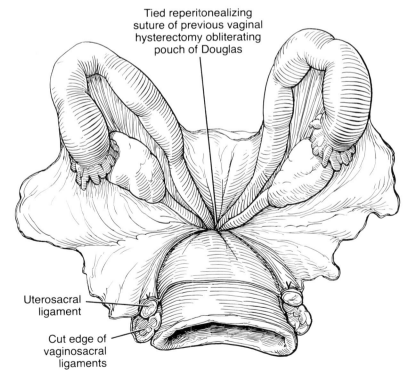

Tied reperitonealizing suture of previous vaginal hysterectomy obliterating pouch of Douglas

Uterosacral ligament

Cut edge of vaginosacral ligaments

Figure 291

Specimen: tubes, ovaries, broad ligament, uterosacral ligament, parametrium, paracervical tissue, paracolpium, and upper vagina.

Pelvic Exenteration

Total abdominal exenteration is currently accomplished in patients with advanced primary or recurrent malignancy involving bowel and bladder but confined to the pelvis. The operation is generally indicated if extirpation of the tumor mass could result in a cure, but occasionally it is performed in selected patients for palliation. Through a lower midline incision (Fig. 292A) extending from the symphysis pubis to the umbilicus, the abdomen is explored to determine operability. Attention is directed at palpating the aortic and pelvic lymph nodes, celiac area, liver, and all peritoneal surfaces. When obvious gross, extra-pelvic malignancy is noted, biopsy is done, immediate frozen-section study is performed, and histologic confirmation of distant metastasis is established.

When none of the findings indicate inoperability, the midline incision is generally extended to the left around the umbilicus to secure wide exposure and accomplish a safe surgical procedure. Patients considered for exenteration have usually received previous irradiation, and the resultant reaction produces a variable degree of pelvic fibrosis and fixation of all

structures. Simple inspection or palpation of the pelvic lymph node–bearing areas, even by an experienced surgeon, may provide little information unless there are large, gross, matted, or fixed areas of metastasis. Even in the previously irradiated patient, one can identify the round ligament, which acts as an indicator and marker for initiation of the incision to open the right broad ligament (Fig. 292B). The ligament is placed under tension and cut, and the peritoneum is incised to open the broad ligament (Fig. 292C). This incision extends laterally to the ovarian vessels to the pelvic brim and medially toward the bladder. With blunt dissection, the areolar tissue of the lateral side wall is entered, and the external iliac artery and vein are exposed. These vessels are followed in the cephalad direction to identify the bifurcation, and the dissection is continued superiorly to the common iliac artery and vein and lower aorta. The ureter is attached to the medial peritoneal leaf of the broad ligament. The ovarian vessels are elevated, clamped, cut, and tied. The pararectal and paravesical spaces are developed in a downward fashion, displacing the bladder, ureter, and rectum medially (Fig. 293A). A similar dissection is done on the patient's left side.

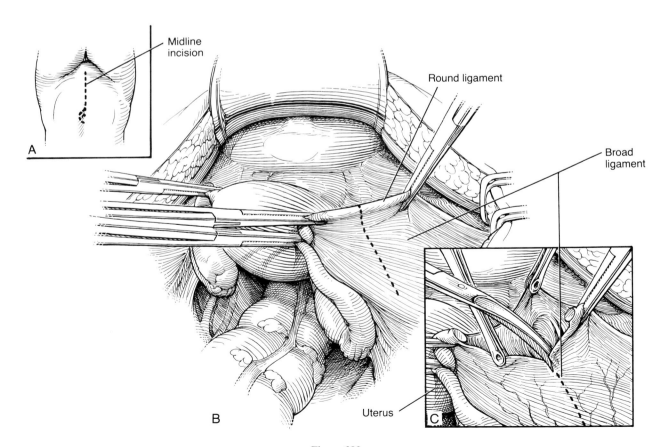

Figure 292

This procedure thus exposes bilaterally the superior pubic ramus, lower end of the obturator vessels, obturator nerves, and lymph nodes, the obturator space, the fascial surface of the obturator internus muscle, and the anterior portions of the levator muscles (Fig. 293*B*). With firm upward and medial traction of the uterus and medial leaf of the peritoneum with its enclosed ureter, the lateral web of tissue extending to the pelvic side wall can be identified. This contains all of the visceral branches of the internal iliac arteries and veins. Care should be taken

that dissection of the pararectal space proceeds medially toward the hollow of the sacrum and away from the internal iliac and lateral sacral veins. When the proper fascial plane has been identified, blunt hand dissection can develop the presacral and pararectal spaces inferiorly to the coccygeal level. Once again, this bloodless plane has, as a rule, been obliterated by previous irradiation and resultant fibrosis. Once the spaces are developed bilaterally, the lateral extent of the central malignancy and its resectability can be determined.

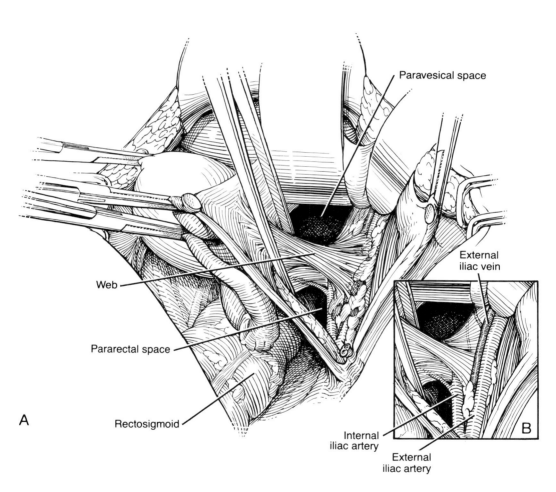

Figure 293

Occasionally, because of extensive fibrosis secondary to pelvic radiation, the customarily easy dissection of the lymph node tissues is considerably more difficult. In fact, it may be difficult to identify lymph node–bearing tissue, which may be sparse. Once the paravesical and pararectal spaces have been established, most of the potential lymph node–bearing tissue that remains has been mobilized with the specimen. After the specimen has been removed, we take additional time at this point in the operation to inspect all the lymph node–bearing areas and to ensure that the major vessels have been ligated and that excellent hemostasis has been obtained.

If at the beginning of the procedure there is a suspicious node on the side wall, we attempt to proceed with a node dissection over the external iliac vessels, which are displaced medially, and over the iliopsoas muscle, which is retracted laterally (Fig. 294). The obturator nerve is identified as it emerges from beneath the iliopsoas muscle. This lymph node–bearing tissue is displaced toward the obturator fossa. A similar dissection is done over the common iliac vessels to the lower portion of the aorta. All of the node-bearing tissue is then sent for histologic study. The anterior division of the internal iliac artery (Fig. 295A and B) (and occasionally of the vein also [Fig. 295C]) is identified, clamped, cut, and ligated with a 0 delayed absorbable suture. The posterior contents of the web are palpated, and the index finger is passed bluntly through the loose areolar tissue beneath the cardinal ligament to allow placement of a long Heaney forceps immediately adjacent to the pelvic side wall (Fig. 296). In the nonirradiated patient, this web is tied with a single 0 delayed absorbable suture. However, in the irradiated patient, the

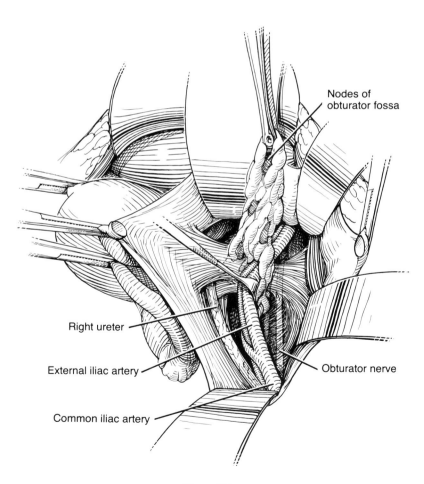

Figure 294

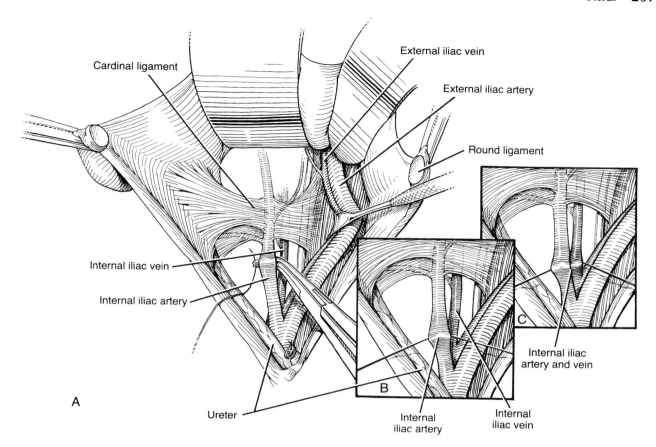

Figure 295

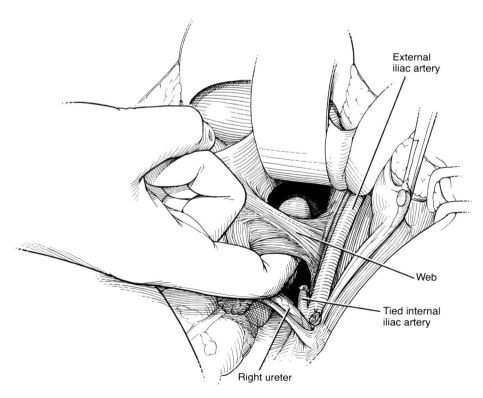

Figure 296

clamp is undersewn and removed, and the pedicle is oversewn to ensure adequate hemostasis (Fig. 297). Care needs to be taken at this phase of the operation to avoid inadvertent trauma to the generous venous network that composes a portion of the web.

Once the lesion is determined to be resectable, the ureters are divided approximately 2 cm below the pelvic brim at approximately the level at which they cross the bifurcation of the iliac vessels (Fig. 298).

We then proceed anteriorly, remove the bladder blade from the Balfour retractor, and enter the space of Retzius, bluntly reflecting the bladder from the back of the symphysis pubis (Fig. 299). Pressure is applied to the bladder and urethra, which permits downward mobilization toward the subpubic arch to the distal urethral area.

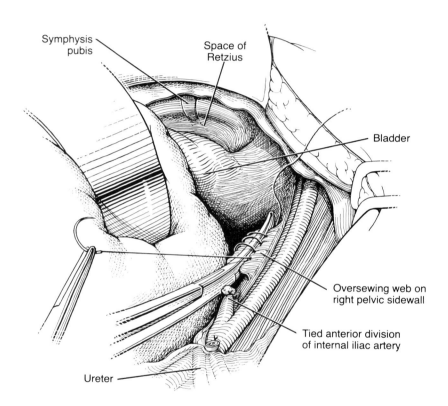

Figure 297

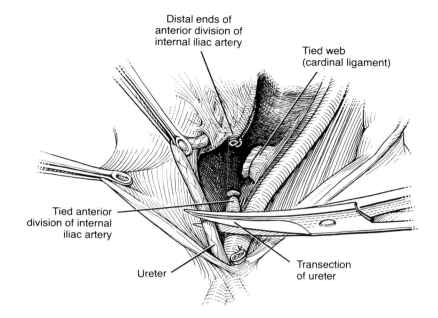

Distal ends of
anterior division of
internal iliac artery

Tied web
(cardinal ligament)

Tied anterior
division of internal
iliac artery

Ureter

Transection
of ureter

Figure 298

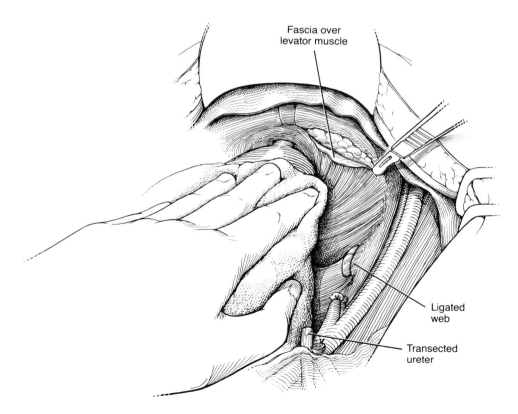

Fascia over
levator muscle

Ligated
web

Transected
ureter

Figure 299

Attention is now directed to the posterior pelvis and the rectosigmoid colon. In most instances, we prefer to preserve the ascending left colic artery, which is usually the first branch off the inferior mesenteric artery. Once the arcuate blood supply of the sigmoid mesentery is established, a point of division is determined (Fig. 300).

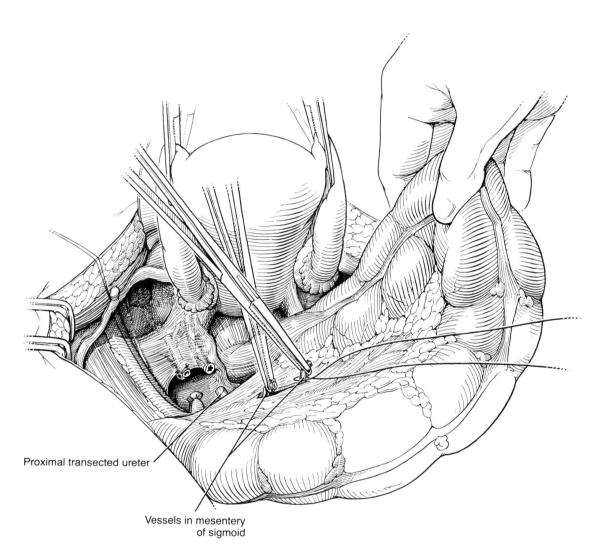

Proximal transected ureter

Vessels in mesentery
of sigmoid

Figure 300

Mobilization of the rectosigmoid colon is begun by incising the parietal peritoneum along the base of the mesosigmoid (Fig. 301*A*). Traction is applied to the sigmoid colon, reflecting it to the left, and the peritoneum is incised to the base of the rectosigmoid (Fig. 301*B*). The sigmoid colon is then reflected to the patient's right side. Again, cephalad traction (to the patient's right) is applied, and the parietal peritoneum is incised to the base of the rectosigmoid. The traction on the sigmoid colon assists in further developing the presacral space, and the loose areolar tissue can be easily elevated with sharp dissection.

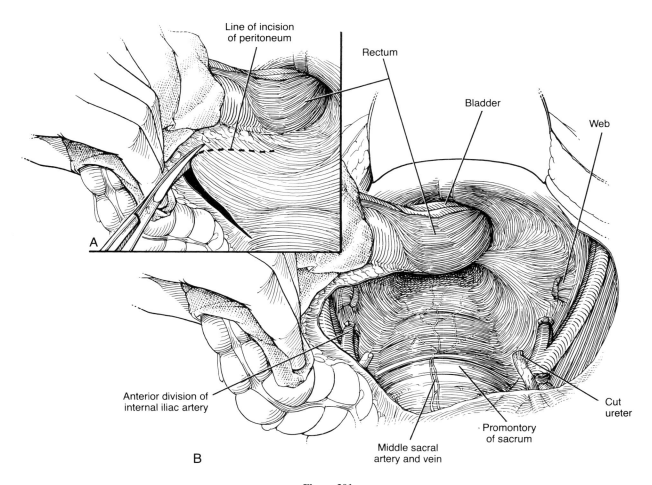

Figure 301

Blunt dissection with the surgeon's right hand further delivers the rectum from the hollow of the sacrum (Fig. 302*A*). This dissection may proceed to the tip of the coccyx, and the surgeon should be constantly aware of the venous plexus overlying the sacrum posterior to the dissecting fingers.

The lateral ligaments of the rectum, which contain the branches of the inferior hemorrhoidal arteries, are clamped, cut, and suture-ligated with a 2-0 delayed absorbable suture (Fig. 302*B*). The colon is then divided between two clamps at the appropriate level, depending on whether the colon is to be used as an end-on colostomy or whether a sigmoid urinary conduit is planned for urinary diversion (Fig. 303).

At this point, the entire specimen has been mobilized except for its attachments to the pelvic floor. If the malignancy does not extend below the lower third of the vagina and the patient is not grossly obese, the exenteration can be completed entirely from the abdominal approach. Under direct vision, the urethra, vagina, and rectum are transected in sequence, and the specimen is removed en bloc (Fig. 304). The venous bleeding from the stump of the urethra is controlled with interrupted 3-0 delayed absorbable suture. The vagina and rectum are closed with two layers of 3-0 delayed absorbable suture. If sufficient

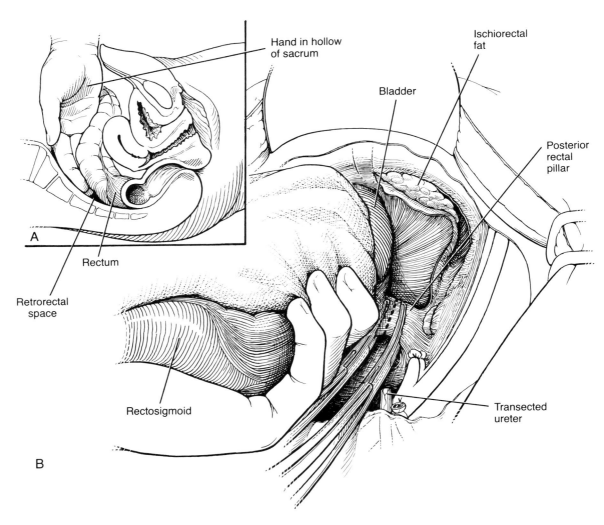

Figure 302

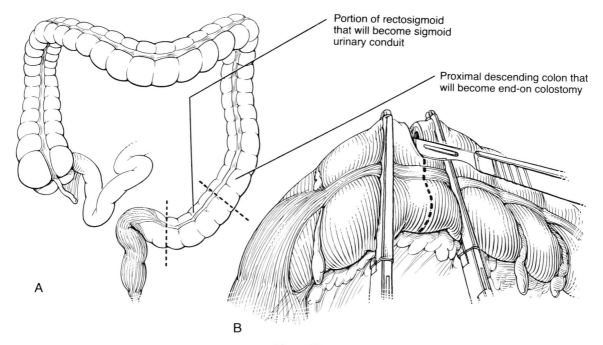

Portion of rectosigmoid that will become sigmoid urinary conduit

Proximal descending colon that will become end-on colostomy

A

B

Figure 303

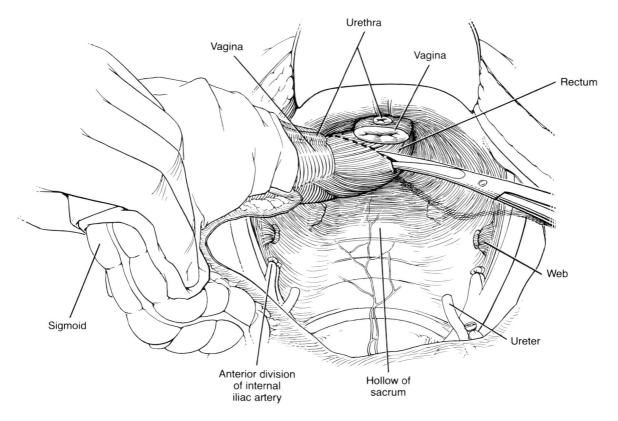

Vagina

Urethra

Vagina

Rectum

Web

Ureter

Sigmoid

Anterior division of internal iliac artery

Hollow of sacrum

Figure 304

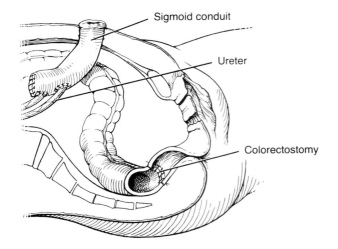

Figure 305

colon remains and the line of resection would not compromise the curability of the operation, a colorectostomy may be accomplished with an inner layer of 3-0 delayed absorbable suture and an outer layer of interrupted 3-0 silk suture (Fig. 305) (or with an intraluminal stapler). The splenic flexure is mobilized, and the descending colon is freed to permit a tension-free anastomosis.

The anterior portion of the levator muscle is incised at the pelvic side wall, where this muscle attaches at the arcus tendineus to the fascia on the obturator internus muscle. This incision exposes the underlying fatty tissue within the ischiorectal fossa. The pubic arch attachments of the pubococcygeal muscle, the pubourethral ligaments, and the urogenital diaphragm are divided. Firm anterior and upward traction on the rectum and on the specimen permits division of the levator muscles from the sacral and coccygeal attachments (Fig. 306*A*).

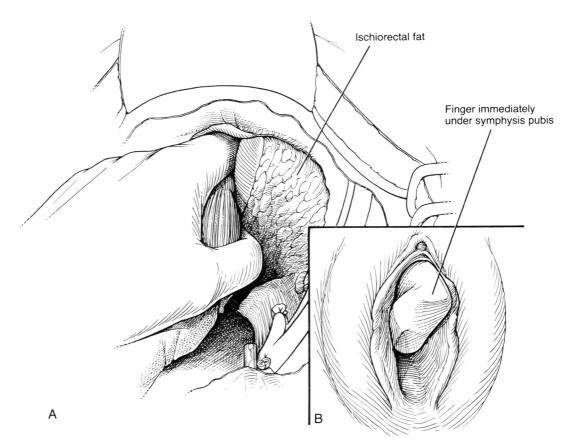

Figure 306

With the use of long scissors, the mucous membrane is divided just above the lateral labia and on each side of the external urethral meatus. The surgeon's left hand grasps the specimen anteriorly at a low level, and one or two fingers are passed under the pubic arch and through the aperture above the urethra (Fig. 306*B*). With traction and finger palpation to identify the external landmarks, the skin can be divided with a long scissors, and the specimen is removed. This should include, in addition to the bladder, uterus, vagina, and rectum, the entire urethral area, vaginal introitus, perineum, and anal canal. Any bleeding from the inferior hemorrhoidal vessels or the ischiocavernous muscles on the inferior pubic rami can be easily controlled by individual interrupted fine absorbable suture. Once the specimen is removed, additional node dissection and meticulous pelvic side wall hemostasis can be accomplished.

When the lower third of the vagina is involved with malignancy, the patient is placed in the modified lithotomy "combined" position at the beginning of the operation, and the drapes are applied to provide perineal access in addition to abdominal wall exposure. Because the levator muscle attachments have already been divided from above, the perineal operation involves little more than a wide elliptic skin incision to mobilize the anal canal, perineum, and labia. The presacral space is entered just anterior to the tip of the coccyx. With a finger passed through this opening to identify the landmarks, the excision can be rapidly accomplished and the viscera then delivered through the perineum (Fig. 307). The rad-

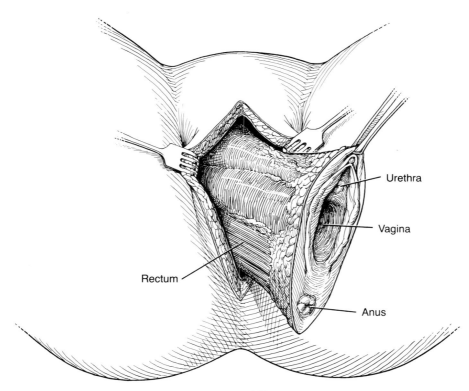

Urethra

Vagina

Rectum

Anus

Figure 307

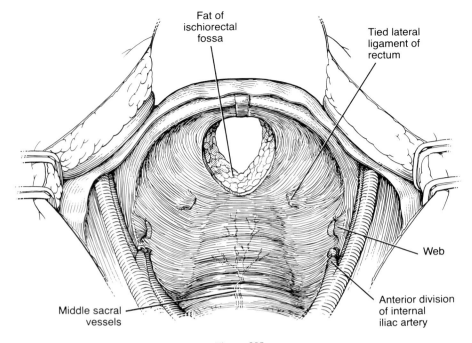

Fat of
ischiorectal
fossa

Tied lateral
ligament of
rectum

Web

Anterior division
of internal
iliac artery

Middle sacral
vessels

Figure 308

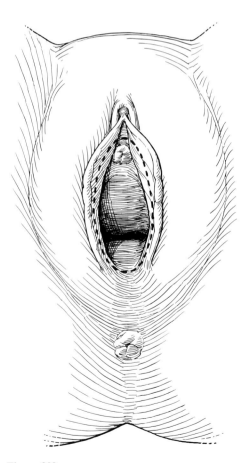

Figure 309

Anterior exenteration—perineal incision.

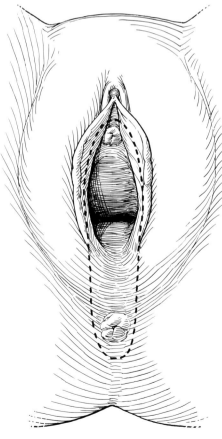

Figure 310

Total exenteration—perineal incision.

icality of the perineal dissection is determined by the extent of disease. Figure 308 shows the pelvic defect as seen through the abdominal incision before construction of a vagina or closure of the perineum. In Figure 309, the rectum is preserved; in Figure 310, the labia are preserved; and in Figure 311, vulvectomy is accomplished with pelvic resection. If a neovagina is not required, the subcutaneous tissues are approximated with absorbable sutures, and the skin is closed with mattress or subcuticular suture to provide accurate skin approximation (Fig. 312). Suction drainage

of the pelvis is accomplished by inserting catheters through the lower abdominal wall, much as described for the Wertheim hysterectomy.

If vaginal function is important, we construct a vagina from perineal flaps hinged posteriorly. (This technique is described later in the text.) An alternative technique is to mobilize the omentum from the lateral portion of the transverse colon to form a mold in which a split-thickness graft is placed as a final step in the exenterative procedure.

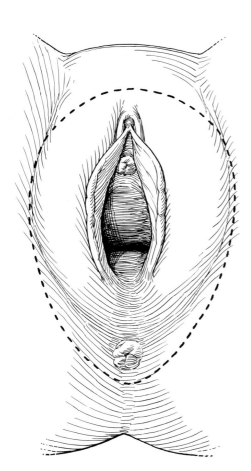

Figure 311
Total exenteration with vulvectomy.

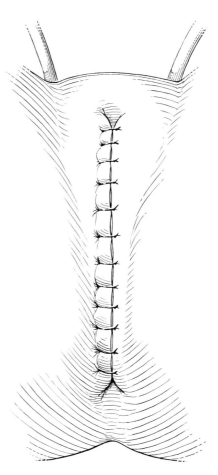

Figure 312
Primary perineal closure.

With total exenteration, the distal sigmoid has already been divided. By transillumination of the sigmoid mesentery, the arcades of the vessels that supply the distal 30 cm of sigmoid are identified. The mesentery of the sigmoid colon is divided just proximal to these vessels, and the bowel is transected (Fig. 313A). The proximal end of the conduit is closed with an inner layer of running 3-0 delayed absorbable suture with an outer layer of interrupted 3-0 silk sutures. A rubber-shod clamp is placed across the distal end of the sigmoid colon that is to become the end-on colostomy (Fig. 313B). The left ureter is always inserted into the sigmoid conduit initially. The distal end of the ureter is incised at the 6-o'clock position for approximately 0.5 cm to increase its diameter and facilitate the anastomosis. The left ureter is mobilized to accomplish a simple end-to-side ureterosigmoidal anastomosis (Fig. 314A). The posterior surface of the bowel segment is identified, and an opening is made into the bowel to approximate the size of the ureter to be transplanted (Fig. 314B). The incision in the colon is made through the taenia (Fig. 315A), after

which the ureteral and intestinal anastomosis is accomplished with six interrupted 4-0 delayed absorbable sutures placed so that the knots are on the outside of the lumen, incorporating a full thickness of the ureter and the bowel (Fig. 315B). After the initial pair of sutures has been tied and tagged, general traction on these maintains good exposure and allows accurate placement of an anterior row of sutures (Fig. 315C).

Before the front row of sutures is placed, a splinting no. 6 self-retaining ureteral catheter may be inserted beginning at the opening of the distal end of the sigmoid conduit and going through the conduit and the distal opening of the taenia of the sigmoid colon into the ureter (Fig. 315D). This catheter is then continued superiorly up the ureter to the renal pelvis, and the distal end of the catheter comes out the end of the sigmoid conduit. The three or four anterior interrupted sutures can now be inserted, and the anastomosis is completed. We prefer to place a second reinforcing anastomotic row of fine 4-0 delayed

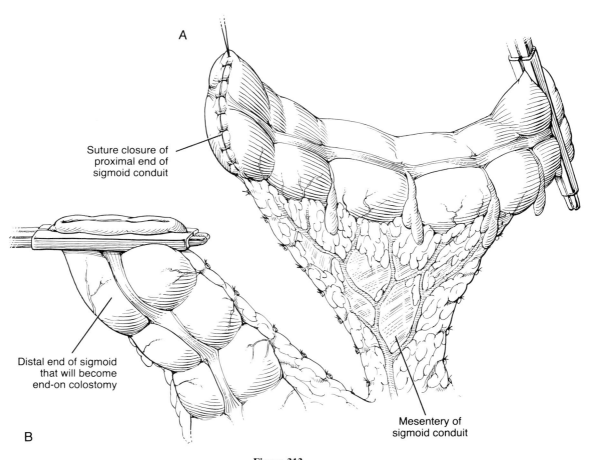

Figure 313
Sigmoid conduit.

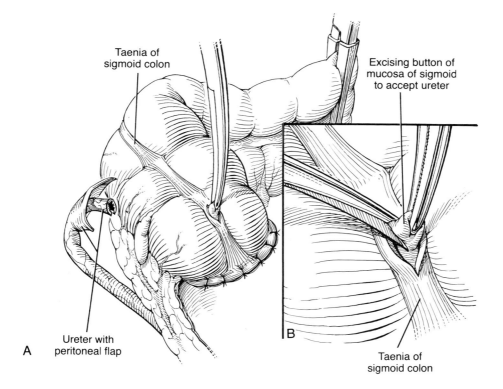

Taenia of
sigmoid colon

Excising button of
mucosa of sigmoid
to accept ureter

A

Ureter with
peritoneal flap

B

Taenia of
sigmoid colon

Figure 314

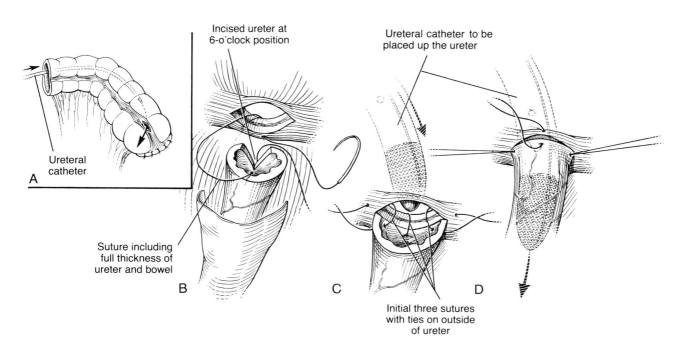

Incised ureter at
6-o'clock position

Ureteral catheter to be
placed up the ureter

Ureteral
catheter

A

Suture including
full thickness of
ureter and bowel

B

C

D

Initial three sutures
with ties on outside
of ureter

Figure 315

absorbable sutures in the button of peritoneum or adventitia of the ureter and in the serosa of the bowel (Fig. 316A). At the time the ureter is initially divided early in the course of the operation, it is advantageous to preserve a significant patch of peritoneum, which will be attached to the ureteral sheath. This peritoneal tissue can be attached to the bowel with interrupted sutures; this maneuver relieves any tension on the previously placed anastomosis (Fig. 316B).

The right ureter is anastomosed in a similar fashion on the inferior surface of the bowel segment, approximately 3 to 4 cm to the right of the previously established left anastomosis. This anastomosis is done in a fashion similar to that just described. If the conduit has been properly created, it can easily be delivered through the previously assigned location on the anterior abdominal wall. There should be no redundancy of the ureters that could lead to a kinking-type obstruction, nor should there be tension on the conduit or its attached ureters. It is preferable to have the conduit slightly longer than necessary rather than too short. Any excessive redundancy to the conduit, once it is brought through the abdominal wall, can be corrected with excision of the distal end.

The external stoma for the distal end of the sigmoid conduit is located on the right side of the abdominal wall. Generally, it is placed through the lateral edges of the rectus muscle and positioned an equal distance between the anterior superior iliac spine and the costal margins sufficiently lateral to the umbilicus to allow room for application of the faceplate of the watertight appliance. If the patient is very obese or has previous abdominal scars or extensive radiation changes, placement of the stoma may have to be altered to accommodate these conditions. As with the colostomy stoma, a button of skin approximately 3 cm is excised (Fig. 317A), and the underlying fascia is incised (Fig. 317B) sufficiently to a two-finger diameter (Fig. 318A). If the sigmoid conduit has a large amount of fat, the opening may necessarily be enlarged. Further consideration should be taken if the abdominal wall is unusually thick, because a scissoring-type effect is produced as the patient changes from a recumbent to a standing position. The stoma is matured with interrupted sutures that fix a full thickness of the bowel to the subcuticular margins of the skin (Fig. 318B to D). The previously designated location for the colostomy is identified; the colostomy is located at an equal distance between the umbilicus and the anterior superior iliac spine, the skin is elevated and excised, and the underlying fascia is incised in the same fashion as was done for the ileal conduit. The distal end of the colon is brought through the abdominal wall and matured with eight interrupted 2-0 delayed absorbable sutures. Infrequently, in the very obese patient, we keep the rubber-shod clamp on the distal end of the colon several days to establish its proper location, after which the excess is resected and the maturing is accomplished at the bedside with the patient under local anesthesia.

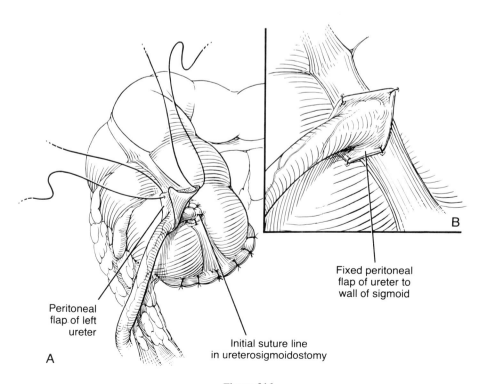

Peritoneal flap of left ureter

Initial suture line in ureterosigmoidostomy

Fixed peritoneal flap of ureter to wall of sigmoid

A

B

Figure 316

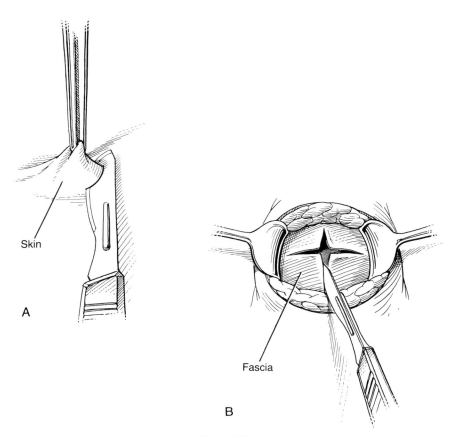

Skin

Fascia

A

B

Figure 317

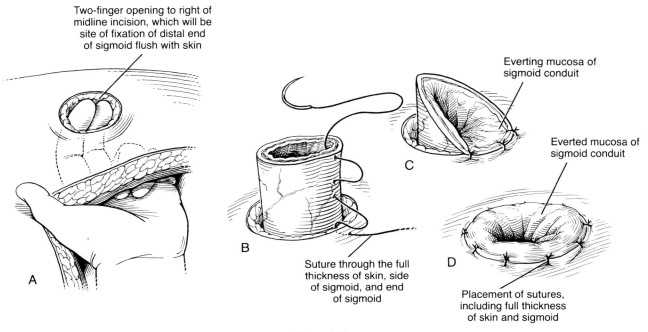

Two-finger opening to right of
midline incision, which will be
site of fixation of distal end
of sigmoid flush with skin

Everting mucosa of
sigmoid conduit

Everted mucosa of
sigmoid conduit

Suture through the full
thickness of skin, side
of sigmoid, and end
of sigmoid

Placement of sutures,
including full thickness
of skin and sigmoid

A

B

C

D

Figure 318

We prefer to use an omental pedicle to cover the pelvic floor. When the omentum is adequate, a viable omental pedicle can be created in a very simple fashion (Fig. 319A), merely by dividing the omentum on the left side at the level of the attachment to the transverse colon. The omental pedicle can be laid down in the midline, anterior to the small intestine between the two stomas and immediately beneath the abdominal incision. It is sutured to the obturator internus muscle and the pubic rami and symphysis pubis anteriorly, and a few sutures attach it to the presacral fascia posteriorly (Fig. 319B). This technique provides a covering for most of the pelvic floor and presents a clean peritoneal surface on which the small bowel can prolapse. In patients without satisfactory omentum, we cover the raw pelvis with absorbable mesh fixed in place with fine absorbable sutures (Fig. 320). The abdominal incision is closed (Fig. 321). The stoma of the conduit (right side) is generally a few centimeters higher than the colostomy on the left side.

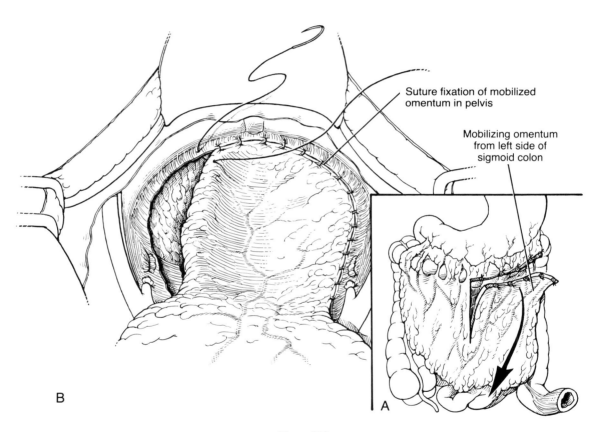

Suture fixation of mobilized omentum in pelvis

Mobilizing omentum from left side of sigmoid colon

B

A

Figure 319

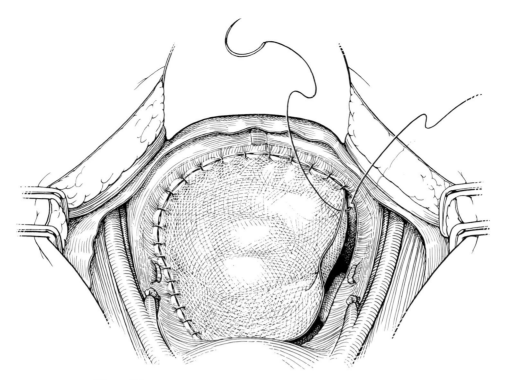

Figure 320
Suture placement of patch of absorbable mesh over raw pelvis.

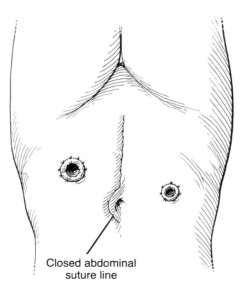

Closed abdominal
suture line

Figure 321

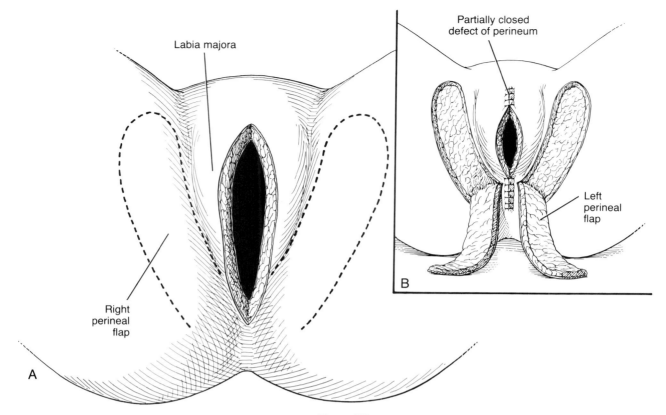

Figure 322

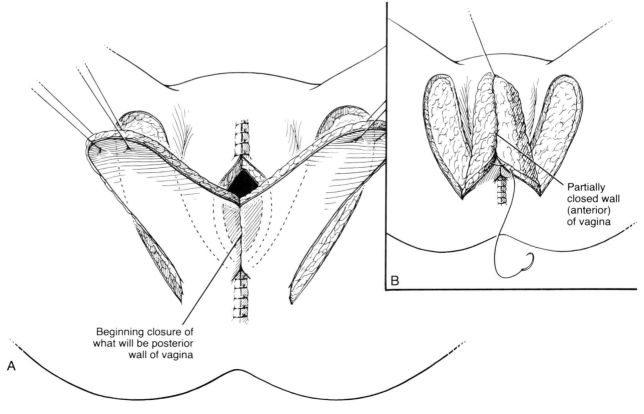

Figure 323

When indicated, a neovagina is constructed from the skin and subcutaneous tissue harvested from the non–hair-bearing areas just lateral to the labia majora (Fig. 322A). The skin flaps are approximately 15 cm by 6 cm, and the most inferior skin margin is at the level of the inferior aspect of the perineal resection (Fig. 322B). The upper aspect of the flaps contains skin and an appropriate amount of subcutaneous tissue. The fascia over the adductor longus and adductor magnus muscle is included with the flap to thus preserve the vessels of the pudendal artery, which is the blood supply of the neovagina. The edges of the flaps are approximated with a running 4-0 subcuticular suture to bring the medial edges of the flaps together, and this suture is continued about the distal end of the flap (Fig. 323) to bring the lateral edges together; the pocket thus formed is lined by skin and covered with subcutaneous tissue. The neovagina is inserted into the defect in the perineum, and the groin incision is closed (Fig. 324A). From within the abdominal cavity, the apex of the coned perineal flaps (newly constructed vagina) is sutured with interrupted 2-0 delayed absorbable suture to the connective tissue and fascia in the hollow of the sacrum (Fig. 324B). The omentum is then placed over the vagina, and the abdominal incision is closed.

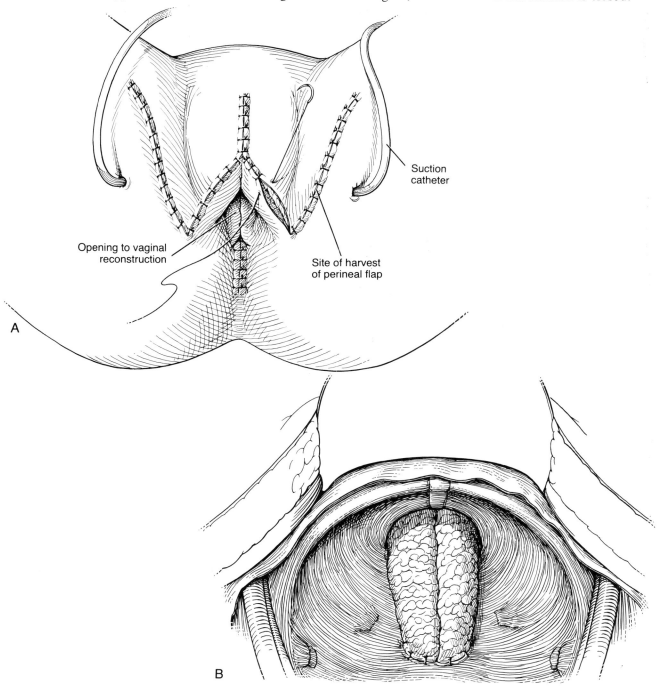

Suction catheter

Opening to vaginal reconstruction

Site of harvest of perineal flap

A

B

Figure 324

Anterior Exenteration with Ileal Conduit

Anterior exenteration includes radical removal of the uterus, pelvic lymph node dissection, total cystectomy, and partial or total vaginectomy. It is used for patients in whom the malignancy has spread anteriorly to involve the lower urinary tract but has not extended to the colon or rectum. Careful evaluation of the extent of the malignancy is required to differ-

entiate patients curable by anterior exenteration from those who require total exenteration.

The incision is the same as that used for total exenteration (Fig. 325A), and abdominal exploration is also the same. The round ligament is clamped, cut, and tied, and the broad ligament is opened (Fig. 325B and C). The pararectal and paravesical spaces are developed as described for total exenteration (Fig. 326). The pelvic node dissection (Fig. 327), ligation

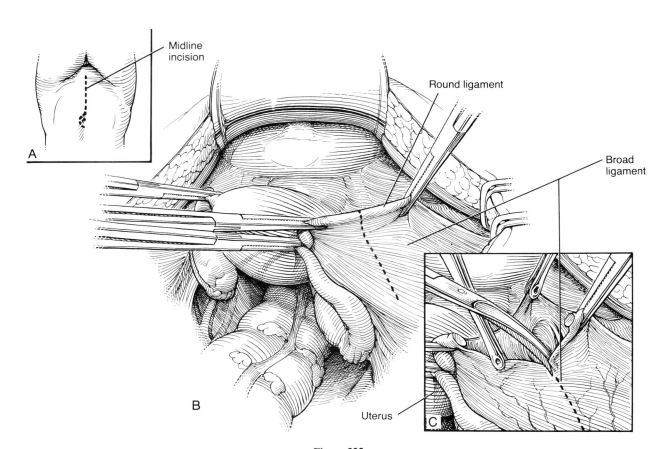

Figure 325

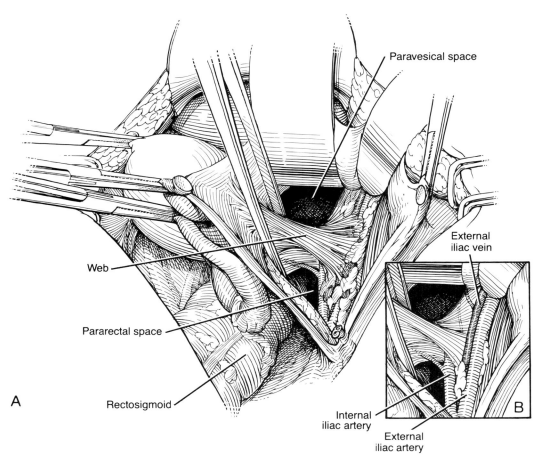

Paravesical space

External
iliac vein

Web

Pararectal space

Internal
iliac artery

External
iliac artery

Rectosigmoid

A

B

Figure 326

Nodes of
obturator fossa

Right ureter

External iliac artery

Obturator nerve

Common iliac artery

Figure 327

227

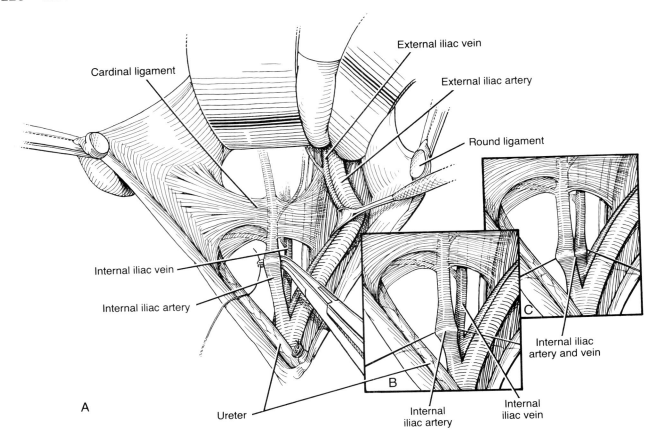

Cardinal ligament

External iliac vein

External iliac artery

Round ligament

Internal iliac vein

Internal iliac artery

Ureter

Internal iliac artery and vein

Internal iliac artery

Internal iliac vein

A

B

C

Figure 328

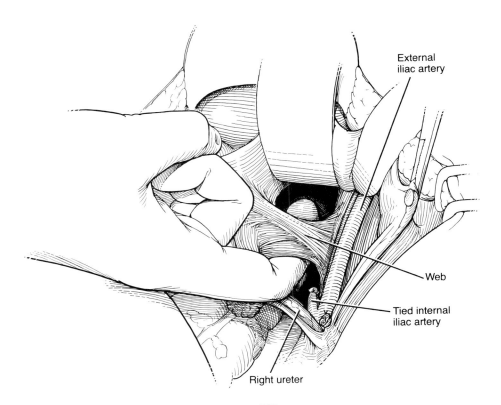

External iliac artery

Web

Tied internal iliac artery

Right ureter

Figure 329

of the anterior division of the internal iliac vessels (Fig. 328), and identification of the web (Fig. 329) and its fixation (Fig. 330) are also accomplished in

the manner described for total exenteration. Once operability is determined, the ureter is transected at the same level and in a fashion similar to that de-

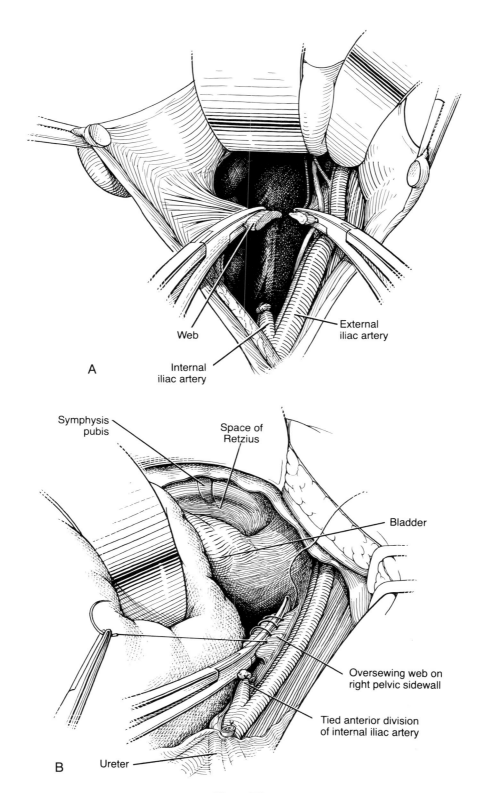

Figure 330

scribed for total exenteration (Fig. 331). The perito- neum is reflected from the back of the symphysis pubis, and the loose areolar tissue is freed all the way to the level of the external urethral meatus. At this point, the uterus is sharply drawn anteriorly and superiorly toward the feet of the patient to place the uterosacral ligaments and peritoneum of the pouch

of Douglas on tension. The peritoneum is incised, and the rectovaginal septum is easily separated with sharp and blunt dissection (Fig. 332) to reflect the rectum posteriorly. The uterosacral and vaginosacral ligaments are clamped, cut, and suture-ligated (Fig. 333). Any indication of tumor extension in this area dictates conversion of the procedure to a total exen-

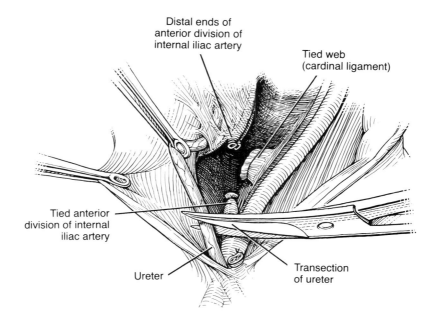

Distal ends of
anterior division of
internal iliac artery

Tied web
(cardinal ligament)

Tied anterior
division of internal
iliac artery

Ureter

Transection
of ureter

Figure 331

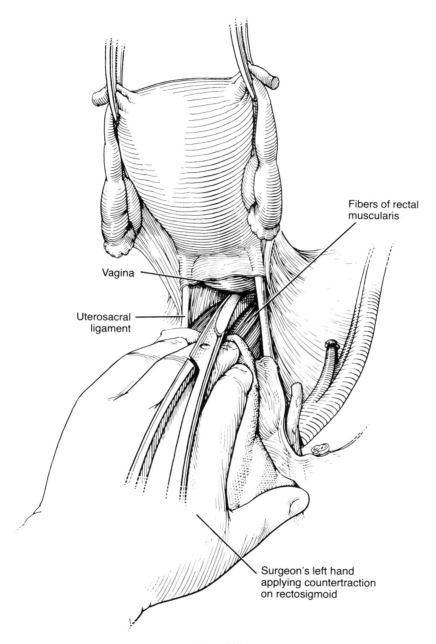

Fibers of rectal
muscularis

Vagina

Uterosacral
ligament

Surgeon's left hand
applying countertraction
on rectosigmoid

Figure 332

teration. Constant cephalad traction with the sponge-covered fingers of the surgeon's left hand on the rectosigmoid and countertraction on the uterus aid in accurate and bloodless dissection of the rectum from the posterior vagina to the introitus. The lateral paravaginal tissue and lateral rectal pillars are clamped, cut, and tied. The specimen now is entirely free of the rectum down to the levator plate. The uterus is pulled toward the head of the patient, and with the gauze-covered finger of the surgeon's left hand applying traction to the bladder and urethra, the urethra is transected superiorly to the attachments of the pubourethral ligaments. The vagina is transected next, after which transection of the posterior wall of the vagina creates a connection to the space previously developed during dissection of the rectum from the posterior vaginal wall (Fig. 334A). The specimen is excised (Fig. 334B). The distal segment of urethra is oversewn, and the vagina may be closed. If vaginal function is important, the short segment of

urethra and vagina may be removed through the perineal approach, and the vagina is reconstructed as described for total exenteration.

After complete hemostasis is accomplished, additional node dissection is done, depending on the degree to which it was accomplished before resection of the specimen.

Attention is now directed to the terminal ileum to begin construction of the ileal conduit (Fig. 335). Approximately 8 to 10 cm from the cecum, the vascular arcade is ideally suited and requires resection of a few vessels to isolate the proper segment of ileum. Once the segment has been established and its blood supply secured, the conduit is set aside, and intestinal continuity is reestablished with an end-to-end anastomosis of the ileum. This is accomplished with an inner layer of 3-0 delayed absorbable suture and an outer layer of 3-0 interrupted silk sutures.

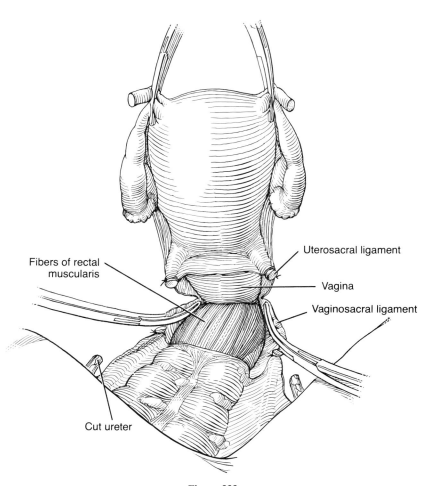

Fibers of rectal muscularis

Uterosacral ligament

Vagina

Vaginosacral ligament

Cut ureter

Figure 333

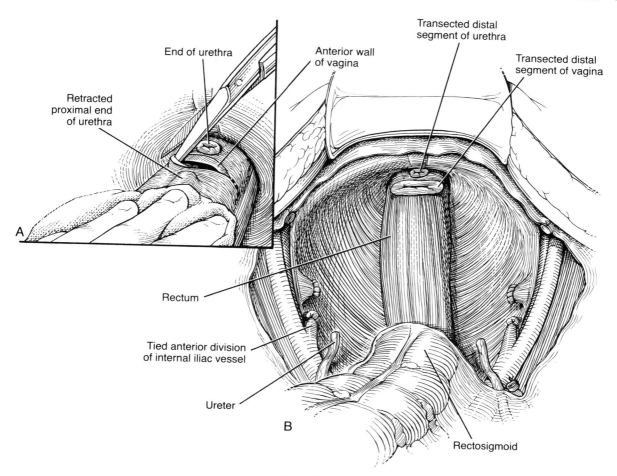

Retracted
proximal end
of urethra

End of urethra

Anterior wall
of vagina

Transected distal
segment of urethra

Transected distal
segment of vagina

A

Rectum

Tied anterior division
of internal iliac vessel

Ureter

B

Rectosigmoid

Figure 334

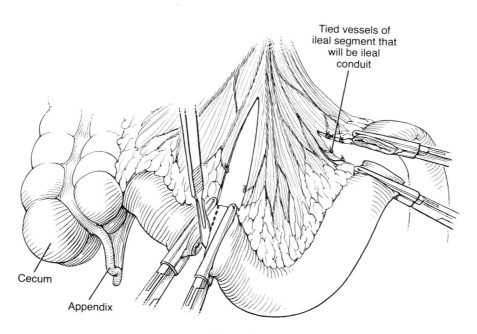

Tied vessels of
ileal segment that
will be ileal
conduit

Cecum

Appendix

Figure 335

The anastomosis is performed as follows (Fig. 336). Two silk corner sutures are placed through the serosa and underlying muscularis (Fig. 336*A*), and each is tagged with a straight clamp. The posterior (sero-muscular) silk sutures are now placed between the corner silk sutures so that, when tied, the knots are on the outside of the anastomosis. All sutures are tied, and each is transected; the corner silk sutures are left tagged with straight clamps. The inner circumferential and running 3-0 delayed absorbable sutures are placed (Fig. 336*B*), apposing the mucosa and the submucosal layers of each lumen. After the posterior and the anterior inverting portions of the anastomosis have been completed (Fig. 336*C*), the rubber-shod clamps are removed. The anterior (seromuscular) silk sutures are now placed, tied, and cut (Fig. 336*D*). The mesenteric defect is closed with a running 3-0 delayed absorbable suture (Fig. 336*E*). Some surgeons have thought that palpation of the anastomotic lumen is important to demonstrate that it will accept the full tip of a finger and thus ensure that it is widely patent.

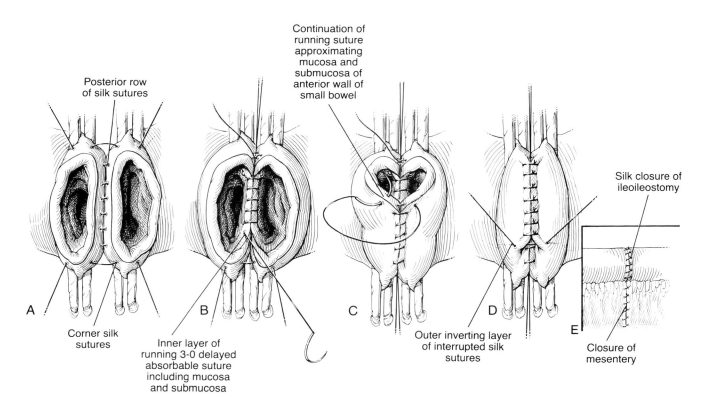

Figure 336

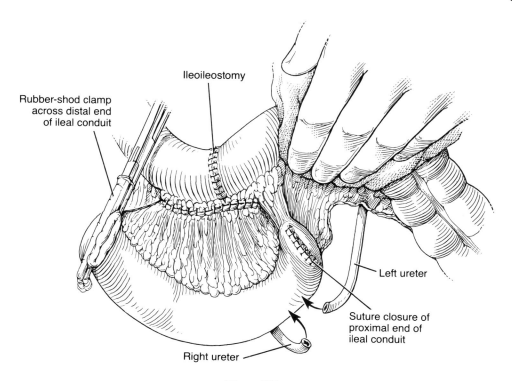

Ileoileostomy

Rubber-shod clamp
across distal end
of ileal conduit

Left ureter

Suture closure of
proximal end of
ileal conduit

Right ureter

Figure 337

The ileal conduit is constructed next. The proximal
end of the ileal conduit is closed with an initial layer
of running 3-0 delayed absorbable suture, placed in
an extramucosal fashion to include the muscularis;
this closure results in perfect approximation of the
mucosal edges. The second-layer suture is accomplished with interrupted 3-0 silk sutures, inverting the
initial suture line (Fig. 337). The sites for ureteral
anastomosis to the ileal conduit are selected on the
antimesenteric surface of the ileum. A small circular
button of the ileum is excised, and entrance into the
bowel is identified with the passage of a small amount
of bile-stained liquid. The ureters are fixed to the
ileum with interrupted 3-0 delayed absorbable sutures
in a manner similar to that described for construction
of the sigmoid conduit with total exenteration. The
anastomosis is accomplished in two layers. The proximal end of the ileal conduit is sutured to the retroperitoneum to reduce any possibility of traction on
the ileum, which would result in disruption of the
ureteroileal anastomosis. The distal end of the ileum
is then brought through the abdominal wall at the
previously designated site, at an equal distance between the anterior superior iliac spine and the umbilicus. Careful selection of the proper location, with
consideration of previous scars or any factors that
would complicate the watertight seal, must be done
at this time. The redundant sigmoid colon is replaced
in the pelvis (covering the operative site), and the
incision is closed in the customary fashion (Fig. 338).

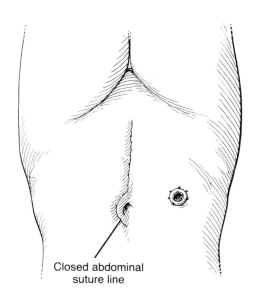

Closed abdominal
suture line

Figure 338

Posterior Exenteration

The same difficult decisions regarding the extent of operation are involved in the select group of patients in whom adequate clearance of the primary malignancy can be accomplished by radical removal of the uterus and vagina with resection of the rectum and preservation of the urinary tract. Obviously, the decision regarding the extent of operation depends on the local extent of the malignancy, which may be ambiguous in the irradiated patient. The final decision rests heavily on the judgment of the surgeon. Posterior exenteration is usually used in the management of lesions of the colon and for an occasional posteriorly situated primary vaginal malignancy or malignancies of the vulva, which require a combined posterior exenteration and vulvectomy. This operation also is associated with the added burden of having a significant deleterious effect on the bladder, which may become completely atonic as a result of the

radical resection of the pelvic structures. The operation consists of radical removal of the uterus, parametrium, and paracolpium with excision of the vagina, rectosigmoid, and rectum. It may or may not include a perineal resection of the anus, and it may or may not require total vaginectomy. Again, the extent of the operation is based on the judgment of the surgeon. Usually, a sizable portion of the rectum is removed with the specimen; however, occasionally there is sufficient normal rectum distal to the resected specimen to permit a primary end-to-end anastomosis of the sigmoid or descending colon to the rectal stump. In the irradiated patient, a proximal loop colostomy may be indicated to "protect" the anastomosis. This can be closed as a delayed secondary procedure.

The surgical approach is through the same incision as described for total exenteration (Fig. 339). Development of the pararectal and paravesical spaces

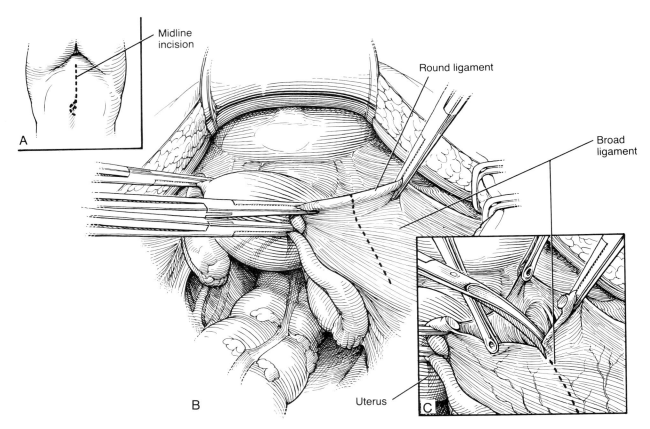

Figure 339

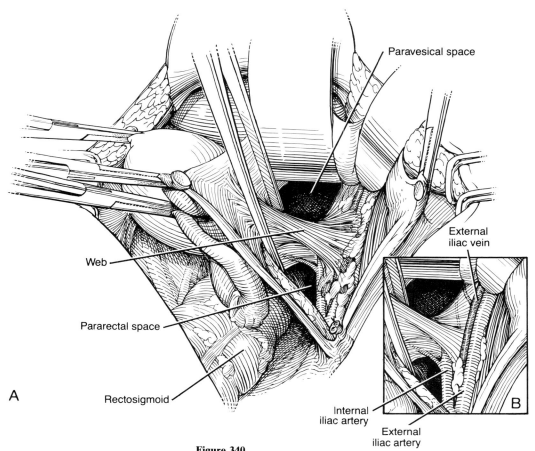

Paravesical space

External
iliac vein

Web

Internal
iliac artery

Pararectal space

External
iliac artery

A

Rectosigmoid

B

Figure 340

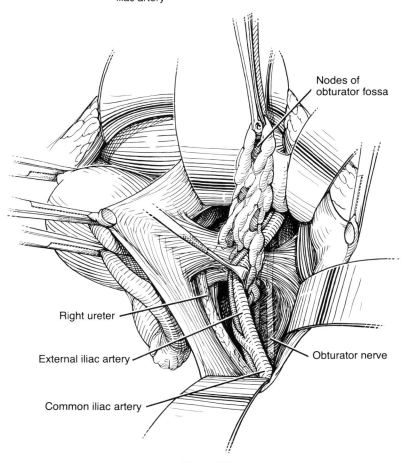

Nodes of
obturator fossa

Right ureter

External iliac artery

Obturator nerve

Common iliac artery

Figure 341

237

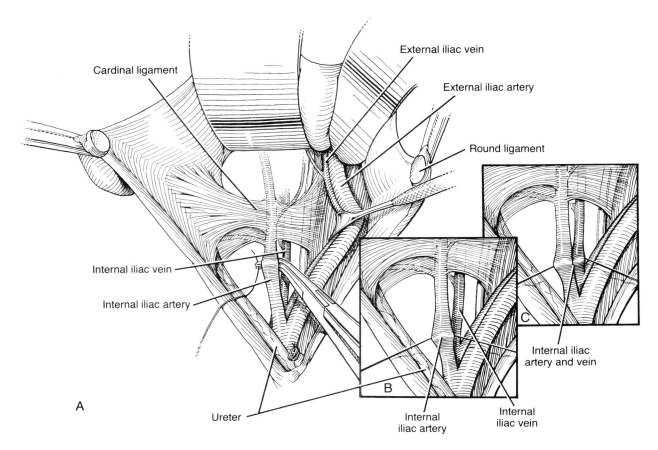

Cardinal ligament

External iliac vein

External iliac artery

Round ligament

Internal iliac vein

Internal iliac artery

Ureter

Internal iliac artery

Internal iliac vein

Internal iliac artery and vein

A

B

C

Figure 342

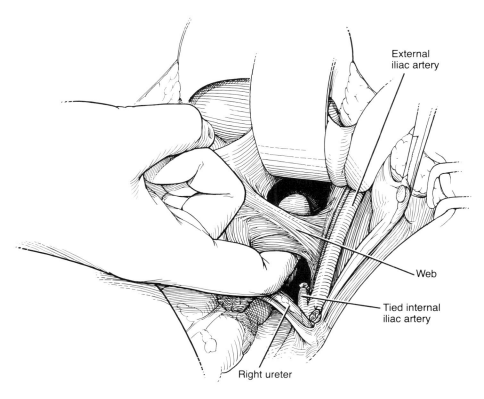

External iliac artery

Web

Tied internal iliac artery

Right ureter

Figure 343

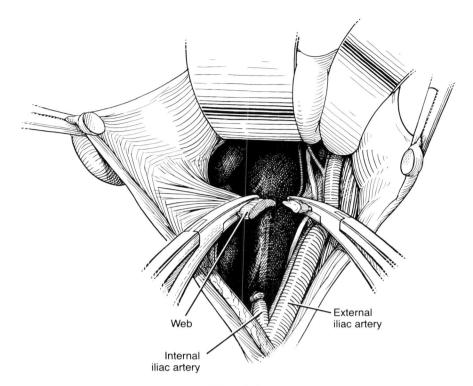

Web

External
iliac artery

Internal
iliac artery

Figure 344

(Fig. 340), the pelvic node dissection (Fig. 341), and the division of the internal iliac artery (Fig. 342) and web (Figs. 343 to 345) are also the same.

The radical resection of the uterus is the same as that described for total exenteration except that the ureters are preserved and they are freed, as is the bladder, from the anterior surface of the uterus, cervix, and vagina. The surgeon exerts tension on the

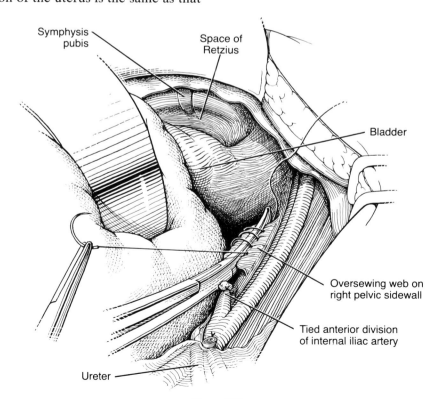

Symphysis
pubis

Space of
Retzius

Bladder

Oversewing web on
right pelvic sidewall

Tied anterior division
of internal iliac artery

Ureter

Figure 345

sigmoid colon with cephaloanterior traction and incises the peritoneum at the base of the mesosigmoid, using air dissection to develop the natural plane posterior to the sigmoid colon and rectum and yet anterior to the presacral vascular plexus (Fig. 346*A*). As the surgeon applies appropriate traction on the junction of the rectum and sigmoid, the base of the mesocolon is similarly lifted on traction (Fig. 346*B*). Having delineated and opened the natural cleavage plane, the surgeon then uses scissors to lift in a side-to-side fashion, pushing the areolar tissue out of the way and effectively completing the mobilization of

the posterior medial sigmoid colon and upper rectum. With similar traction applied to the sigmoid colon toward the patient's right, the surgeon incises along Toldt's white line, sweeping the lateral peritoneal attachments off the sigmoid and rectum as the ipsilateral ureter is visualized. This maneuver effectively frees the sigmoid and rectum laterally. With the left hand pulling on the rectosigmoid anteriorly and toward the patient's feet, the surgeon slides the right hand gently over the presacral veins and, with finger dissection in a caudal direction, to the levator ani (Fig. 347). Then, the lateral midrectal attachments

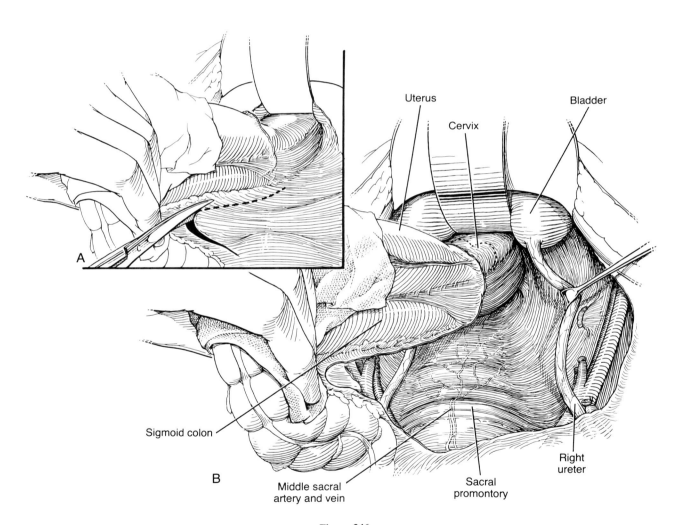

Figure 346

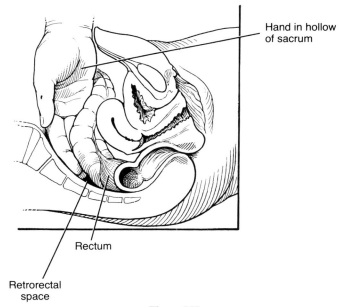

Hand in hollow
of sacrum

Rectum

Retrorectal
space

Figure 347

are identified bilaterally and clamped, cut, and tied. Exerting the same traction on the sigmoid, the first assistant applies countertraction with a Harrington retractor to hold the bladder and lower ureters in the opposite direction. The surgeon then frees the anterior wall of the vagina from the back of the bladder in a fashion sufficient to give adequate clearance to the underlying malignancy, after which the vagina is entered and, under direct vision, is incised to remove the necessary portion of the vagina with the specimen containing the rectal involvement. The bowel is transected at a level necessary for adequate clearance, which may mean a total excision of the vagina and rectum accomplished with a perineal phase (Fig. 348).

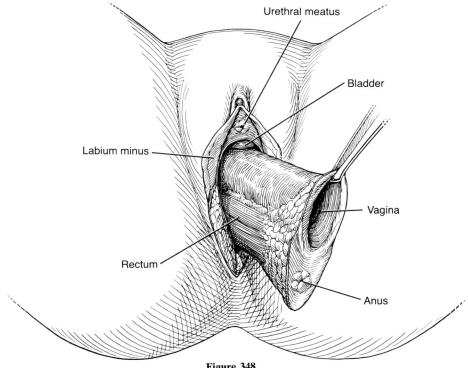

Urethral meatus

Bladder

Labium minus

Vagina

Rectum

Anus

Figure 348

Vaginal reconstruction is accomplished as already described, as indicated for the individual patient. If it is possible to do an adequate resection and leave an adequate stump of rectum, the anastomosis may be accomplished with an end-to-end anastomosis. The anastomosis is accomplished with an inner layer of 3-0 delayed absorbable suture and an outer layer of interrupted 3-0 silk suture. Selected patients may need a protecting proximal colostomy, which is closed as a secondary procedure at a later date. For patients in whom anastomosis is not possible, an end-on colostomy is established at the preassigned position with an equal distance between the left anterior superior iliac spine and the umbilicus (Fig. 349). The colostomy is matured with eight interrupted sutures that include a full thickness of skin, a small bite of the side of the colon, and the full thickness of the colon; this procedure results in direct mucosal cutaneous approximation. If the surgeon believes that it is necessary to prevent tension on the stoma, additional sutures may be taken from the peritoneal surface to include a significant bite in the side of the colon and fix it to the adjacent peritoneum and muscle with interrupted 3-0 delayed absorbable sutures. Particularly in the obese patient, this technique may assist in reducing any potential tension on the mucosal cutaneous suture line.

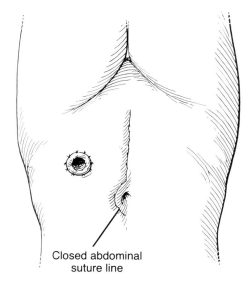

Closed abdominal
suture line

Figure 349

Adnexa

Ovarian Cystectomy

A large group of benign ovarian cysts of multiple histologic varieties lend themselves to ovarian cystectomy. Such cysts may vary significantly in size, although the same principles are followed in their removal. Care must be taken to preserve adequate ovarian tissue where it is thinly spread over a centrally located ovarian cyst. In such circumstances, reconstitution of the affected ovary must be accomplished with perfect hemostasis, generally performed with two or three separate layers.

When the abdomen is entered, fluid is immediately obtained from the posterior cul-de-sac for cytologic analysis, and abdominal exploration is done in the customary fashion. The ovarian cyst is exposed with the surgeon's left hand; it is lifted from the pelvis, and a linear incision is made through the capsule with a scalpel (Fig. 350). Occasionally, the capsule is extremely thin; if so, care must be taken to avoid

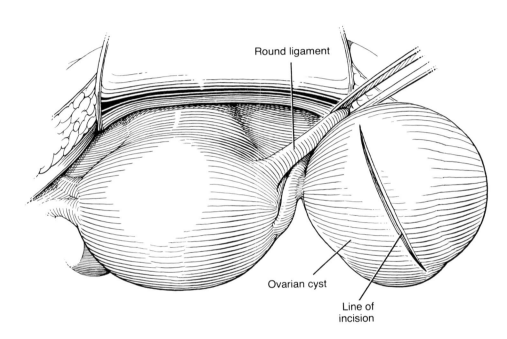

Round ligament

Ovarian cyst

Line of incision

Figure 350

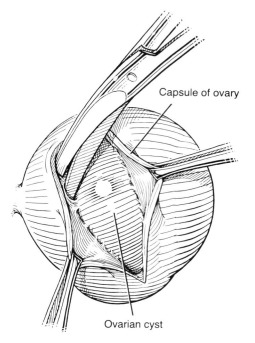

Capsule of ovary

Ovarian cyst

Figure 351

entering the ovarian cyst. The cut edge of the ovarian capsule is then placed under traction, and the cyst is separated from the bed of the ovary with sharp dissection with scissors (Fig. 351). The process continues until the cyst is completely enucleated. Generally, bleeding is minimal and is easily controlled with light cautery or single interrupted 4-0 or 5-0 delayed absorbable suture. Beginning deep in the hilus of the ovary, hemostasis is further established with a running lock suture or interrupted 4-0 or 5-0 delayed absorbable sutures in reconstruction of the ovary (Fig. 352A). The second layer is accomplished similarly, after which the capsule is closed with either running locked suture or interrupted 5-0 sutures (Fig. 352B).

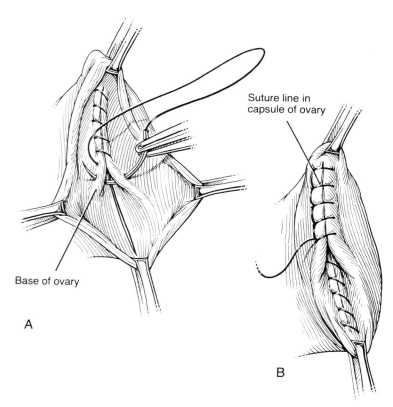

Suture line in capsule of ovary

Base of ovary

A

B

Figure 352

Right Salpingo-oophorectomy

Usually, because of benign cystic conditions, complications of benign cysts (e.g., torsion, rupture, or hemorrhage), and, less commonly, ovarian malignancy, a salpingo-oophorectomy, individual salpingectomy, or oophorectomy may be done as the condition dictates. Because the size of the adnexal mass and the degree of involvement and fixation of surrounding structures vary significantly, changes in the approach may vary. The round ligament is always present and acts as an excellent guide to structures in the pelvis (Fig. 353). The round ligament is clamped and cut (Fig. 353B), the broad ligament is entered (Fig. 353C), and the external iliac artery and vein are identified. The external iliac artery is followed supe-

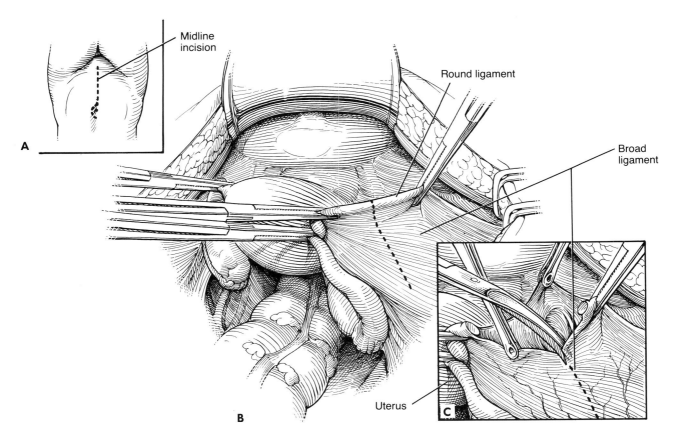

Figure 353

riorly to the point at which the ureter is identified as it crosses the superior surface of this vessel. Once the ureter is identified, the surgeon passes the index finger through the peritoneum, lifting the infundibulopelvic ligament from the underlying ureter (Fig. 354). The position of the ureter is checked again before placement of a Kocher clamp across the infundibulopelvic ligament, after which the pedicle is clamped, cut, and

tied with a single 2-0 delayed absorbable suture. As the uterus is approached, the suspensory ligament, mesosalpinx, ovarian ligament, and fallopian tube are transected (Fig. 355A). These structures may be taken in two or three separate clamps, after which the tissue is cut and tied with single 2-0 delayed absorbable suture. This approach permits removal of the adnexal mass en bloc. The distal end of the round ligament

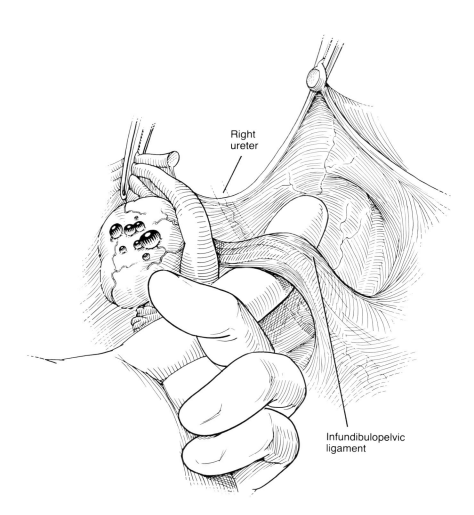

Right ureter

Infundibulopelvic ligament

Figure 354

(its proximal end still originates from the right pelvic side wall) is approximated to the cornual portion of the uterus with a single 2-0 delayed absorbable suture. The pedicle adjacent to the uterus (containing the fallopian tube and ovarian ligament) is suture-ligated immediately adjacent to the uterus with a single 2-0 delayed absorbable suture. The pelvis is then carefully

reperitonealized beginning at the infundibulopelvic ligament; the edges of the parietal peritoneum are approximated with a running 3-0 delayed absorbable suture all the way to the cornual area of the uterus. The entire operative site is thus placed completely in an extraperitoneal position (Fig. 355*B*).

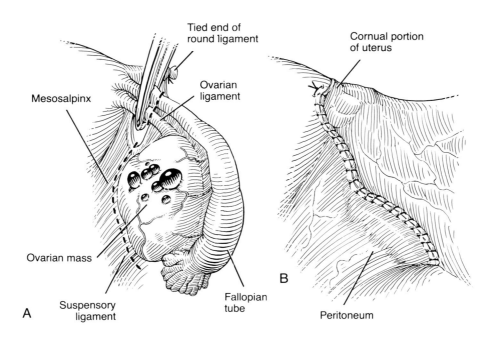

Figure 355

Left Salpingo-oophorectomy

Salpingo-oophorectomy that involves the left ovary frequently is complicated by involvement of the ovary with the sigmoid colon. In the procedure shown, the uterus and right tube and ovary had been removed previously. Now an 18-cm left adnexal mass has developed, exposed here through a low midline incision (Fig. 356). The mass is covered with the mesentery of the sigmoid colon, the blood vessels of which are identified as they course over the underly-ing tumor. The peritoneum lateral to the sigmoid colon is incised with countertraction on its inferior edge; the peritoneum is placed under tension, incised under direct vision, and freed from the lateral edge of the sigmoid colon and the underlying ovarian tumor (Fig. 357). Near the superior edge of the tumor as it abuts the sacrum, the external iliac artery, internal iliac artery, and left ureter are identified, after which the infundibulopelvic ligament can be safely clamped, cut, and ligated (Fig. 358).

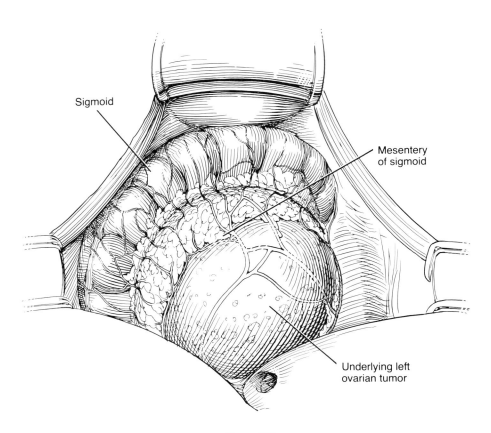

Figure 356

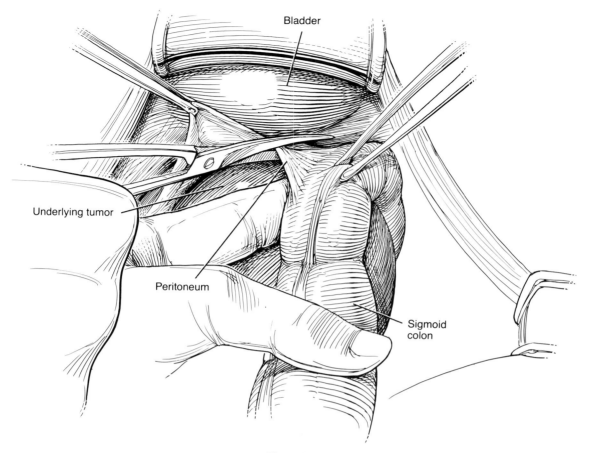

Figure 357

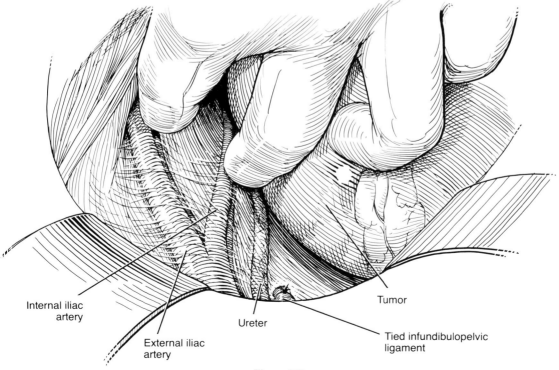

Figure 358

Appropriate traction on the lateral surface of the cystic tumor aids in identifying the ureter, which can be seen as it courses along the lateral inferior surface of the mass (Fig. 359). The peritoneum separating the ureter from the ovarian mass is incised at its junction lateral to the tumor (Fig. 360). Traction is applied to the cut edge of the peritoneum such that the longitudinal blood supply of the ureter within the ureteral sheath is not damaged. Countertraction applied to the tumor in a medial direction permits sharp, accurate dissection that frees the ureter from the left lateral surface of the ovarian mass. With the major vessels of the left pelvis (left common iliac artery and vein, internal iliac artery and vein) and left ureter freed, the surgeon carefully inserts the left hand and with blunt dissection lifts the tumor from the hollow of the sacrum (Fig. 361). The tumor can thus be removed intact, the ureter having been freed throughout its entire pelvic course. The bladder is reflected from the anterior surface of the tumor, and the sigmoid is reflected from its superior and medial surfaces.

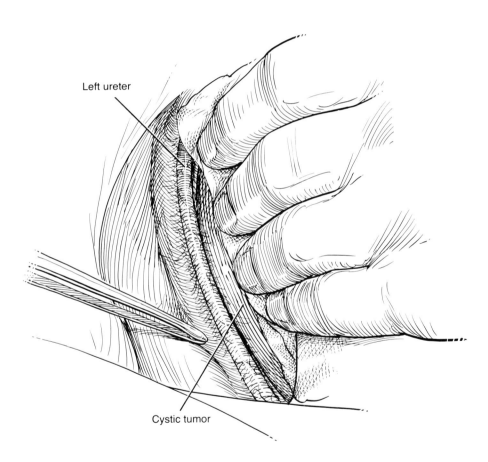

Figure 359

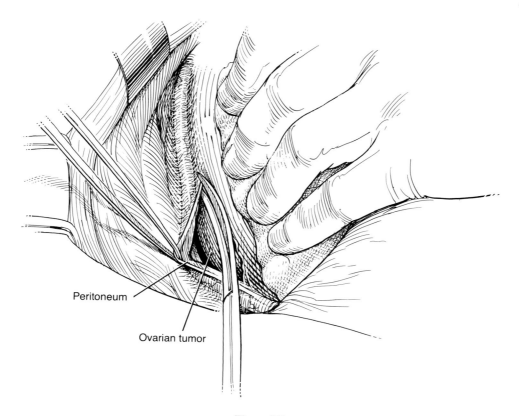

Peritoneum

Ovarian tumor

Figure 360

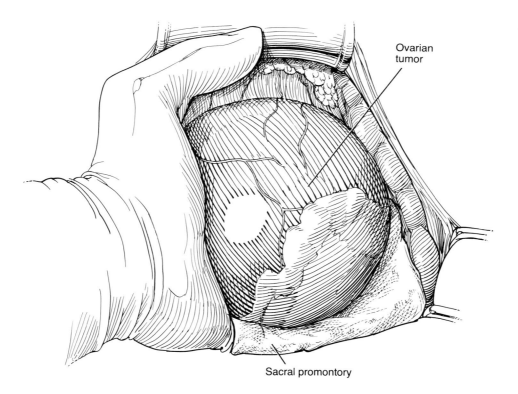

Ovarian
tumor

Sacral promontory

Figure 361

With the tumor removed, hemostasis is carefully obtained, the ureter is examined throughout its pelvic course, and the sigmoid colon with its intact mesentery is replaced along the left pelvic side wall to cover the denuded operative site (Fig. 362). A suction catheter can be placed at the site of the tumor resection and brought out through a separate stab wound to reduce the possibility of hematoma formation. Accurate dissection with insistence on identification and, when necessary, mobilization of contiguous structures and meticulous hemostasis permit safe resection of an adnexal mass with minimal potential for injury.

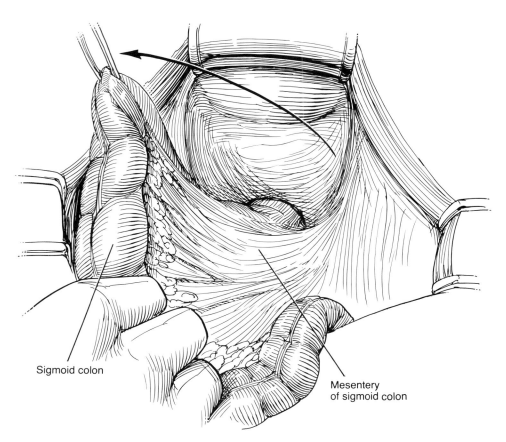

Sigmoid colon

Mesentery of sigmoid colon

Figure 362

Salpingectomy: Excision of Hydrosalpinx

Salpingectomy is done with decreasing frequency as new methods of management, specifically of ectopic pregnancy, are developed. Occasionally, this procedure may be indicated in patients with inflammatory disease or unilateral hydrosalpinx. In the procedure shown, a large hematosalpinx that had undergone torsion and necrosis necessitated salpingectomy. A Kocher clamp placed across the corner of the uterus, including the round ligament and the proximal end of the fallopian tube, assists in exposing the diseased tube. A Kocher clamp may aid in elevating the tube and thus allow accurate placement of small Kocher clamps across the mesosalpinx; this approach permits surgical excision of the tube and leaves a small pedicle of the mesosalpinx, which is tied in an interrupted fashion with 4-0 delayed absorbable suture (Fig. 363). Peritoneal covering is reestablished with a running 4-0 delayed absorbable suture to reduce the chances of adhesions to the normal ovary, which is left in place (Fig. 364).

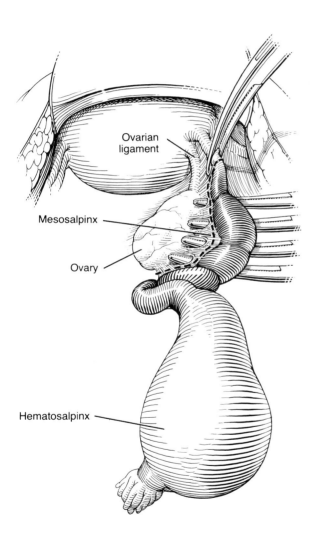

Figure 363

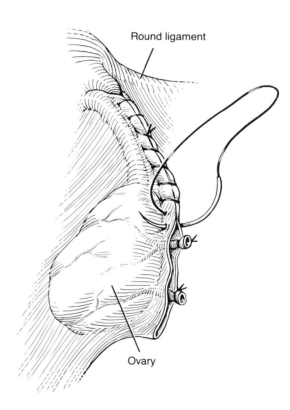

Figure 364

Prolapsed Fallopian Tube

Prolapse of a fallopian tube through the vaginal vault is an unusual complication of abdominal or vaginal hysterectomy (Fig. 365A). The fimbriated end of the fallopian tube prolapsing through the vault has much the same appearance as, and may be misinterpreted as, granulation tissue in the suture line after hysterectomy. The patient may have watery discharge, which is frequently blood-tinged, in association with lower abdominal pain. Any suspected granulation tissue that is exquisitely tender should be removed and sent for histologic study to be sure it is not the fimbriated end of a fallopian tube. Also, a small probe can be inserted into the lumen and up the tube to establish the diagnosis. The exquisite tenderness makes office management of a prolapsed tube somewhat difficult. Success has been obtained with light cautery, but we prefer a transvaginal excision.

An elliptic incision is made in the vaginal wall surrounding the tube, after which traction is applied to the specimen and the underlying tissues are mobilized. This approach permits delivery of the tube through the apex of the vagina (Fig. 365B); the tube is clamped and cut, and the base is ligated and permitted to retract into the abdomen. The vaginal mucosa is then approximated with fine 3-0 delayed absorbable suture (Fig. 365C).

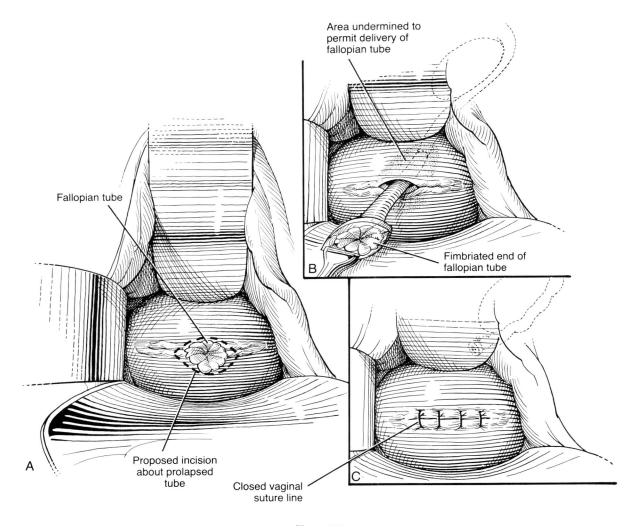

Figure 365

Ovarian Remnant Syndrome

The ovarian remnant syndrome is an unusual complication of bilateral oophorectomy; it usually occurs when oophorectomy is done in combination with hysterectomy. The patient often presents with pain, with or without a definable pelvic mass. Pathologic study of the excised mass reveals ovarian tissue frequently associated with functional or pathologic cystic disease. Most patients present with pelvic pain of highly variable quality—chronic or cyclic pain with periodic sharp, stabbing exacerbations. A palpable mass or thickening is identifiable in most patients. The wider availability and use of ultrasonography and computed tomography have improved the accuracy of diagnosis, and these techniques aid in detecting the nonpalpable but symptomatic mass.

We favor operative excision with identification of the ureter in an extraperitoneal position, beginning above the level of the previous operation. The round ligament is clamped and cut. The broad ligament is entered, and the ureter is identified; the infundibulopelvic ligament can then be safely clamped, cut, and tied (Fig. 366). In some patients, we develop the pararectal and paravesical spaces and the anterior division of the internal iliac vessels, which are clamped, cut, and suture-ligated (Fig. 367). This approach "sets up" the operation and facilitates dissection of the ureter, which is reflected laterally away

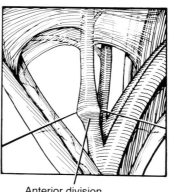

Anterior division
of internal iliac artery

Figure 367

from the medial surface of the peritoneum, which is removed en bloc with the ovarian remnant. With a large Deaver retractor in the paravesical space pulling inferiorly and with a large curved clamp on the medial leaf of the peritoneum pulling posteriorly and medially, the ureter can be dissected; dissection begins at the pelvic brim and proceeds to the entrance of the ureter into the bladder.

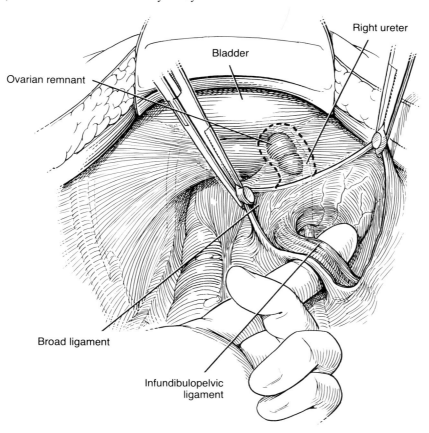

Figure 366

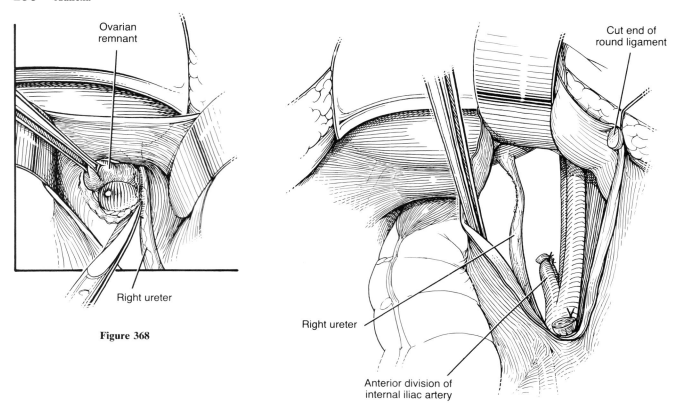

Ovarian
remnant

Right ureter

Figure 368

Cut end of
round ligament

Right ureter

Anterior division of
internal iliac artery

Figure 369

The dissection is kept close to the ureter; tension is applied to the mass and to its peritoneal covering to provide countertraction that facilitates sharp dissection of the ureter (Fig. 368). Attention is now focused on complete dissection of the ureter, rather than on excision of the mass, to free it from all its peritoneal attachments to the point at which it enters the bladder. After this step is accomplished, the ovarian remnant is completely excised with its contiguous peritoneum and surrounding tissues. After this dissection, the ureter is "hanging free" from the pelvic brim all the way to its entrance into the bladder (Fig. 369). If there is significant ureteral trauma or if a ureteral stent would help delineate the ureter, an

extraperitoneal retropubic cystotomy can be performed, the ureteral orifice identified, and a no. 6 ureteral stent passed up the ureter in a retrograde fashion. In Figure 370, a nephrectomy was required because of ureteral obstruction and total destruction of the left kidney. A portion of the specimen demonstrates the immediate apposition and obstruction of the ureter by the ovarian remnant. In most patients and in all those undergoing reoperation, a suction catheter drain is used extraperitoneally to prevent fluid collection. Successful excision of the mass is associated with prompt relief of symptoms and few complications.

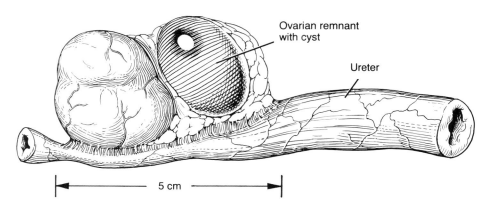

Ovarian remnant
with cyst

Ureter

5 cm

Figure 370

Ovarian Carcinoma

The surgeon must be not only skilled in pelvic surgery but also technically capable of removing metastatic lesions involving upper abdominal organs. The exent of the operation required varies with the stage, cell type, and grade of the malignancy. The conventional operation, largely applicable to low-stage lesions, consists of total abdominal hysterectomy, bilateral salpingo-oophorectomy, omentectomy, and appropriate biopsies to establish accurate staging. A primary cytoreductive operation includes all the phases of the conventional effort in addition to resection of other organs involved by the malignancy in order to obtain total removal of the tumor or at least a maximal reduction of tumor volume. Not infrequently, resection of segments of the large or small bowel and portions of the urinary tract and pelvic and abdominal wall structures is required. Palliative procedures may be needed for relief of bowel obstruction or other complications of widespread malignancy, but frequently major resection is required.

The 5-year survival rate of patients with advanced ovarian malignancy has not improved significantly during the past 25 years, despite more aggressive operations, use of radiation therapy, and advances in chemotherapy. However, occasionally a patient who is thought to have inoperable disease may be cured; in many more patients, debulking may improve the quality of remaining life. Anyone with experience in ovarian malignancy (Fig. 371) is aware that, because of its tendency to invade surrounding structures, the most logical and effective approach is a retroperitoneal dissection beginning on the pelvic side walls.

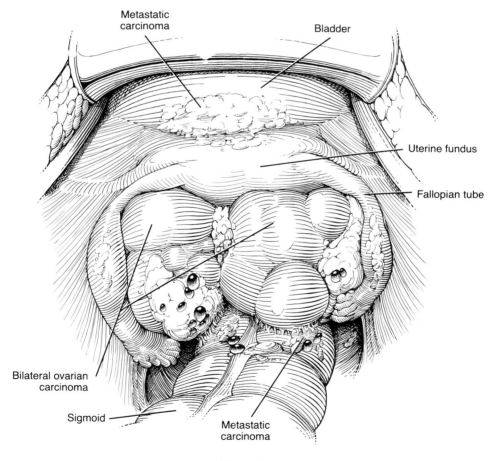

Metastatic carcinoma

Bladder

Uterine fundus

Fallopian tube

Bilateral ovarian carcinoma

Sigmoid

Metastatic carcinoma

Figure 371

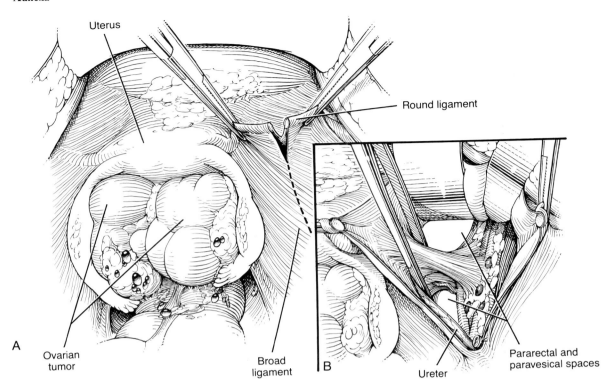

Uterus

Round ligament

A

Ovarian tumor

Broad ligament

B

Ureter

Pararectal and paravesical spaces

Figure 372

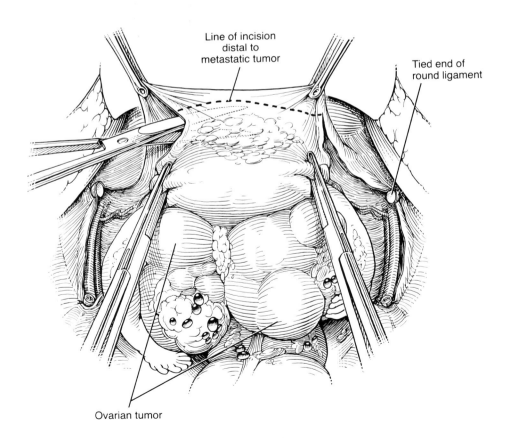

Line of incision distal to metastatic tumor

Tied end of round ligament

Ovarian tumor

Figure 373

The procedure is initiated by clamping, cutting, and tying the round ligament and opening the broad ligament to identify the ureter (Fig. 372A). The infundibulopelvic ligament is clamped, cut, and tied. The ureter is followed inferiorly to the point at which it is crossed by the uterine vessels, which are clamped, cut, and divided; in some patients we prefer to clamp, cut, and tie the anterior division of the internal iliac artery and develop the pararectal and paravesical spaces (Fig. 372B). The ureter is then mobilized laterally and separated from the medial leaf of the

parietal peritoneum. A similar dissection is done on the left side.

Frequently, invasion of the tumor in the vesicouterine fold requires a wide excision of the peritoneum over the dome of the bladder (Fig. 373). With appropriate traction on the bladder toward the patient's feet and with countertraction with the gauzed fingers of the surgeon's left hand, the muscularis of the bladder is separated from the peritoneum and anterior surface of the uterus, cervix, and vagina (Fig. 374). The

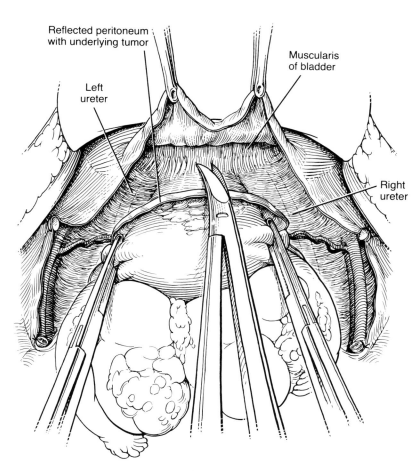

Figure 374

muscularis of the bladder and the lower portions of the ureter are then mobilized laterally with sharp and blunt dissection to free the pillar of the bladder from the anterior lateral surface of the uterus and cervix. In Figure 371, it is apparent that the ovarian tumors are densely fixed into the posterior cul-de-sac and involve the anterior surface of the rectosigmoid, the lateral side walls laterally, and the back of the uterus anteriorly.

In preparation for an en bloc resection of the sigmoid colon, the surgeon grasps the sigmoid colon in the gauzed fingers of the left hand, applying traction up and to the patient's left side (Fig. 375A). At the level of the pelvic brim, the ureter is again identified, and the peritoneum along the root of the mesentery is incised toward the hollow of the sacrum down to the point at which the ovarian tumor is fixed to the sigmoid colon. A similar dissection is accomplished on the left side of the sigmoid colon by the surgeon applying traction with the gauzed fingers of the left hand, taking the sigmoid colon to the patient's right and superiorly. The peritoneum is again incised, and the ureter is identified laterally. With appropriate traction on the sigmoid colon, the loose areolar connection between the back of the sigmoid colon and the front of the sacrum is separated, and this is further mobilized by the surgeon's inserting the right hand behind the rectosigmoid, lifting the bowel from the hollow of the sacrum, and at the same time applying traction with the left hand on the sigmoid colon (Fig. 375B).

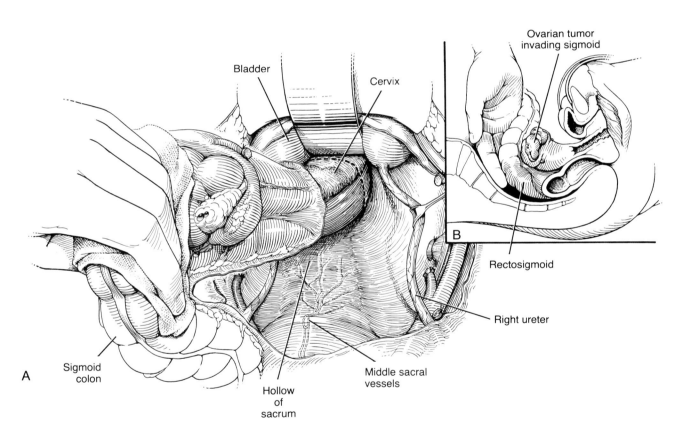

Figure 375

At this point, the tumor is free from the ureters laterally at the level of the pelvic brim, from the hollow of the sacrum posteriorly, and from the bladder and lower ureters anteriorly. In Figure 376A, there is sufficient mobilization of the entire specimen, and a wide Deaver retractor is placed behind the bladder to apply traction toward the feet of the patient. Countertraction is applied to the anterior surface of the uterus with the gauzed fingers of the surgeon's left hand, and the vagina is entered (Fig. 376A). The anterior vaginal wall is incised at the 12-o'clock position. The opening is extended laterally to the patient's right and left, and the wide Deaver retractor is used to lift the base of the bladder and the lower portions of the ureter out of the way. As the posterior wall of the vagina is incised, a tenaculum is placed on the proximal cut edge of the vagina, and traction is applied toward the patient's head. Fre-

quently, the posterior wall of the vagina can be separated easily from the underlying anterior wall of the rectum superiorly in order to gain additional length of the rectum, which permits an anastomosis at a higher level. A rubber-shod clamp is placed across the mobilized lower rectum; the bowel is transected; the appropriate mesenteric vessels are clamped, cut, and tied; and the entire specimen is rolled superiorly out of the pelvis (Fig. 376B). This technique permits placement of the rubber-shod clamp on the distal end of the descending colon and sigmoid colon, and the specimen can then be removed en bloc. Careful hemostasis is then obtained. The splenic flexure is mobilized, and the descending colon is freed up sufficiently to accomplish an end-to-end anastomosis with the remaining rectal stump. This is done with an inner layer of running 3-0 delayed absorbable suture and an outer layer of interrupted

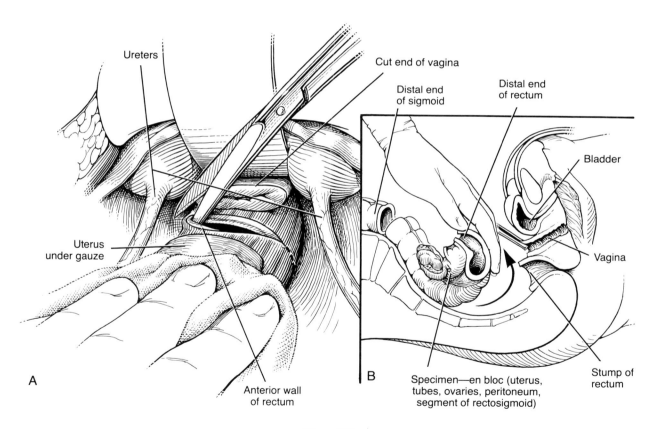

Figure 376

3-0 silk sutures. The vagina is closed in two layers with 3-0 delayed absorbable sutures (Fig. 377). Two large Jackson-Pratt drains are placed in the hollow of the sacrum and brought out through stab wounds lateral to the midline incision. The rest of the procedure is accomplished in the customary fashion, consisting of an omentectomy and removal of as much tumor as possible.

Certainly, the most aggressive operation should be performed when all or nearly all of the gross tumor can be excised. This is accomplished without regard to the size of the largest metastatic deposit or the degree of ascites present. The procedure continues with individual removal of any sizable tumor deposits about the stomach, spleen, margins or segments of the liver, and retroperitoneal structures, even if morbidity could be increased as a result. This approach is worthwhile in patients who are cured as a result of the surgical procedure and in many other patients who derive considerable palliative benefit.

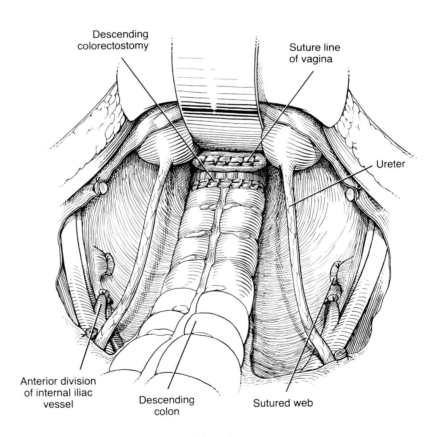

Descending colorectostomy

Suture line of vagina

Ureter

Anterior division of internal iliac vessel

Descending colon

Sutured web

Figure 377

Urinary Tract

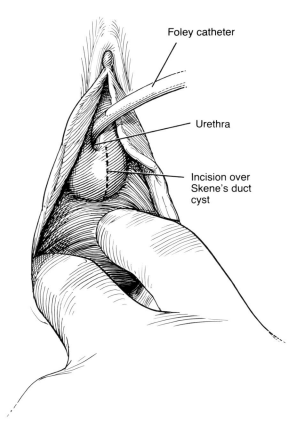

Foley catheter

Urethra

Incision over Skene's duct cyst

Figure 378

Skene's Duct Cyst

Paraurethral (Skene's) duct cysts may present laterally and caudally to the urethra and may cause urinary symptoms (frequently, spraying of the urinary stream), although they are usually not more than 2 cm in diameter. Their constant site of origin usually differentiates them from urethral diverticula and wolffian remnant cysts, but they may extend peripherally beneath the skin of the vestibule so that the diagnosis is not immediately obvious. The incision is made in the mucosa of the vagina over the cyst (Fig. 378). The mucosa is mobilized laterally, and the cyst is excised, keeping the incision adjacent to the wall of the cyst to avoid entering the lumen of the urethra (Fig. 379*A*). After excision of the cyst, the urethral supporting tissues are approximated with fine suture, and the vaginal mucosa is closed; care is taken not to place any suture deep enough to enter the urethral lumen (Fig. 379*B*).

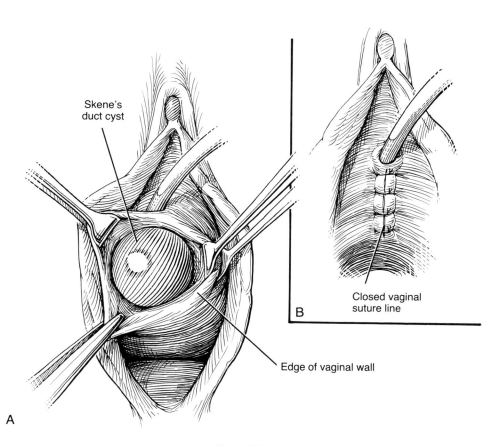

Skene's duct cyst

Closed vaginal suture line

B

Edge of vaginal wall

A

Figure 379

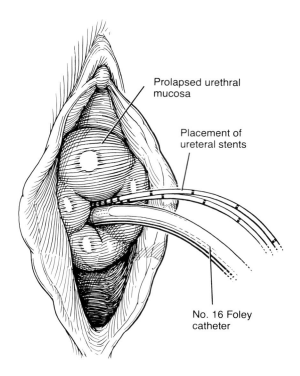

Figure 380

Prolapsed Urethral Mucosa

Prolapse of edematous urethral mucosa occasionally is of sufficient degree to require surgical excision. In Figure 380, the ureteral orifices were located at the bladder neck. During excision, each anchoring suture is placed as the mucosa is freed (Fig. 381). Thrombosed veins are visible in the cut edge of the prolapsed segment as it is held laterally; thus, there is comparatively little bleeding with the procedure. The tissues are very edematous and friable. Generally, six sutures are sufficient in this situation (Fig. 382). If the sutures are not placed in their proper positions, the mucosa has a tendency to retract superiorly and is thus difficult to secure once the thrombosed tissue is removed.

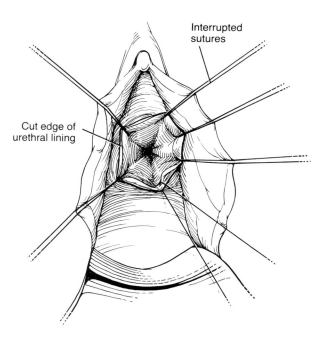

Figure 382

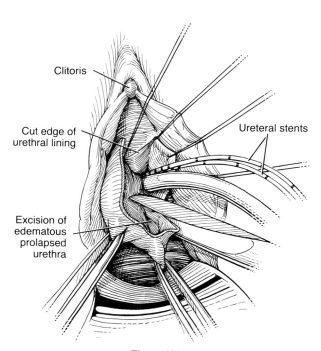

Figure 381

Diverticulum of the Urethra

Most repairs of diverticula are tedious and difficult and are associated with more loss of blood than one would expect from a small lesion. The potential for development of a serious complication depends on the size and number of the diverticula, the degree of inflammation, the viability of the tissues, and the position of the ostium in relation to the floor of the urethra and bladder neck. The resection of multiple, large, multiloculated, or saddle-shaped diverticula can require extensive dissection about the floor of the urethra at the bladder neck and the lower trigone. In these conditions, the placement of ureteral catheters before operation can facilitate identification of the ureters and reduce the risk of damage during dissection. Actual or potential destruction or fixation of the smooth muscle of the urethra and bladder neck produced both by the expanding inflammatory mass and by the trauma associated with excision of the diverticulum can result in urethral fistula or stress urinary incontinence. Accurate reconstruction of the urethra and its supporting structures in combination with perfect hemostasis and antibiotic therapy for control of the infectious process substantially reduces the frequency of these potentially disabling complications.

Figure 383 shows the relative position of a diverticulum of the midurethra. A vertical incision is made in the vaginal wall (Fig. 384), the underlying cervicopubic (periurethral) fascia is exposed, and the lateral

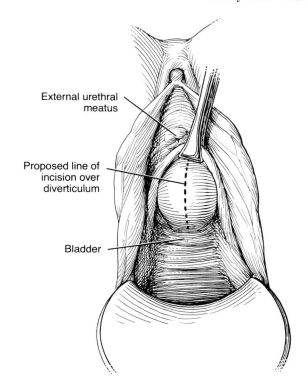

Figure 384

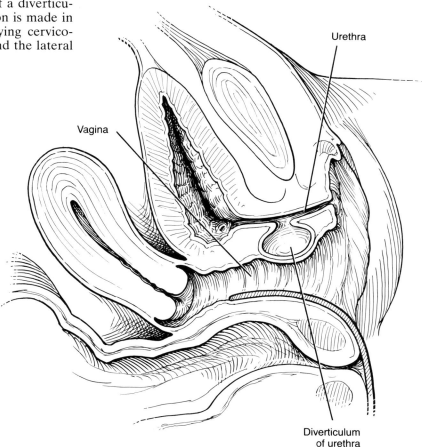

Figure 383

vaginal wall flaps are mobilized laterally to the descending pubic rami (Fig. 385A). A similar incision is made in the fascia, which is mobilized laterally to expose the underlying diverticulum (Fig. 385B). The dissection must be sharp, accurate, and meticulously accomplished. The preoperative placement (coiling) of a ureteral catheter within the diverticulum to distend its wall, if this can be accomplished, may enhance the identification and dissection of the diverticulum.

Not infrequently, the diverticulum is in immediate apposition to or even perforating the cervicopubic fascia, and it can be easily identified (and perhaps even inadvertently entered) during dissection. Depending on the size of the diverticulum, it may have loculations containing various amounts of urine, purulent material, necrotic debris, and even small stones; such loculations or septa should be incised.

If the diverticulum is entered, the surgeon may insert the index finger within the diverticulum and place a broad Allis forceps on its rim with gentle traction, which aids in dissection with scissors to ensure total

excision (Fig. 386). Occasionally, the sac of the diverticulum extends laterally and upward around the urethra. Rarely, it may extend into the retropubic space, where the urethral orifice enters the roof of the urethra. In this instance, the dissection is continued as far superiorly as possible, at which point the neck of the diverticulum is simply transected and permitted to retract; no attempt is made to close the defect. In some patients, the diverticulum is saddle-shaped, extending around the entire urethra or bladder neck; in these cases, extensive dissection of the lower trigone or major portion of the urethral floor is required.

The urethra is reconstructed in a linear direction over a no. 12 Foley Silastic catheter with interrupted 4-0 delayed absorbable sutures placed in an extramucosal position (Fig. 387A). Occasionally, the opening in the urethra is more appropriately closed (to prevent tension on the suture line) in a transverse direction. The suture is inserted through the muscular coat of the urethra but does not penetrate or enter the urethral lumen (Fig. 387B).

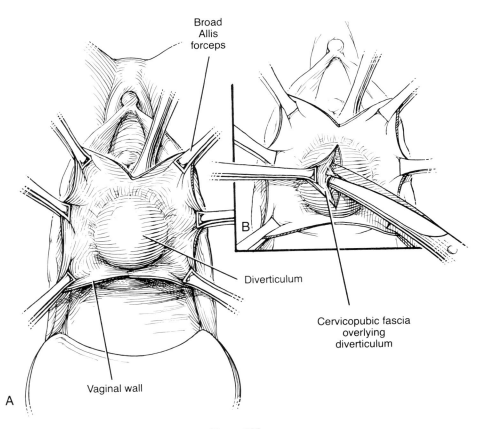

Broad
Allis
forceps

Diverticulum

Cervicopubic fascia
overlying
diverticulum

Vaginal wall

A

B

C

Figure 385

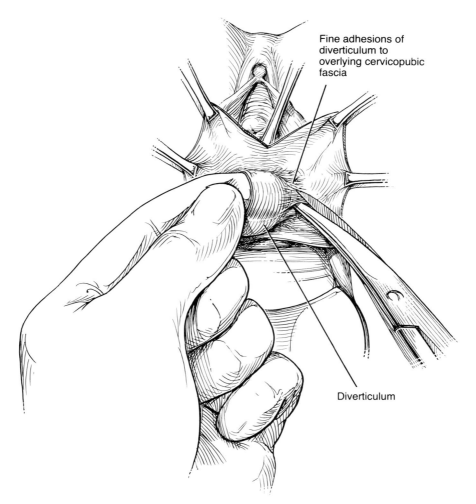

Fine adhesions of
diverticulum to
overlying cervicopubic
fascia

Diverticulum

Figure 386

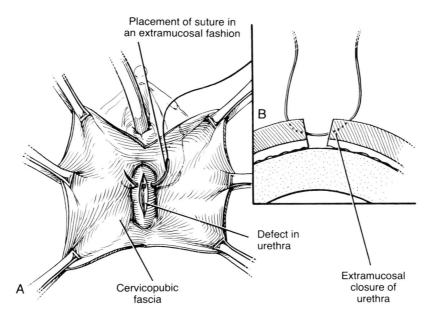

Placement of suture in
an extramucosal fashion

B

Defect in
urethra

Extramucosal
closure of
urethra

A

Cervicopubic
fascia

Figure 387

After the urethral defect is repaired, the cervicopubic fascia is imbricated in a side-to-side ("vest-over-pants") fashion with interrupted 3-0 delayed absorbable sutures (Fig. 388). By providing two additional supporting layers and avoiding superimposed suture lines, this method appears to diminish the possibility of fistula formation. In addition, it provides good support for the proximal urethra and the bladder neck. Complete hemostasis must be ensured as each layer is closed. This can be accomplished with fine interrupted sutures and judicious electrocoagulation. The vaginal wall is closed with 3-0 delayed absorbable suture material (Fig. 389). A urethral catheter is left in place for 4 to 7 days postoperatively. In some cases, the complexity of the repair may require that the catheter be retained longer or that a suprapubic catheter be used by itself or in combination with a urethral catheter.

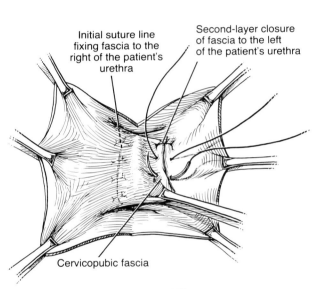

Initial suture line fixing fascia to the right of the patient's urethra

Second-layer closure of fascia to the left of the patient's urethra

Cervicopubic fascia

Figure 388

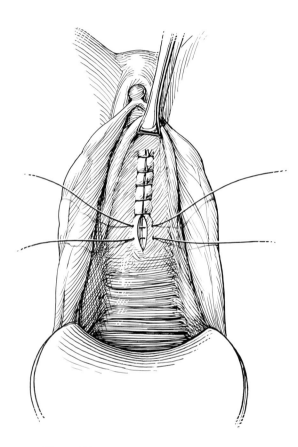

Figure 389
Partially closed suture line of vaginal mucosa.

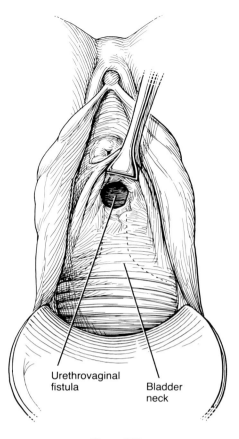

Urethrovaginal
fistula   Bladder
neck

Figure 390

Urethrovaginal Fistula

Depending on its location, a simple urethrovaginal fistula may not cause symptoms and may not require surgical repair. However, most urethrovaginal fistulas are associated with some leakage, and operative repair is required. The reconstruction is relatively simple, and yet success depends on meticulous attention to details during each phase of the operation. In Figure 390, the broken line indicates the junction of the urethra and the bladder neck, and the urethrovaginal fistula is located at the junction of the lower and middle thirds of the urethra. A vertical incision is made in the anterior vaginal wall, extending up and around the margins of the urethral defect (Fig. 391A). The vaginal mucosa is separated from the underlying cervicopubic fascia laterally to the descending pubic ramus (Fig. 391B). Infrequently, mo-

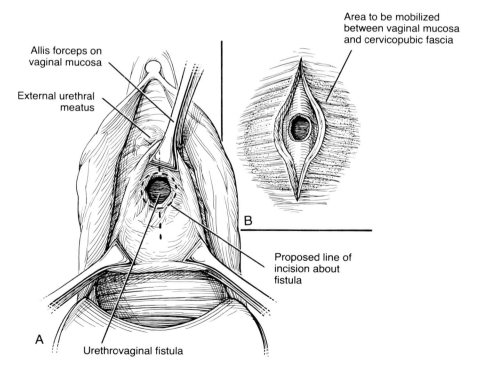

Allis forceps on
vaginal mucosa

External urethral
meatus

Area to be mobilized
between vaginal mucosa
and cervicopubic fascia

B

Proposed line of
incision about
fistula

A

Urethrovaginal fistula

Figure 391

bilization is continued laterally into the retropubic space as well as posteriorly in order to free completely the entire trigone and lower segments of the base of the bladder and proximal portions of the urethra. Sufficient mobilization is required to provide a tension-free closure of the reconstructed urethra. The edges of the wall of the urethra are accurately approximated with interrupted fine (4-0) delayed absorbable sutures placed in an extramucosal position (Fig. 392A). The initial suture line is inverted with a second suture line that incorporates the adjacent cervicopubic fascia and picks up a portion of the underlying tissue to obliterate dead space and aid in complete hemostasis (Fig. 392B). The vaginal suture line is approximated with interrupted 4-0 delayed absorbable sutures (Fig. 393).

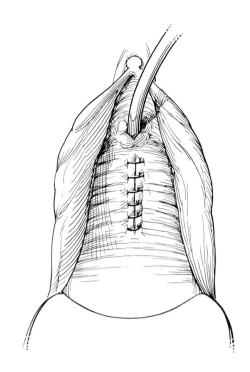

Figure 393
Enclosed vaginal suture line with Foley catheter in place.

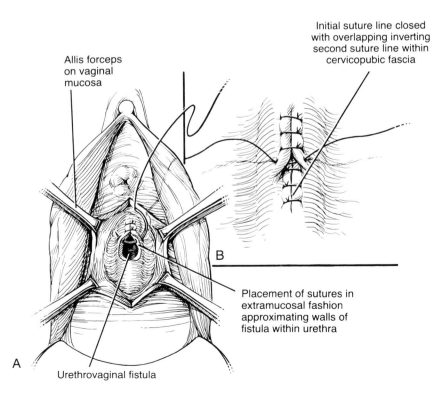

Allis forceps on vaginal mucosa

Initial suture line closed with overlapping inverting second suture line within cervicopubic fascia

B

Placement of sutures in extramucosal fashion approximating walls of fistula within urethra

A

Urethrovaginal fistula

Figure 392

Linear Loss of the Floor of the Urethra

In patients who have a linear urethrovaginal fistula (loss of a major portion of the urethra; in the procedure illustrated here, the distal two thirds of the floor of the urethra is lost), urethral reconstruction may be more difficult, and urinary continence, even in what appears to be a well-constructed urethral tube, may not be predictable. The basic principles of the repair are the same as those for "simple" urethrovaginal fistula. An incision is made in the anterior vaginal mucosa adjacent to the margin of the defect, with wide mobilization of the vaginal wall laterally to or past the descending pubic ramus (Fig. 394). The anatomic defect may appear to be rather extensive;

however, the actual loss of urethral tissue and muscle may be minimal. The injury results in retraction of the uninvolved musculature into the urethral roof, which is usually intact in affected patients. The retraction of the urethral musculature may be comparable to a similar type of retraction that occurs in the perineal muscles and anal sphincter with unrepaired fourth-degree tears. After the vaginal mucosa is mobilized laterally, a small portion of the roof of the remaining urethra is mobilized in preparation for reconstruction of a new urethral tube (Fig. 395). The remaining urethral roof should provide the patient with a contractile (albeit narrow) urethra; the reconstructed tube is of necessity of small caliber. This size offers some advantage and may result in urinary control.

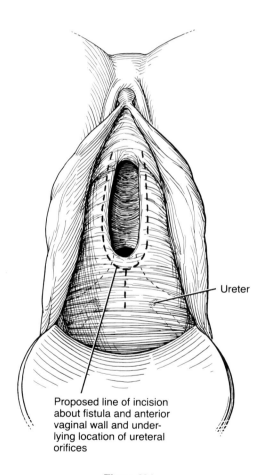

Ureter

Proposed line of incision about fistula and anterior vaginal wall and underlying location of ureteral orifices

Figure 394

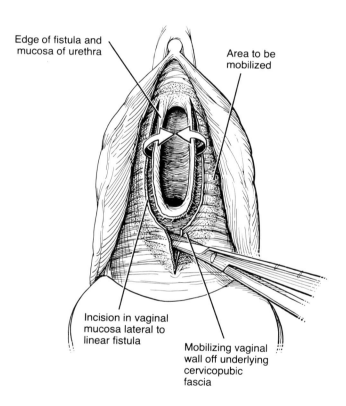

Edge of fistula and mucosa of urethra

Area to be mobilized

Incision in vaginal mucosa lateral to linear fistula

Mobilizing vaginal wall off underlying cervicopubic fascia

Figure 395

Usually, a no. 8 or no. 10 urethral catheter is placed in the bed of the roof of the urethra; this permits accurate approximation of the freed edges of the roof of the urethra in reconstruction of the tube (Fig. 396*A*). The sutures are placed in an interrupted fashion with 4-0 delayed absorbable suture positioned extramucosally. This initial suture line reconstructing the urethra is inverted with a second layer approximating the periurethral tissues to aid in support of the initial suture line (Fig. 396*B*). The third layer of sutures is placed in the cervicopubic fascia to plicate the urethra and bladder neck area further (Fig. 396*C*). Figure 397*A* shows the third layer tied and closure of the vaginal wall, which in this case was approximated free of tension (Fig. 397*B*).

In patients who have a slough of the entire floor of the urethra and including the bladder neck and the base of the bladder, reconstruction of a continent urethra may be more difficult. The surgical repair is initiated with a vertical incision in the anterior vaginal wall extending close to either edge of the defect, after which the vaginal mucosa is separated from the underlying cervicopubic fascia far laterally to provide for the possibility of reconstruction of a tension-free urethral tube (Fig. 398).

What later will be the second row of sutures is initially placed under direct vision to permit large, more secure portions of the supporting tissue to be obtained without fear of entering the urethra. The insertion of a finger into the open bladder neck ensures accurate identification and location of the ureters during the snug plication of the bladder neck (Fig. 399). Once these sutures are placed in the supporting tissues, they are tagged laterally.

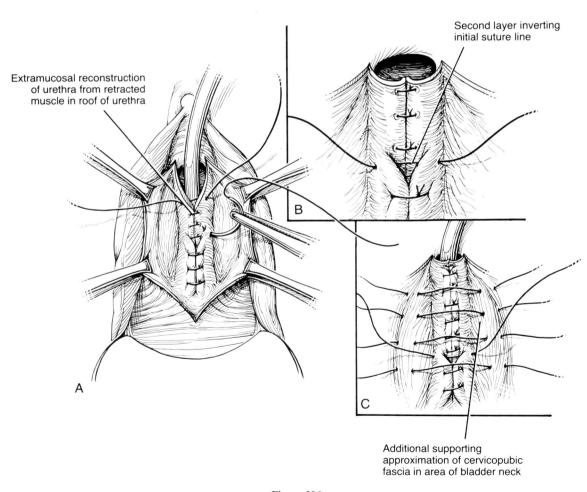

Extramucosal reconstruction of urethra from retracted muscle in roof of urethra

Second layer inverting initial suture line

Additional supporting approximation of cervicopubic fascia in area of bladder neck

Figure 396

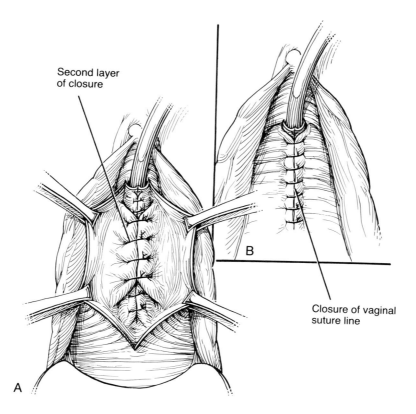

Second layer
of closure

Closure of vaginal
suture line

A

B

Figure 397

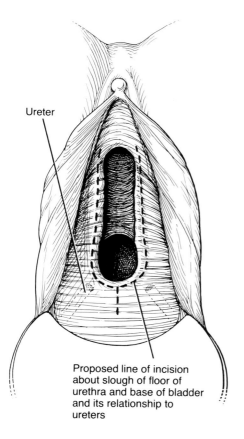

Ureter

Proposed line of incision
about slough of floor of
urethra and base of bladder
and its relationship to
ureters

Figure 398

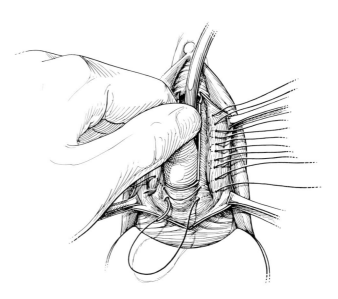

Figure 399

Finger in bladder to aid in placement of deep suture line of bladder
neck (second layer).

The urethral tube is reconstructed in the manner already described, and care is taken to approximate the edges of the urethral mucosa accurately without entering the future urethral lumen. These sutures are then tied with 4-0 delayed absorbable suture, following which the previously placed sutures (including those at the bladder neck and the base of the bladder) are tied to result in a second layer of closure of the urethra (Fig. 400). If further supporting sutures of the cervicopubic fascia can be placed, this step is also accomplished at this time (Fig. 401).

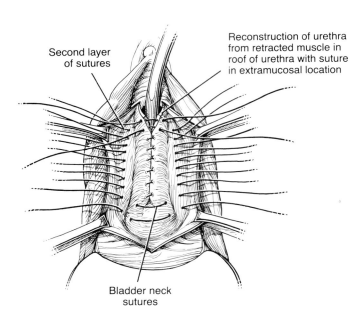

Figure 400

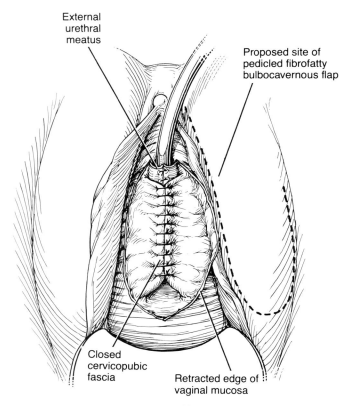

Figure 401

Usually, patients with linear loss of the urethral floor have loss of a significant portion of the anterior vaginal wall, and thus approximation of the wall of the vagina cannot be accomplished without undue tension (Fig. 401). In these cases, the size of the defect is accurately evaluated, and an appropriate tongue of tissue from the labium majus is identified to be incised and swung into the vagina to replace the anterior vaginal wall. This fibrofatty, bulbocavernous flap is usually hinged anteriorly, but depending on the nature of the defect, it may be hinged posteriorly. The flap is developed, and the small venous bleeders in the subcutaneous tissues are suture-ligated or cauterized as necessary. The most distal portion of the flap (that deepest into the vagina) is secured initially with full-thickness interrupted 3-0 delayed absorbable sutures (Fig. 402). Care is taken to suture the labial flap to the edge of the vagina in an accurate way to promote primary healing. At the point at which the flap approximates the urethral meatus, it has a tendency to "hide" the meatus and may need to be tailored accordingly.

The site of the graft is closed with an initial layer of subcutaneous sutures, which permits closure of the skin edges of the labium with 4-0 delayed absorbable suture in a tension-free fashion (Fig. 403). A small suction catheter has been placed under the labial graft, between the graft and the reconstructed urethra. This is brought out through a stab wound laterally and usually is removed in 3 to 4 days. Despite adequate vesical neck plication and satisfactory elevation and support of the reconstructed urethra, what appears to be an anatomically sound urethra may not provide satisfactory urinary control. In approximately 50% of patients, a delayed second-stage modified Marshall-Marchetti-Krantz type of bladder neck elevation may be required for urinary control.

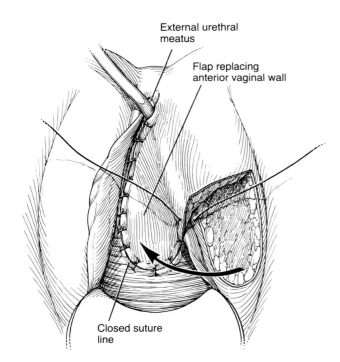

External urethral meatus

Flap replacing anterior vaginal wall

Closed suture line

Figure 402

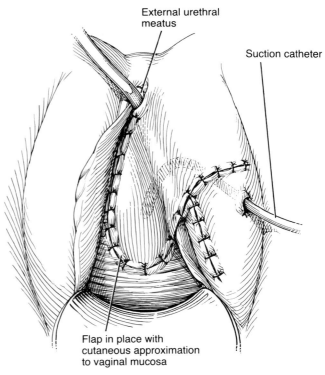

External urethral meatus

Suction catheter

Flap in place with cutaneous approximation to vaginal mucosa

Figure 403

Vesicovaginal Fistula

Vaginal Repair

A vesicovaginal fistula with its constant odorous, scalding, unimpeded leakage of urine is one of the most devastating surgical complications that occur in women. Surgical treatment of benign conditions causes approximately 90% of vesicovaginal fistulas in our experience; "simple" total abdominal hysterectomy is the causative procedure in 70% of these patients. The point at which the fistula first becomes symptomatic is determined to a major degree by its cause, site of origin, and method of catheter drainage. Immediate leakage after operation probably represents an unrecognized perforation or laceration of the urinary tract. In most patients, leakage of urine is noted between the second and the tenth postoperative days; undoubtedly, this is a result of various degrees of trauma and precarious placement of clamps or sutures, followed by devascularization, necrosis, and invariably delayed development of a fistula. In addition, complications such as infection and hematoma formation, resulting from compression with additional devascularization and necrosis, may lead to delayed fistula formation.

The usual fistula resulting from an operation is located on the posterior wall of the bladder (Fig. 404), above the interureteric ridge just in front of or involving the scar of the closure of the vaginal vault (Fig. 405).

With a weighted speculum holding down the posterior vaginal wall, the vaginal mucosa in the region of the fistula is exposed and the mucosa is incised, usually in a transverse fashion (Fig. 406A). Sufficient vaginal mucosa is separated from the underlying cervicopubic fascia to permit later tension-free closure of the tissues. Traction is applied to the scar tissue encircling the fistula, and countertraction is placed on the edges of the vaginal mucosa to facilitate accurate undermining of the vaginal wall, as denoted by the fine stippled area on Figure 406A.

Figure 406B shows the scar tissue immediately about the fistulous tract still attached to the underlying bladder, with the mobilized vaginal mucosa separated from the underlying cervicopubic fascia. Traction is

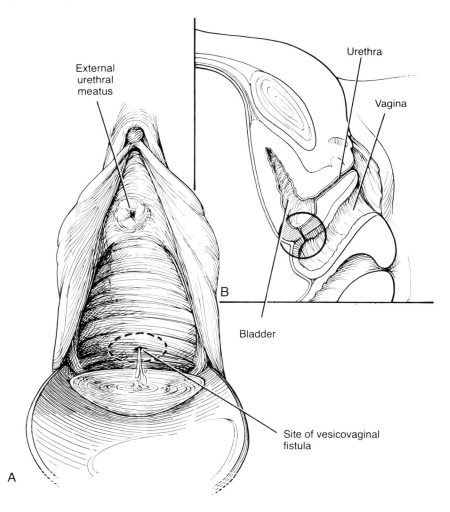

External urethral meatus

Urethra

Vagina

B

Bladder

Site of vesicovaginal fistula

A

Figure 404

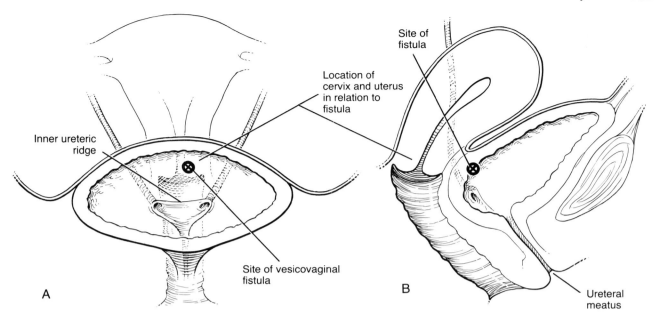

Inner ureteric
ridge

Location of
cervix and uterus
in relation to
fistula

Site of
fistula

Site of vesicovaginal
fistula

Ureteral
meatus

A

B

Figure 405

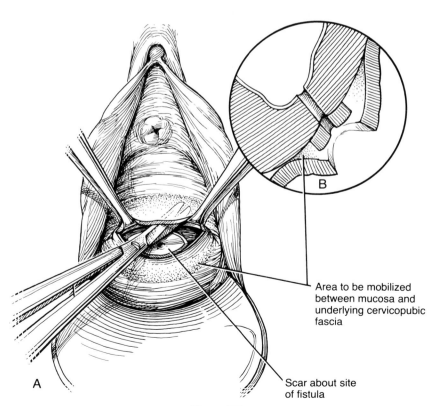

Area to be mobilized
between mucosa and
underlying cervicopubic
fascia

Scar about site
of fistula

A

B

Figure 406

applied to this scar tissue encircling the fistula, and with sharp dissection, the fistulous tract (full thickness) is excised (Fig. 407A). A relatively small, scarred fistulous opening is thus converted into a fresh injury (albeit a larger fistula) with healthy tissue and healthy blood supply (Fig. 407B).

With excellent exposure provided with Deaver retractors, the initial suture line consisting of 4-0 delayed absorbable sutures is placed in an extramucosal fashion extending lateral to the fistulous opening (Fig. 408A). All sutures are placed, after which they are tied in the order of their placement, resulting in an accurate approximation of the edges of the bladder

mucosa. Figure 408B shows the tied suture with accurate edge-to-edge placement of the mucosa of the bladder; the suture within the wall of the bladder is in an extramucosal position.

The initial suture line is then inverted with a second suture line of similar suture placed in a similar fashion (Fig. 409A); this further supports the initial suture line and provides excellent hemostasis. Figure 409B shows inversion of the initial suture line with a second layer placed in the muscularis of the bladder. Each suture line inverting its previous suture line is placed approximately 3 to 4 mm lateral to the initially closed suture line.

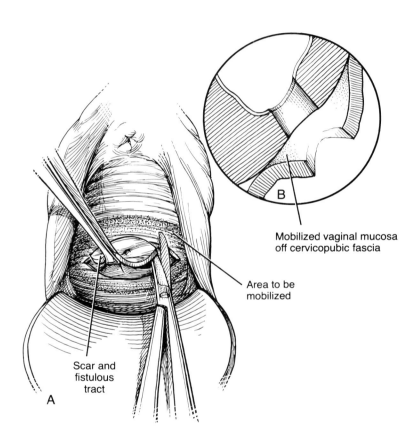

Mobilized vaginal mucosa off cervicopubic fascia

Area to be mobilized

Scar and fistulous tract

A

Figure 407

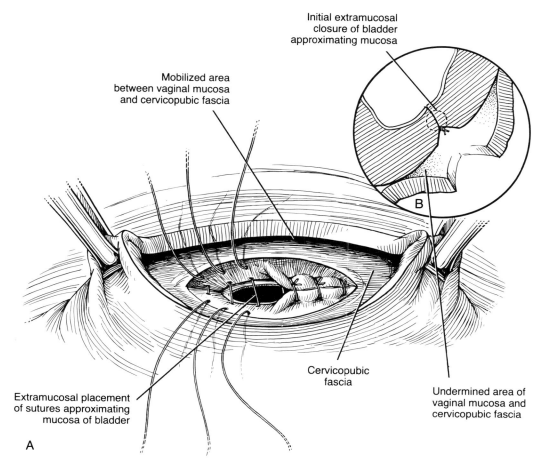

Initial extramucosal
closure of bladder
approximating mucosa

Mobilized area
between vaginal mucosa
and cervicopubic fascia

B

Extramucosal placement
of sutures approximating
mucosa of bladder

Cervicopubic
fascia

Undermined area of
vaginal mucosa and
cervicopubic fascia

A

Figure 408

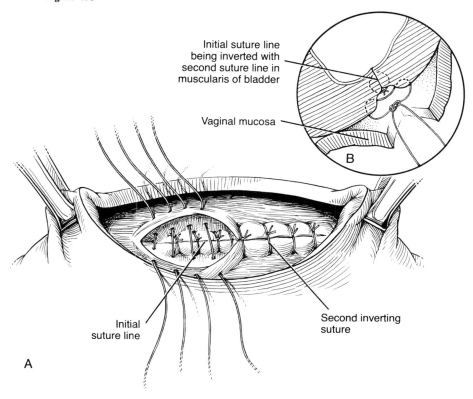

Initial suture line
being inverted with
second suture line in
muscularis of bladder

Vaginal mucosa

B

Initial
suture line

Second inverting
suture

A

Figure 409

Occasionally, the peritoneum can be pulled from the posterior surface of the bladder through the cul-de-sac overlying the previously placed two layers within the bladder; this acts as an additional layer of closure for the fistulous opening (Fig. 410). The vagina is then closed, usually in a transverse fashion; this closure further imbricates the previously closed suture lines (Fig. 411).

Figure 412 shows the approximate position of the fistula high on the posterior vaginal wall above the interureteric ridge, with two or three layers of suture within the wall of the bladder, each inverting the prior layer with peritoneum pulled down over the fistulous opening, and with a separate closure of the vagina.

In the nonirradiated patient with a postoperative vesicovaginal fistula, our experience indicates that the tissue has a good blood supply, minimal edema and infection, little evidence of previous suture material, and readily identifiable cleavage planes for the dissection at about 8 to 10 weeks after the formation of a fistula (or a previous failed repair). This condition permits wide mobilization and adequate dissection to allow accurate approximation of the tissues without tension on the suture lines. Nevertheless, we are certain that some fistulas may be successfully managed by early operation (e.g., obstetric lacerations and some of the fistulas diagnosed a few hours after operation).

From the patient's standpoint, the vaginal approach is easier, safer, and more comfortable. The size and number of fistulas or previous operative repair does not necessarily preclude the vaginal approach. Regardless of the approach chosen, the basic fundamentals of successful repair remain the same: wide mo-

bilization of the tissues surrounding the fistulous tract with excision of the scarred epithelialized fistulous tract, a layered closure using extramucosal delayed absorbable sutures free of tension, and a second and a third inverting suture line within the wall of the bladder with a layered closure of the vaginal wall that is free of tension and provides excellent hemostasis. Careful attention should be given to obliteration of dead space and minimization of potential infection. When possible, the peritoneum from the back and dome of the bladder is sutured between the bladder and vaginal suture lines.

Successful fistula repair of the bladder requires sound surgical judgment during the operation and postoperative period; any tension or manipulation of the suture line must be avoided. Adequate bladder drainage with a large-caliber catheter urethrally or suprapubically, or both, is mandatory. Overdistention of the bladder because of obstruction, blood, or mucus can be prevented by hourly charting of the urine output and appropriate use of irrigation. Some surgeons have recommended early removal of the urethral catheter for treatment of simple vesicovaginal fistula. Although this may be acceptable for some patients, we are unable to predict with certainty for which patients this would be appropriate. As a result, we customarily provide catheter drainage for at least 7 days, and in selected patients, for a few weeks.

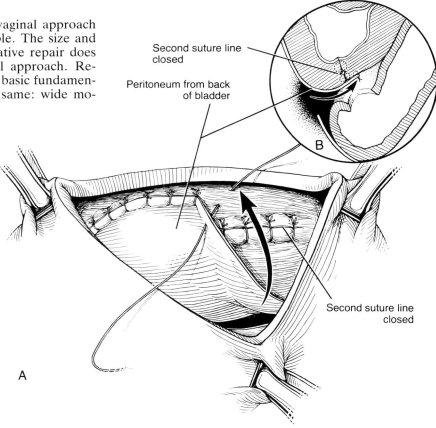

Second suture line closed

Peritoneum from back of bladder

B

Second suture line closed

A

Figure 410

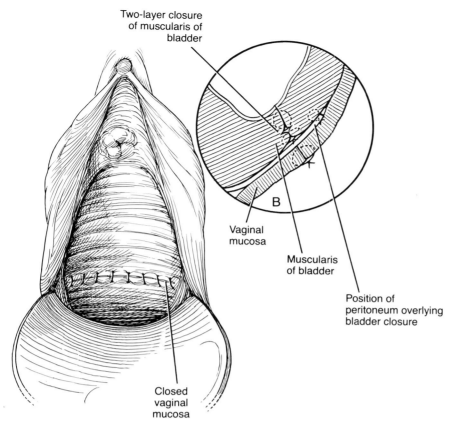

Two-layer closure
of muscularis of
bladder

B

Vaginal
mucosa

Muscularis
of bladder

Position of
peritoneum overlying
bladder closure

Closed
vaginal
mucosa

Figure 411

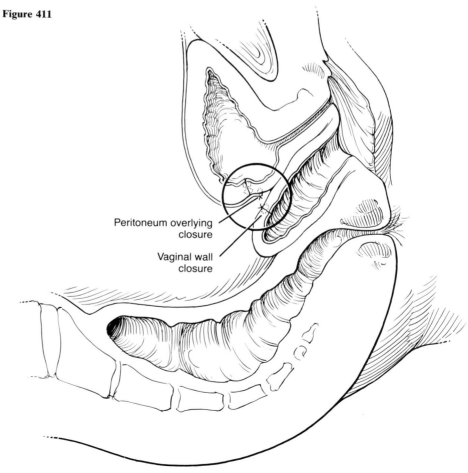

Peritoneum overlying
closure

Vaginal wall
closure

Figure 412

Abdominal Repair

Although most repairs are done vaginally (more than 80%), specific indications for an abdominal repair are the presence of a large vesicovaginal fistula in proximity to the ureter and difficulty obtaining adequate exposure with the vaginal route, even with the use of the Schuchardt incision. When an abdominal approach is chosen (because of the proximity of the ureter or adherent segment of bowel), we prefer the transperitoneal approach, which permits mobilization of the base of the bladder and ureter (usually with an indwelling ureteral catheter) such that an accurate and safe repair can be accomplished under excellent visibility.

Through a lower midline incision (and in this case with a ureteral stent placed through the cystotomy incision), the back wall of the bladder is separated from the front wall of the vagina (Fig. 413A). A pack placed in the vagina preoperatively results in vaginal distention and facilitates countertraction, which assists dissection. Traction exerted by the surgeon's fingers in the bladder and countertraction on the vagina facilitate sharp, accurate separation of these two surfaces (Fig. 413B). The posterior wall of the

bladder is elevated, and the rim of the fistulous tract in the bladder to the vagina is excised. In the procedure shown, the opening in the vaginal wall is being closed in a transverse extramucosal fashion with running 3-0 delayed absorbable suture. Figure 414A shows the initial extramucosal closure of the vaginal portion of the fistula. It is being inverted with a second running suture of similar material (Fig. 414B); this incision commences and extends 0.5 cm beyond the original fistulous opening. Occasionally, the defect lends itself more appropriately to a vertical closure; the basic principles—approximation in an extramucosal fashion that is free of tension, excellent hemostasis, and inversion by each suture line of the previously closed suture line—are applied.

Figure 415, a view through the cystotomy, shows the interior of the initial suture line, which is closed in an extramucosal fashion that approximates the edges of the fresh mucosal injury with no sutures within the interior of the bladder. This subcuticular-like closure permits approximation of the edges of the mucosa, direct visualization of the ureteral orifices, and palpation of the intramural portion of the ureter to ensure that it is not included in the suture line. As seen from the posterior wall of the bladder, the initial

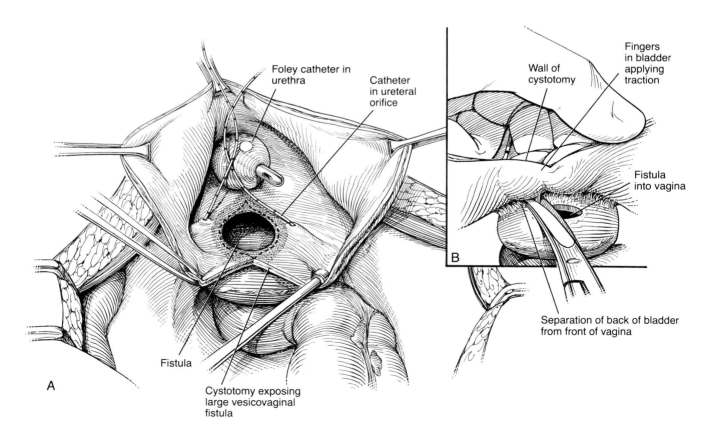

Figure 413

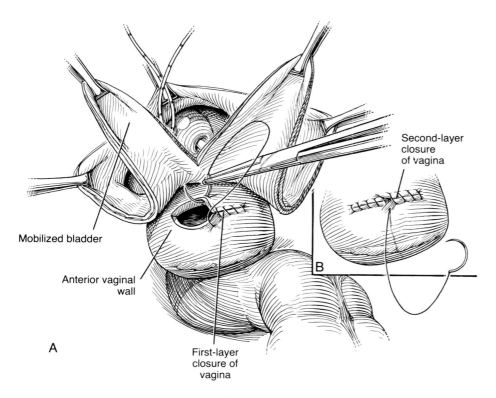

Mobilized bladder

Anterior vaginal wall

Second-layer closure of vagina

First-layer closure of vagina

A

B

Figure 414

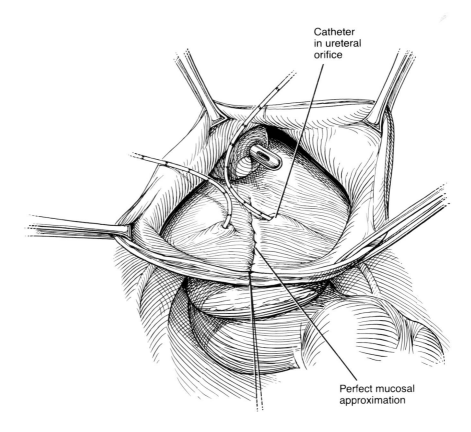

Catheter in ureteral orifice

Perfect mucosal approximation

Figure 415

layer of the approximated mucosa and submucosa of the bladder is closed with a second running layer (3-0 delayed absorbable) suture, begun 1 cm distal to the original suture line and inverting the suture line; again, care is taken so that the intramural portion of the ureter is not included in this suture line (Fig. 416).

Figure 417 is a lateral view showing the two-layer closure of the anterior wall of the vagina with a similar closure of the posterior wall of the bladder. In this case, the peritoneum from the back of the bladder was pulled down over the two suture lines of the posterior wall of the bladder; this suture line was thus separated from the suture line closing the vagina.

In more complex fistulas, it occasionally may be advantageous to mobilize the omentum from the left side of the transverse colon and to fix the omentum into the posterior cul-de-sac (Fig. 418A). It is sutured to the anterior wall of the vagina or the posterior wall of the bladder to thus give additional blood supply and a tissue barrier between the suture lines (Fig. 418B). Catheter drainage may be accomplished with a urethral or suprapubic approach (or both), depending on the circumstances of the repair.

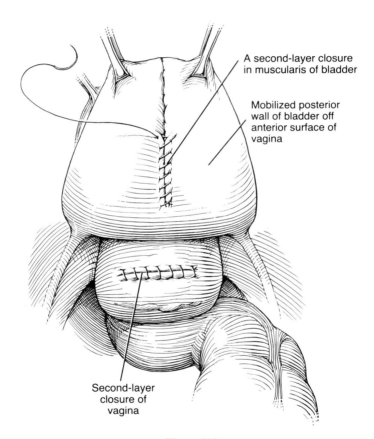

A second-layer closure in muscularis of bladder

Mobilized posterior wall of bladder off anterior surface of vagina

Second-layer closure of vagina

Figure 416

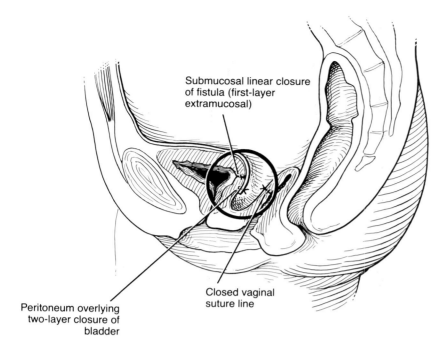

Submucosal linear closure
of fistula (first-layer
extramucosal)

Closed vaginal
suture line

Peritoneum overlying
two-layer closure of
bladder

Figure 417

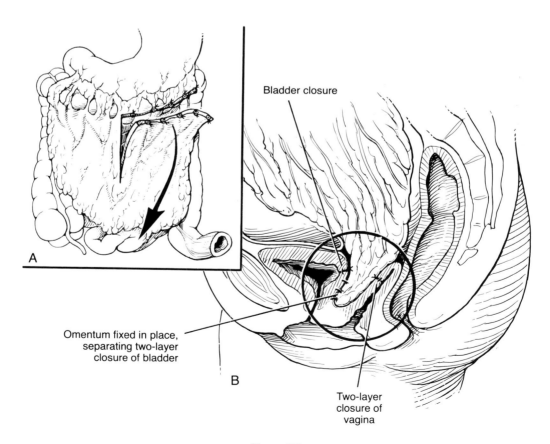

Bladder closure

A

Omentum fixed in place,
separating two-layer
closure of bladder

B

Two-layer
closure of
vagina

Figure 418

Vesicouterine Cervicovaginal Fistula

Patients with vesicouterine fistula may have cyclic hematuria with or without incontinence or repeated urinary tract infection. Most patients have continuous leakage of urine, which on examination is seen to arise from the cervix into the vagina (Fig. 419A).

Most vesicouterine fistulas are sequelae of difficult obstetric or gynecologic problems. In recent years, the most common sequence has been marked adhesions of the bladder occurring after repeated cesarean sections that require tedious dissection, occasionally resulting in unrecognized tear of the bladder wall. Extravasation of urine, superimposed infection, and subsequent dehiscence of the uterine incision constitute the most likely sequence of events in formation of the fistula. Operative repair can usually be accomplished vaginally. However, in selected patients, an abdominal approach may be required.

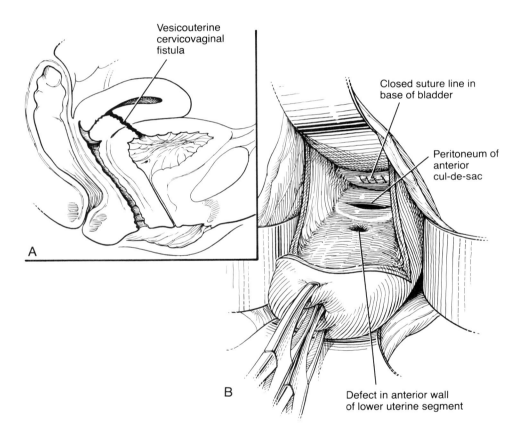

Figure 419

Our usual approach has been to proceed vaginally, separating the bladder from the anterior surface of the uterus, much as is done for vaginal hysterectomy. The bladder is mobilized superiorly and laterally to permit excision of the fistulous tract, generally cephalad to the interureteric ridge on the posterior wall of the bladder. The fistula is closed with two separate layers of 3-0 delayed absorbable suture in the manner already described for vesicovaginal fistula (Fig.

419*B*). The peritoneum from the back of the bladder is pulled over the suture line in the bladder and fixed in place with interrupted 3-0 delayed absorbable sutures (Fig. 420). The opening in the wall of the uterus is freshened, and the wall of the uterus is closed with a single layer of similar suture. The space is irrigated, excellent hemostasis is obtained, and the vagina is resutured to the anterior surface of the cervix and lower uterine segment.

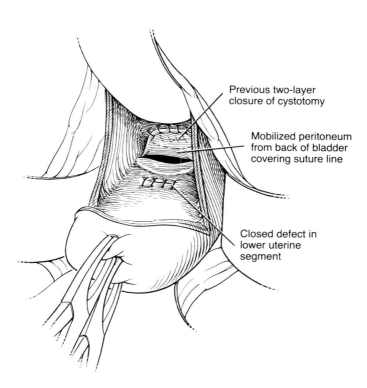

Previous two-layer closure of cystotomy

Mobilized peritoneum from back of bladder covering suture line

Closed defect in lower uterine segment

Figure 420

Modified Marshall-Marchetti-Krantz Operation

Various surgical procedures—vaginal plications, suprapubic suspensions, slings, and combinations or variations of these procedures—are advocated for the management of primary and recurrent urinary stress incontinence. No single procedure is universally effective, but each has advantages for selected patients.

To control urinary stress incontinence successfully, any procedure must narrow the patulous bladder neck by tightening the musculofascial planes through which the urethra passes. The procedure results in a high retropubic position of the bladder neck, which pre-

vents rotational descent of the proximal urethra (Fig. 421). The permanence of the operation is determined by the quality of the tissues used for urethrovesical support, by the quality of the smooth muscle comprising the urethra and bladder neck, and by the surgeon's ability and experience.

In patients who undergo the modified Marshall-Marchetti-Krantz procedure, a small midline incision is made from the symphysis pubis superiorly for approximately 10 cm (Fig. 422A) (a similar exposure could be obtained through a transverse incision in the properly selected patient). A curved forceps is used for blunt mobilization of the loose areolar tissue on either side of the midline vein (Figs. 422B and 423), which is elevated, clamped, cut, and tied.

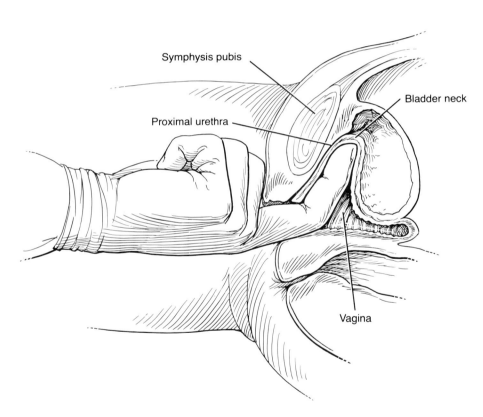

Figure 421
Preoperative positioning of bladder neck and proximal urethra.

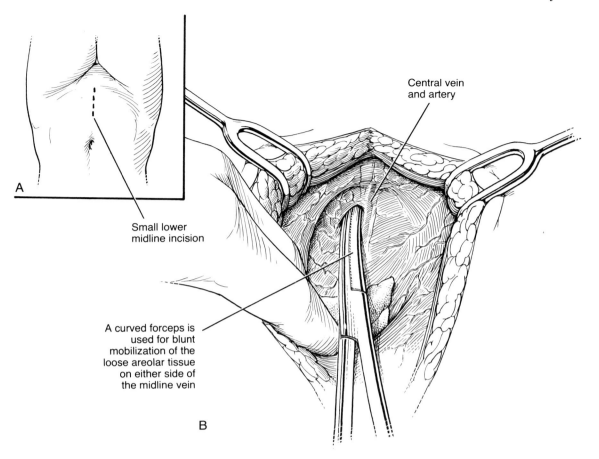

Central vein and artery

Small lower midline incision

A curved forceps is used for blunt mobilization of the loose areolar tissue on either side of the midline vein

A

B

Figure 422

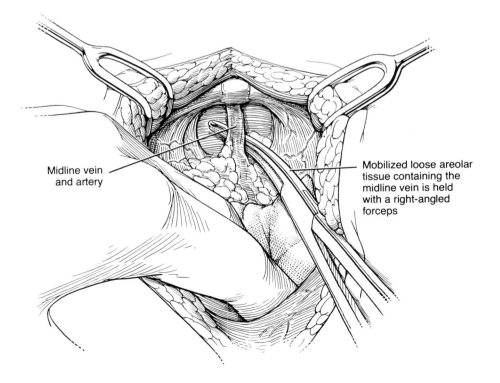

Midline vein and artery

Mobilized loose areolar tissue containing the midline vein is held with a right-angled forceps

Figure 423

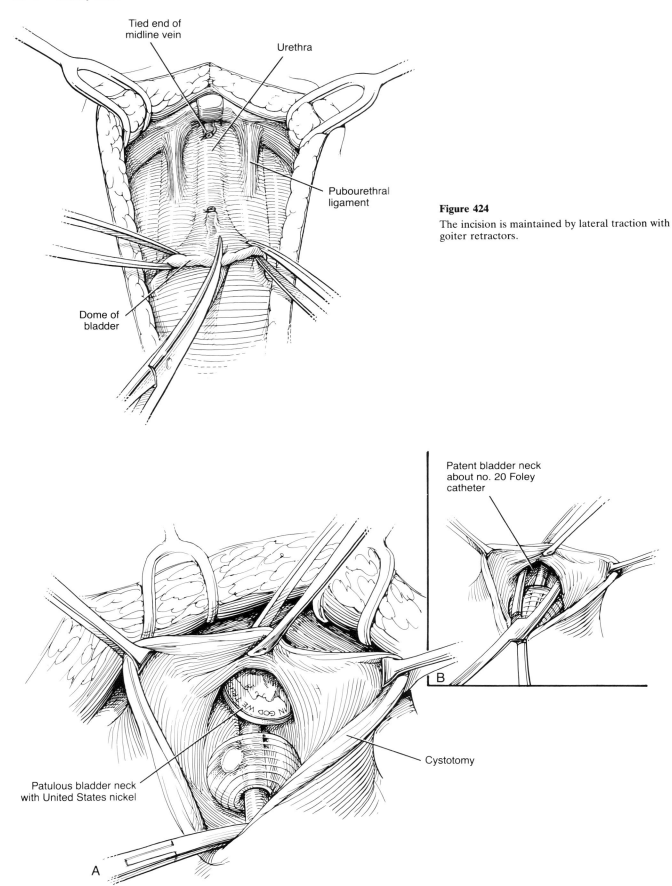

Tied end of
midline vein

Urethra

Pubourethral
ligament

Dome of
bladder

Figure 424

The incision is maintained by lateral traction with
goiter retractors.

Patent bladder neck
about no. 20 Foley
catheter

B

Cystotomy

Patulous bladder neck
with United States nickel

A

Figure 425

With removal of the loose areolar tissue, the underlying fascia and the right and left pubourethral ligaments (thick, white condensations of the fascia) can easily be identified. The dome of the bladder is elevated with Russian forceps, and a 3-cm incision is made in the midline, 2 to 3 cm superior to the bladder neck (Fig. 424).

The cystotomy allows direct inspection and palpation of the bladder neck and proximal urethra. Through the cystotomy, the patulous, funnel-shaped bladder neck is easily identified. In Figure 425A, a United States nickel placed in the bladder neck demonstrates the degree of patulence. A curved forceps can be used to define the open bladder neck (Fig. 425B). The surgeon inserts the left hand into the vagina with the index and middle fingers on either side of the catheter. The no. 22 Foley catheter may be palpated by the surgeon's right index finger to help define the lateral borders of the urethra (Fig. 426).

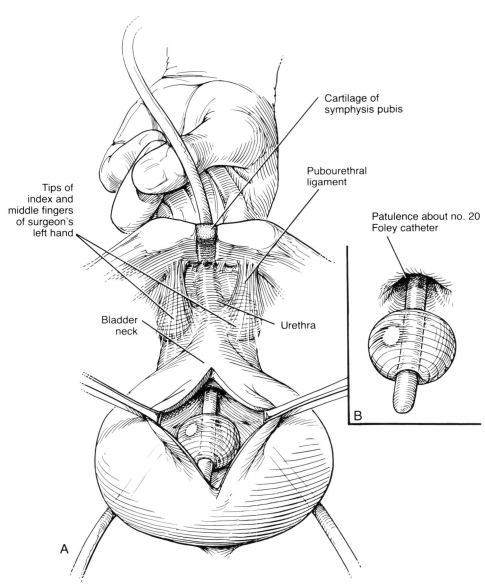

Figure 426

The Russian forceps outlines the location of the catheter within the urethra (Fig. 427). On the patient's right side, the posterior pubourethral ligament is identified, and the first suture is inserted through the posterior pubourethral ligament using a permanent 0 suture on a no. 6 Mayo needle approximately 2 to 3 mm lateral to the urethra.

The surgeon's left hand elevates the anterior vaginal wall toward the symphysis pubis to determine where the suture should be placed such that when it is tied the vaginal wall will be fixed to the back of the symphysis pubis free of tension. The suture on the no. 6 Mayo needle is placed securely and deeply into the fibrocartilage of the symphysis pubis (not the periosteum) (Fig. 428). A lighter-weight needle might break with penetration of the symphysis pubis. The suture is tagged but not tied.

The needle is placed initially just lateral to the urethra on the opposite side to come up through the posterior pubourethral ligament (Fig. 429); later, it is fixed at a location similar to that of its sister suture in the cartilage of the symphysis pubis. The surgeon's fingers elevate the anterior vaginal wall to assist in proper identification of a tension-free fixation to the back of the symphysis pubis. The first suture of the second set is placed approximately 0.5 cm distal to the bladder neck on the right side of the urethra. The second companion suture is placed at the same level on the left side of the urethra, incorporating essentially a full thickness of the anterior vaginal wall (approximately 0.5 cm distal to the bladder neck). The needle is then placed in the appropriate location in the cartilage of the symphysis pubis and tagged. With the bladder open, the surgeon can evaluate the location of the higher suture set in relation to the bladder neck.

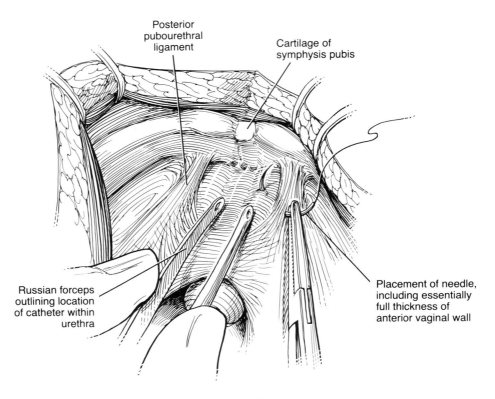

Figure 427

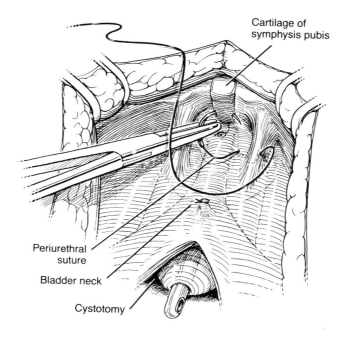

Cartilage of symphysis pubis

Periurethral suture

Bladder neck

Cystotomy

Figure 428

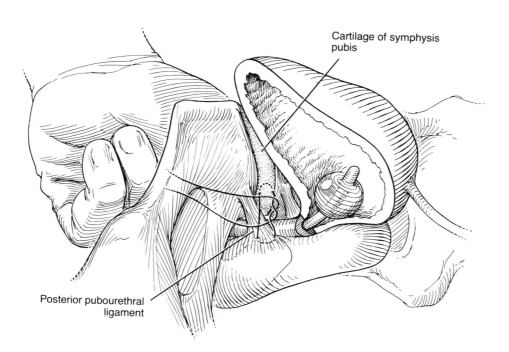

Cartilage of symphysis pubis

Posterior pubourethral ligament

Figure 429

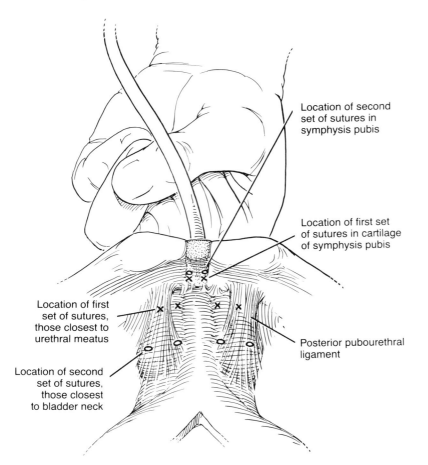

Location of second
set of sutures in
symphysis pubis

Location of first set
of sutures in cartilage
of symphysis pubis

Location of first
set of sutures,
those closest to
urethral meatus

Location of second
set of sutures,
those closest
to bladder neck

Posterior pubourethral
ligament

Figure 430
Relative position of sets of sutures on either side
of urethra.

In general, two sets of 0 permanent sutures, one on either side of the urethra firmly fixed into the cartilage of the symphysis pubis, prove sufficient. In Figure 430, the x's on either side of the urethra show the placement of the suture through the vaginal wall adjacent to the urethra, which will be fixed to the x located on the cartilage of the symphysis pubis. The o's show the location of the second set of sutures; each side corresponds to its future placement in the symphysis pubis just cephalad to the previously placed x suture. Each suture includes almost the entire thickness of the anterior vaginal wall, approximately 2 to 3 mm lateral to the urethra (Fig. 431).

Each suture is tied in the order in which it was placed; this technique restores the bladder neck to its normal patency and fixes the vagina in perfect approximation to the back of the symphysis pubis (Fig. 432). The paravaginal tissues are snugly pulled about the urethra (Fig. 433). After the second set of sutures (those closest to the bladder neck) are tied, the bladder neck assumes a high retropubic position (Fig. 434).

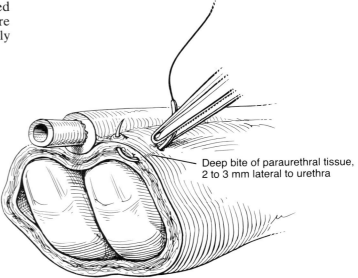

Deep bite of paraurethral tissue,
2 to 3 mm lateral to urethra

Figure 431

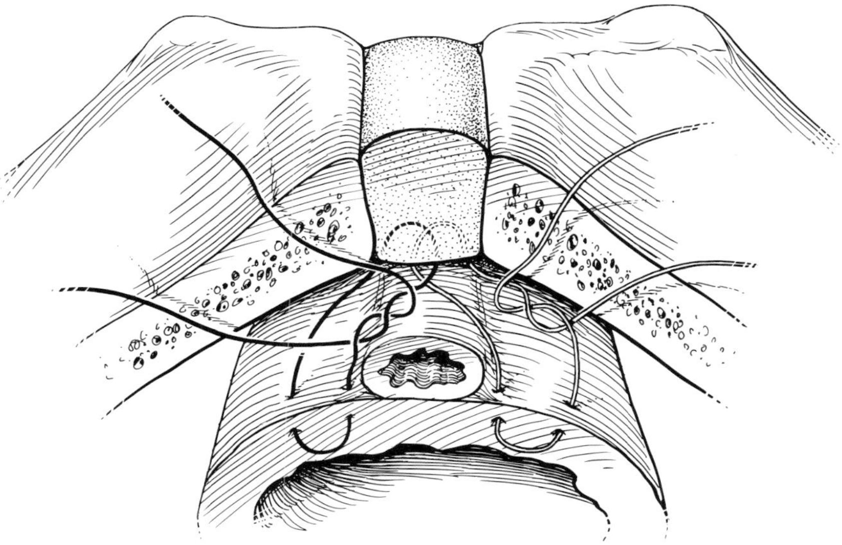

Figure 432

Suture 2 to 3 mm lateral to urethra and almost a full thickness of the vagina.

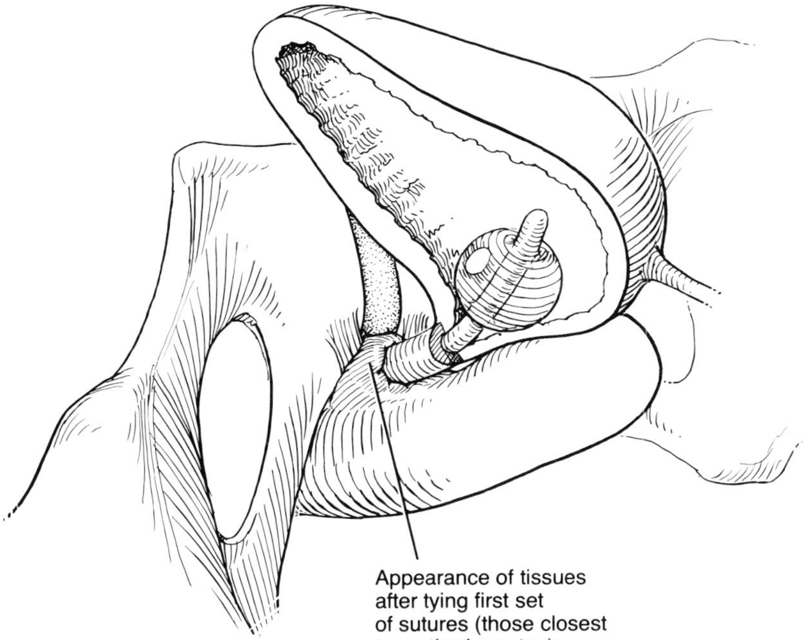

Figure 433

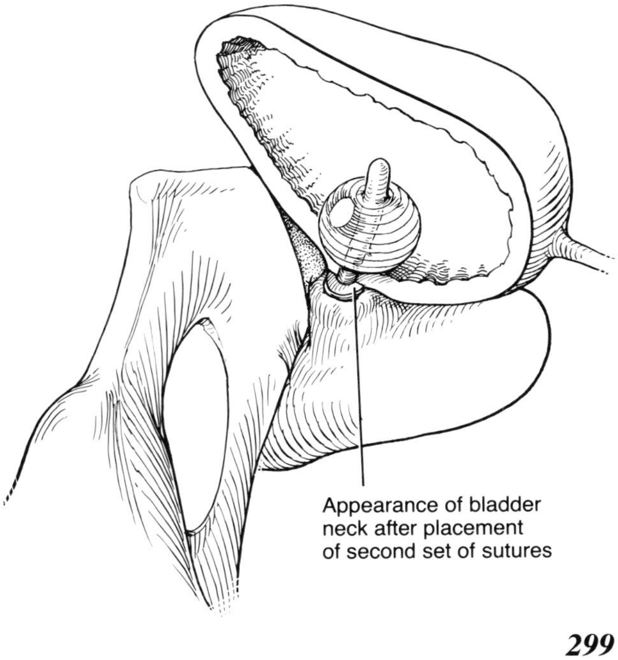

Appearance of tissues after tying first set of sutures (those closest to urethral meatus)

Figure 434

Appearance of bladder neck after placement of second set of sutures

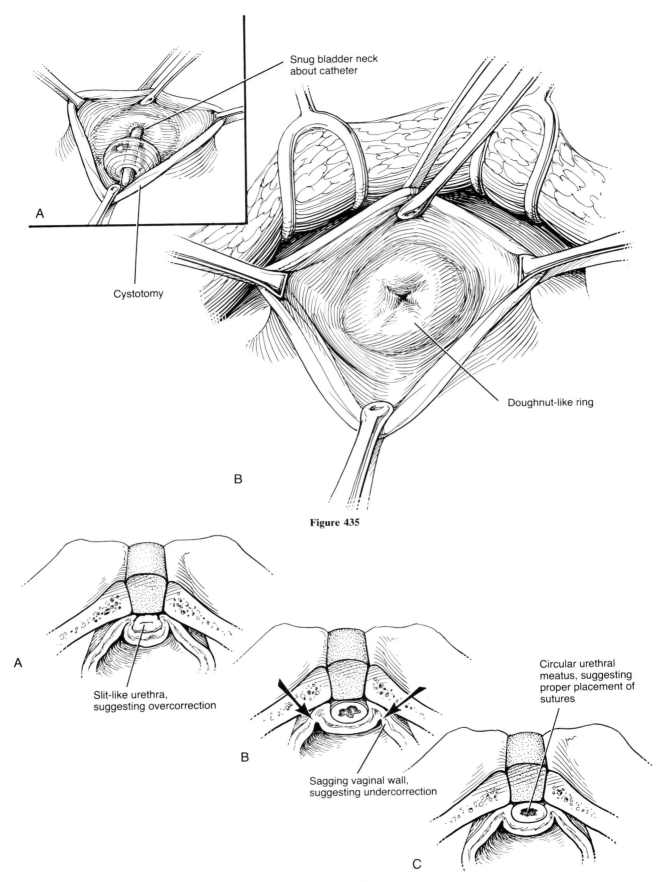

A

Snug bladder neck
about catheter

Cystotomy

Doughnut-like ring

B

Figure 435

A

Slit-like urethra,
suggesting overcorrection

B

Sagging vaginal wall,
suggesting undercorrection

Circular urethral
meatus, suggesting
proper placement of
sutures

C

Figure 436

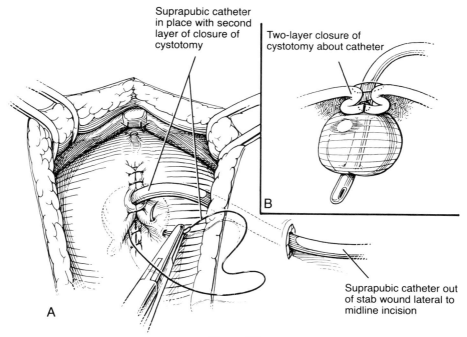

Suprapubic catheter in place with second layer of closure of cystotomy

Two-layer closure of cystotomy about catheter

B

Suprapubic catheter out of stab wound lateral to midline incision

A

Figure 437

With a no. 20 Foley catheter in place, a sphincter or washer-like ring can be noted about the catheter (Fig. 435*A*). When the balloon is punctured and the Foley catheter is removed, the doughnut-like ring of peri-urethral supporting tissues about the bladder neck can be seen (Fig. 435*B*). One can inspect and palpate the snugly closed bladder neck, which feels much like the contracted anus of a newborn infant. If the sutures are properly placed, the bladder neck does not have a slit-like appearance (which represents sutures obstructing the urethra) (Fig. 436*A*) nor is it too loose

such that there is a sagging of the walls (Fig. 436*B*). Rather, it is circular, and this configuration represents perfect approximation (Fig. 436*C*).

A single Foley catheter with a 5-ml balloon is inserted through the cystotomy, which is closed with two layers of running 3-0 delayed absorbable suture (Fig. 437*A*). The initial suture may or may not penetrate the mucosa (Fig. 437*B*). The second suture merely inverts the initial suture line. Because the incision is in the dome of the bladder, it may be closed with a single full-thickness layer, either interrupted or running.

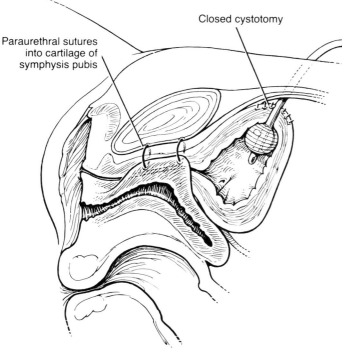

Closed cystotomy

Paraurethral sutures into cartilage of symphysis pubis

The catheter is brought out through a stab wound lateral to the midline incision so that the skin incision does not override the incision in the bladder. The abdominal incision is closed in the customary fashion. At the completion of the procedure, the paraurethral tissues are snugly placed about the urethra, and the bladder neck is thus in a high retropubic position, fully corrected from its previous patulous state (Fig. 438).

Figure 438

Urinary Tract Injury

Even with sufficient surgical experience, injury to the urinary tract can and does occur. With all dissections, the contiguous structures subject to injury must be exposed. This step not only avoids injuries to the ureter and bladder but also facilitates recognition of any urinary tract injuries at the time of operation (an equally important consideration). Injuries do occur that are followed by an uneventful postoperative course and are never recognized. In this patient, the tied ureter (and silent nephrectomy) is discovered at a later operation (Fig. 439). With recognition and adequate repair, problems such as fistula formation and serious morbidity can be avoided. The type of operative repair is determined by the degree of trauma and the location of the injury.

Bladder Injury

Most injuries to the bladder occur during abdominal hysterectomy or cesarean section (Fig. 440). Once the injury is identified, we generally prefer to proceed with the operation in the proper plane of dissection, with the plan that the cystotomy would be repaired after completion of the hysterectomy and during the reconstructive phase of pelvic repair. If the injury is repaired immediately, the otherwise satisfactory bladder repair could be disrupted during the rest of the dissection necessary for hysterectomy or cesarean section.

In the procedure shown in Figure 441, the uterus is removed, and traction is applied to the corners of the vagina to aid in any additional mobilization of the bladder that may be necessary to provide a tension-free closure of the cystotomy. The cystotomy is closed in two separate extramucosal layers with 3-0 delayed absorbable suture (Fig. 441A). The peritoneum from the back of the bladder is pulled down to cover the suture line in the bladder and separate it from the underlying suture line of the vagina (Fig. 441B). The urethral or suprapubic catheter is left in place a sufficient time to ensure primary closure of the injury.

Ureteral Injury

Rather commonly, the ureteral sheath can be significantly traumatized and thus result in potential interruption of the longitudinal blood supply to the ureter. When only a short segment is damaged, it can be simply repaired with a few (one or two) interrupted 5-0 delayed absorbable sutures. The sutures are placed through the sheath and do not involve the underlying longitudinal vessels. If a large segment of the ureteral sheath has been traumatized, it is preferable to reflect the bladder, open its dome, and insert a splinting ureteral catheter in a retrograde fashion up the ureter with the distal segment remaining in the bladder (Fig. 442). Appropriate repair is accomplished with 5-0 delayed absorbable suture. After a sufficient time, the ureteral catheter can be removed through the cystoscope.

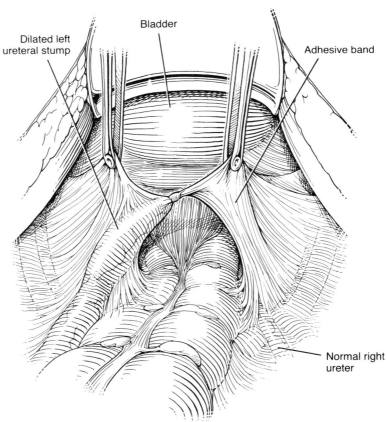

Figure 439

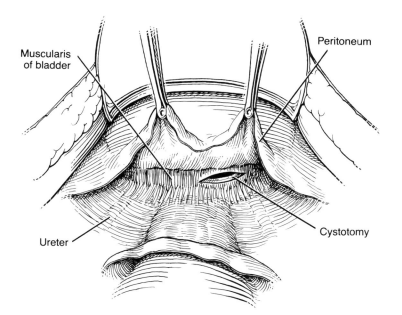

Muscularis of bladder

Peritoneum

Ureter

Cystotomy

Figure 440

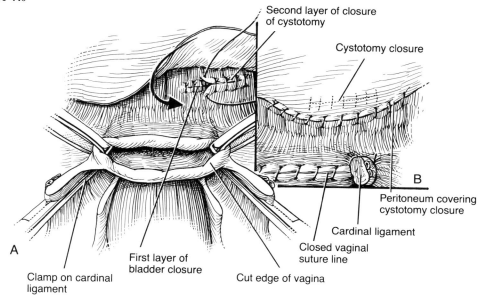

Second layer of closure of cystotomy

Cystotomy closure

Clamp on cardinal ligament

First layer of bladder closure

Cut edge of vagina

Closed vaginal suture line

Cardinal ligament

Peritoneum covering cystotomy closure

A

B

Figure 441

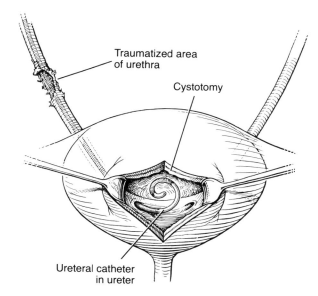

Traumatized area of urethra

Cystotomy

Ureteral catheter in ureter

Figure 442

Ureteroneocystostomy

Ureterovaginal fistulas and most ureteral injuries that occur with gynecologic procedures usually result from injuries close to the bladder. For these, we prefer an open technique of ureteroneocystostomy that includes a direct mucosal approximation of ureter to bladder. The particular site of the fistula or the area of trauma is resected, and the distal segment of ureter just adjacent to the bladder is tied with a single 2-0 delayed absorbable suture. The distal end of the proximal ureter is mobilized (with the adjacent peritoneum), and care is taken not to damage the sheath or longitudinal blood supply. The distal end of the proximal ureter is incised vertically in the 6-o'clock position for a distance of approximately 5 mm. A fine suture is placed through the distal end of the ureter; it is used to assist in delivery of the ureter into the bladder. A finger is inserted inside the open bladder to tent up the bladder wall and indicate the most accessible area on the posterior lateral wall for insertion of the ureter (Fig. 443).

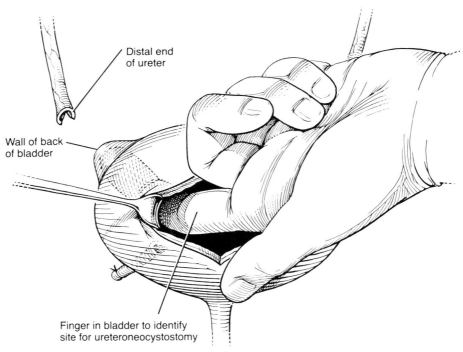

Distal end
of ureter

Wall of back
of bladder

Finger in bladder to identify
site for ureteroneocystostomy

Figure 443

A 1-cm opening is dissected directly through the full thickness of the bladder by a spreading action of the dissecting scissors. A curved forceps is then passed inside the bladder out through the opening in the bladder wall, where it grasps the previously placed suture. Traction on the suture delivers the ureter within the bladder (Fig. 444*A*). From inside the bladder, five or six interrupted 4-0 delayed absorbable sutures are used to anastomose the full thickness of the spatulated ureter to near full thickness of the bladder in a mucosa-to-mucosa approximation (Fig. 444*B*). Three or four interrupted sutures of the same material are placed in the peritoneum, incorporating the peritoneal flap of the ureter with the muscularis and serosa of the bladder to reinforce the repair and reduce any potential tension on the mucosal approximation (Fig. 444*C*). We prefer to then pass a self-retaining ureteral catheter with its most proximal end lodged in the renal pelvis and its distal end free within the bladder. This is generally left in place 10 to 14 days or longer, depending on the individual circumstances. The bladder is drained with a suprapubic Foley catheter brought out through an anterior cystotomy, which is then closed with two layers of running 3-0 delayed absorbable suture. Appropriate suction drainage and reperitonealization are accomplished in the customary fashion.

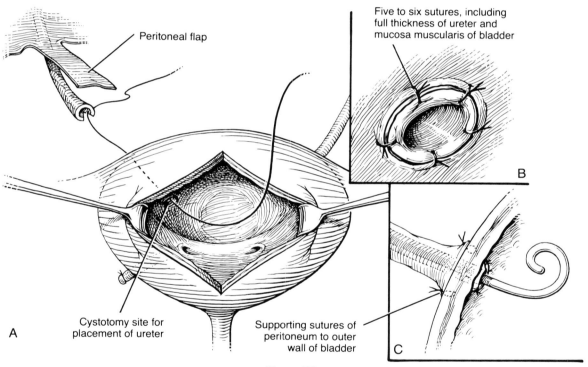

Peritoneal flap

Five to six sutures, including full thickness of ureter and mucosa muscularis of bladder

B

A

Cystotomy site for placement of ureter

Supporting sutures of peritoneum to outer wall of bladder

C

Figure 444

Ureteroureterostomy

When the ureter has been divided at a high level, it may not lend itself to ureteroneocystostomy. Ureteroureterostomy becomes the procedure of choice. If the ureter is small, a slight spatulation (4 mm) on both ends facilitates an anastomosis and thus enlarges its diameter. The anastomosis is accomplished in a single layer of interrupted 5-0 delayed absorbable sutures (Fig. 445A). After placement of three full-thickness interrupted sutures on the posterior wall, a ureteral catheter is passed up the ureter with the distal end of the catheter passed down the ureter into the bladder. The anastomosis then is completed over the ureteral stent (Fig. 445B). The catheter is left in place for a sufficient time, depending on the circumstances. The anastomotic site is drained with an extraperitoneal suction catheter lateral to the midline incision. Appropriate follow-up includes intravenous pyelography to ensure satisfactory healing and long-term function.

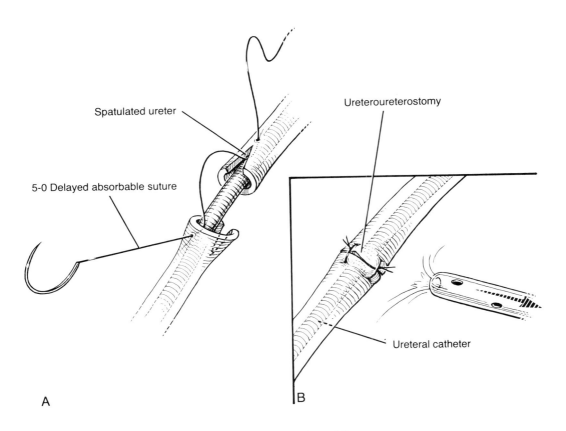

Spatulated ureter

Ureteroureterostomy

5-0 Delayed absorbable suture

Ureteral catheter

A

B

Figure 445

Ureteroneocystostomy

With Bladder Extension

Occasionally, a ureteral fistula may be so high or the trauma to the ureter such that the bladder must be freed from the back of the symphysis pubis and either side wall in order to bridge this gap without tension on the anastomosis. The anterior parietal peritoneum from the lower abdominal wall is incised, and the bladder is displaced posteriorly off the symphysis pubis, much as is done during a modified Marshall-Marchetti-Krantz procedure. If additional length is needed, the parietal peritoneum can be divided laterally above the bladder; this approach thus completely mobilizes one entire side. The bladder is then held in place by interrupted 0 delayed absorbable suture to fix the bladder to the iliopsoas muscle (Fig. 446A). Further length can be obtained by mobilizing the kidney in an inferior direction. The peritoneum is incised lateral to the colon, and the colon is displaced medially. The kidney and upper ureter are displaced downward to a lower level by simply freeing them from the retroperitoneal tissues in the lumbar region (Fig. 446A). To maintain any mobilization acquired, it may be necessary to suture the lower portion of the kidney with a heavy delayed absorbable suture between the capsule and the iliopsoas fascia.

Once the bladder extension and kidney are fixed in place, the ureter is implanted into the bladder (end of the ureter to the side of the bladder) (Fig. 446B). The technique and type of anastomosis are the same as those described for ureteroneocystostomy. Through the cystotomy incision, a small opening is made in the bladder for the end-to-side anastomosis. The fine suture placed through the spatulated distal end of the ureter is grasped with a curved forceps, and with appropriate traction, the suture delivers the ureter within the bladder. From the inside of the bladder, five or six interrupted 4-0 delayed absorbable sutures are used to anastomose the full thickness of

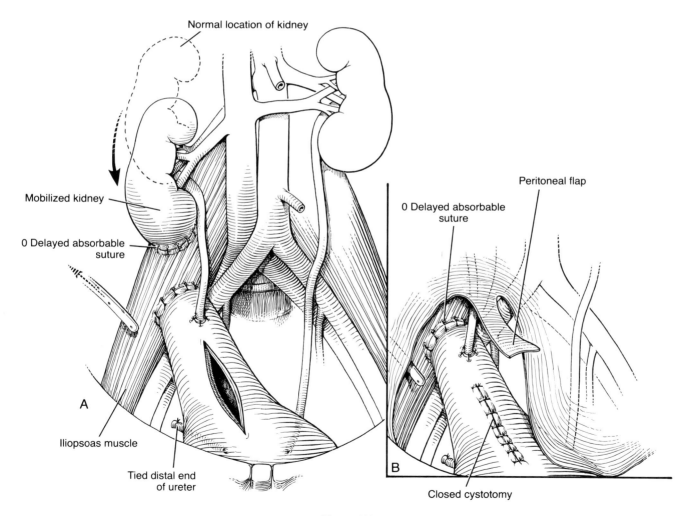

Normal location of kidney

Mobilized kidney

0 Delayed absorbable suture

A

Iliopsoas muscle

Tied distal end of ureter

Peritoneal flap

0 Delayed absorbable suture

B

Closed cystotomy

Figure 446

the spatulated ureter to nearly the full thickness of the bladder in a mucosa-to-mucosa approximation. Three or four interrupted sutures of the same material are placed in the peritoneum about the ureter and fixed to the muscularis and serosa of the bladder to reinforce the repair and reduce any potential tension on the anastomosis.

A self-retaining ureteral catheter (no. 6 F) is passed up the ureter, with the proximal end lodged in the renal pelvis and the distal end free in the bladder. A large extraperitoneal suction catheter is inserted near to but not touching the anastomosis and brought out through a stab wound lateral to the incision. This suction catheter and the urethral catheter draining the bladder are left in place for a sufficient time, which is determined on an individual basis.

With Bladder Flap Extension

If the previously described technique does not permit the bladder to reach the ureter free of tension, then construction of a tube of the bladder flap to bridge the defect must be considered. An obliquely placed flap is outlined on the outside of the bladder (Fig. 447A). This must be widely based superiorly; if care is taken to avoid making the flap too narrow distally, its blood supply should be excellent (Fig. 447B). Generally, an end-to-side, mucosa-to-mucosa approximation can be accomplished as previously described for ureteroneocystostomy (Fig. 447C). The anastomosis is done under direct vision before closure of the long linear defect of the anterior bladder wall produced by creation of the tube. When a peritoneal flap has been preserved along with the upper end of the ureter, this flap can be brought down well over the anterior cystotomy incision and fixed in a position such that it additionally relieves any tension on the anastomosis. A self-retaining ureteral catheter (no. 6 F) is passed up the ureter, with the proximal end in the renal pelvis and the distal end free in the bladder (Fig. 447D).

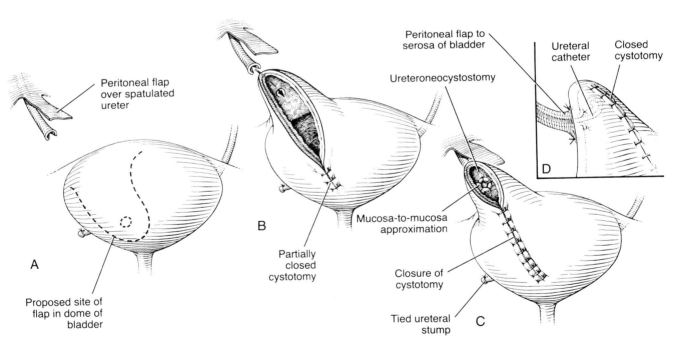

Peritoneal flap over spatulated ureter

Peritoneal flap to serosa of bladder

Ureteral catheter

Closed cystotomy

Ureteroneocystostomy

Mucosa-to-mucosa approximation

Partially closed cystotomy

Closure of cystotomy

Proposed site of flap in dome of bladder

Tied ureteral stump

A

B

C

D

Figure 447

Ureteroileocystostomy

Sometimes the bladder and retroperitoneum are scarred and fixed (from multiple previous operations or the effects of radiation) such that mobility of the bladder is severely restricted. It may be possible to isolate a relatively normal segment of small intestine in which the distal end of the ureter can be anasto-mosed (ureteroileal) in a two-layer closure as an end-to-side anastomosis (end of ureter to side of ileum) and the distal end of the segment of ileum can be anastomosed to the dome of the bladder in a two-layer closure (Fig. 448). This is essentially an ileal conduit anastomosis to the bladder with a single ureter.

In all these anastomoses, we prefer a simple ureteral catheter passed up to the renal pelvis down into the bladder. The catheter is left in place for an appropriate length of time. Drainage of the anastomotic site is essential. A large extraperitoneal suction tube is inserted and left in place for about 10 days or longer if there is any urinary leakage. An excretory urogram is obtained between 2 and 3 weeks after the operation and at 3-month intervals thereafter during the first year to be certain that delayed stricture does not occur.

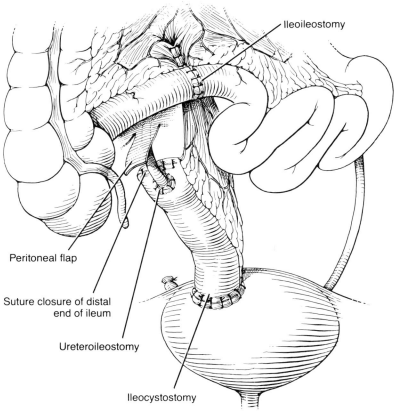

Figure 448

Intestinal Tract

Anal Incontinence

The complexity of the anatomic and physiologic mechanisms responsible for fecal incontinence is well appreciated by those treating patients with this problem. The intact anatomy of the internal anal sphincter, external anal sphincter, and puborectalis division of the levator ani muscle in the female contributes to (and may be essential for) complete anal continence of solid, liquid, and gaseous states (Fig. 449). Disruption of this anatomy, usually secondary to obstetric trauma, may result in some degree of enteric incontinence.

The internal anal sphincter is a thickened, downward continuation of the circular layer of the smooth muscle of the rectum. The external sphincter, composed of striated muscle, surrounds the internal sphincter. The two sphincters are somewhat separated by the conjoint longitudinal layer formed by a merger of the longitudinal layer of the smooth muscle of the rectum and the pubococcygeal fibers of the levator ani muscle. This conjoint layer of muscle fibers is replaced distally by thin fibroelastic fibers that penetrate the distal portions of the sphincters and insert in the anal submucosa and perianal skin. The sphincters encircle the anal canal just distal to the anorectal angle formed by the tonus of the loop of the puborectalis muscle pulling the rectum anteriorly. The puborectalis muscle is considered to be that most medial portion of the pubococcygeal muscle that contributes to neither the conjoint longitudinal layer nor the anal coccygeal raphe but, rather, forms a continent loop around the posterior aspect of the anal rectum. The internal sphincter, which is under anatomic control, is thought to exert most of the resting pressure. The external sphincter is a three-part skeletal muscle sphincter innervated by the inferior rectal branch of the pudendal nerve and the perineal branch of the fourth sacral nerve, and it exerts most of the maximal squeeze pressure. Studies done at our institution reveal the sphincter to be an ellipsoidal cylinder with an anterior length almost equal to its posterior length (that is, it is thickest anteriorly and posteriorly, with some thinning laterally). Probably both the smooth muscle internal sphincter, providing most of the resting pressure of the anal canal, and the fatigable voluntary striated external sphincter, providing most of the squeeze pressure, play important roles and both should be fully repaired when divided. Cylindrical sphincters with a substantial internal sphincteric component suggest that reapproximation of an internal and external sphincter mass of approximately 2 cm thick over a zone at least 3 to 4 cm long would result in a more anatomic repair and perhaps better restoration of the high-pressure zone of the anal canal.

The levator plate is another structure that, in conjunction with the puborectalis muscle, is important for anal continence. It supports the rectum above the level of the anorectal angle, keeping the pressure of the enteric contents as well as changes in intra-abdominal pressure away from the sphincteric complex.

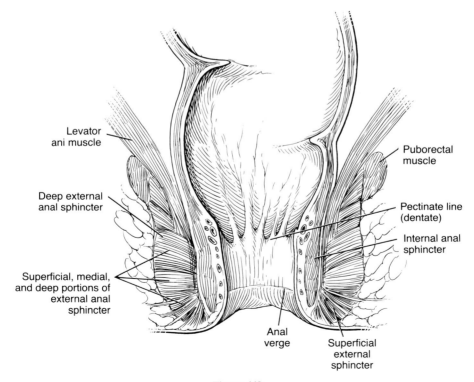

Figure 449

A finger in the rectum identifies a thinned rectovaginal septum with retraction of the external anal sphincter and poor response of the puborectalis muscle (Fig. 450). The corrective operative procedure is as follows. A curvilinear incision is made from the 9- to 12- to 3-o'clock positions through the skin of the perineum, following which a midline incision is made up the vagina (Fig. 451), similar to that accomplished for a posterior colpoperineorrhaphy. The mucosa of the vagina is separated from the anterior wall of the rectum sufficiently laterally and superiorly to provide access to the retracted muscles (Fig. 452). With a finger in the anal canal, those exposed tissues laterally (thought to be retracted bundles of the superficial, medial, and deep portions of the external anal sphincter) are identified with a muscle stimulator (Fig. 453). Usually, these muscles are found in the 3- to 4-o'clock positions on the patient's left side and the 8- to 9-o'clock positions on the patient's right side. If necessary, the curvilinear incision is continued posteriorly to permit dissection to identify contracting muscle that may have retracted back to the 5-o'clock position on the patient's left side or to the 7-o'clock position on the patient's right side.

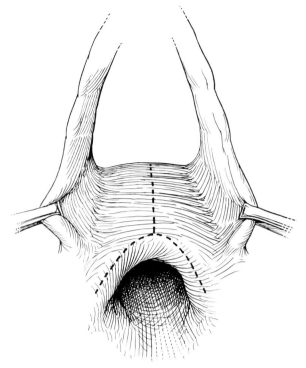

Figure 451
Proposed incision in rectovaginal septum.

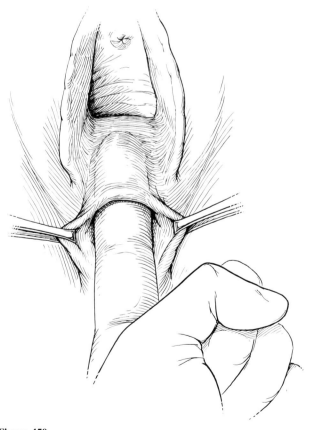

Figure 450
Finger in rectum, demonstrating thin rectovaginal septum with retraction of external anal sphincter.

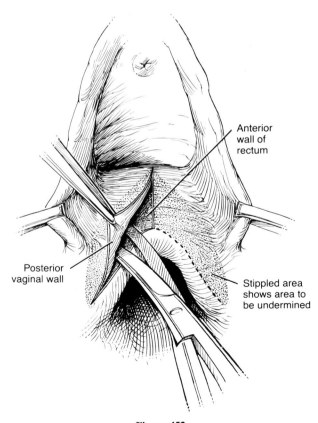

Anterior wall of rectum

Posterior vaginal wall

Stippled area shows area to be undermined

Figure 452

Once the sphincter muscles have been identified, the initial suture is placed at the superior aspect of the incision (that highest on the anal canal). This suture and each subsequent suture used to reestablish muscle continuity are placed in the following fashion. With a finger in the anal canal, the surgeon takes a full and deep bite (with a Mayo needle with a swaged-on 0 monofilament delayed absorbable suture) (Fig. 454*A*), incorporating the contracting muscle bundle (portion of external anal sphincter) on the patient's left side with intervening bites of the anterior rectal wall. This approach thus incorporates a portion of the internal anal sphincter with an equally deep bite on the right side of the anal canal (retracted segments of external anal sphincter) (Fig. 454*B*), after which the suture is elevated and tagged. At this point, the placement of this suture can be evaluated to determine whether the suture, if tied, would severely narrow the introitus and result in dyspareunia. Additional sutures are placed similarly, each incorporating a full and deep bite of the muscle with intervening bites of the anterior rectal wall, after which they are tagged. Usually, four to six sutures are placed before the last suture (that incorporating the most inferior aspect of the external anal sphincter) is reached (covering a distance of 4 to 5 cm). The surgeon then

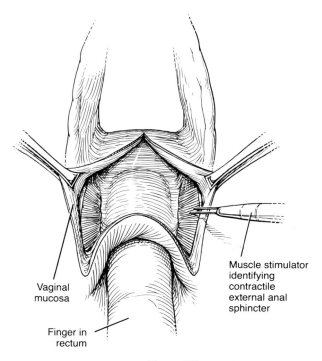

Vaginal mucosa

Muscle stimulator identifying contractile external anal sphincter

Finger in rectum

Figure 453

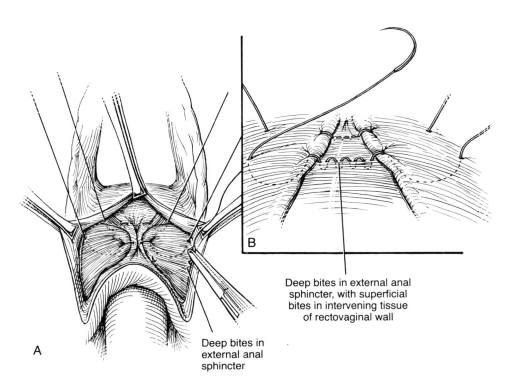

Deep bites in external anal sphincter, with superficial bites in intervening tissue of rectovaginal wall

Deep bites in external anal sphincter

Figure 454

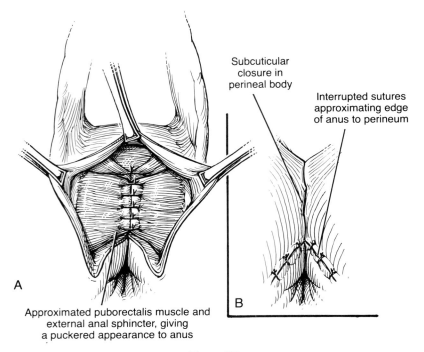

Subcuticular
closure in
perineal body

Interrupted sutures
approximating edge
of anus to perineum

A

B

Approximated puborectalis muscle and
external anal sphincter, giving
a puckered appearance to anus

Figure 455

changes gloves and proceeds to tie the sutures in the order in which they were placed; this method results in approximation of the laterally retracted muscles to the midline, severely narrowing the anal canal (Fig. 455*A*). The highest suture, that including a portion of the puborectalis muscle, is carefully assessed to ensure that the high approximation will not cause dyspareunia. Once the sutures are approximated, the deep muscles of the perineum are approximated, the skin of the perineal body is closed with subcuticular delayed absorbable suture, and the edges of the anal canal are approximated to the skin of the perineum with 4-0 delayed absorbable suture (Fig. 455*B*). The reconstituted anal canal should feel snug around the surgeon's little finger, and the perineal body is returned to its normal length (Fig. 456).

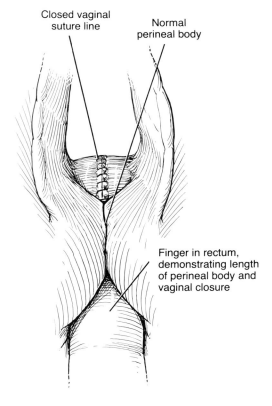

Closed vaginal
suture line

Normal
perineal body

Finger in rectum,
demonstrating length
of perineal body and
vaginal closure

Figure 456

Rectovaginal Fistula

Repair After Obstetric Injury

Repair of rectovaginal fistula is successful if the entire fistulous tract is excised and the rectovaginal septum is accurately approximated free of tension and with perfect hemostasis and minimal resultant infection. Physical examination is essential to confirm the presence of a rectovaginal fistula, to determine the exact size and location of the fistula, and to assess the condition of the anal sphincter. Most often, the fistula is palpable and can be visualized easily by rectovaginal examination and proctosigmoidoscopy. Stool may be seen in the vagina. If the fistula is small, its opening may appear only as a depression or pit-like defect. The gentle use of a probe may be necessary to define the fistula. Ancillary studies may occasionally be necessary to outline the rectovaginal fistula and to exclude underlying diseases, involvement of other parts of the bowel, or fistulas concomitant with other organs. An elusive rectovaginal fistula tract may be identified by placing the patient in the Trendelenburg position and filling the vagina with water while simultaneously inflating the anal canal and rectum with air; the vagina is carefully observed, and bubbles of air are seen passing from the anus or rectum through the fistula into the vagina.

The surgeon's left index finger is inserted in the rectum to aid in identification of the fistula and to assess the area of scarring and the mobility available (Fig. 457).

An incision is made about the fistula to include the scar tissue and also to provide a rim about the fistulous tract on which to apply countertraction for the future mobilization of the vagina from the rectal wall (Fig. 458). (The surgeon's left index finger may remain in the rectum to provide support to the rectal wall as this incision is made.)

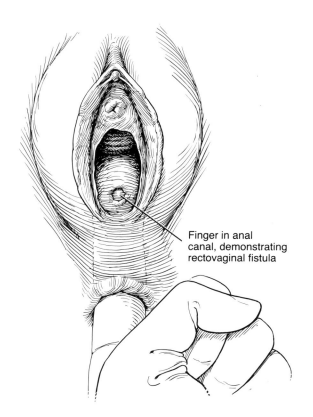

Finger in anal canal, demonstrating rectovaginal fistula

Figure 457

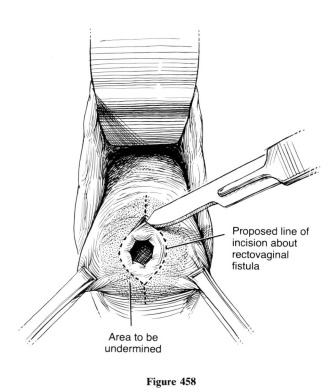

Proposed line of incision about rectovaginal fistula

Area to be undermined

Figure 458

With traction on the vaginal wall and countertraction applied to the edge of the fistulous tract, the vagina is separated from the underlying rectal wall with sharp dissection that proceeds circumferentially; this mobilization permits later approximation of the fresh injury free of tension (Fig. 459).

Once the vaginal walls are widely mobilized from the underlying rectum, the entire fistulous tract is excised, including a small rim of rectal mucosa, to convert the fistula to a fresh injury (Fig. 460).

With the surgeon's left index finger lifting and supporting the anterior rectal wall, the initial sutures are placed extramucosally, including a portion of the muscularis and submucosa, with 3-0 delayed absorbable sutures. Figure 461 shows the suture being tied. However, we frequently place all the sutures throughout the length of the fistula, after which they are individually tied in the order in which they were placed. The initial suture line begins and is extended a full 5 to 8 mm above and below the site of the fistulous tract.

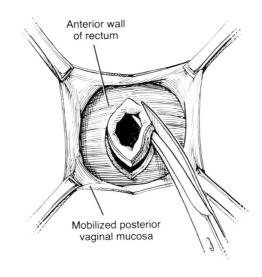

Anterior wall of rectum

Mobilized posterior vaginal mucosa

Figure 460

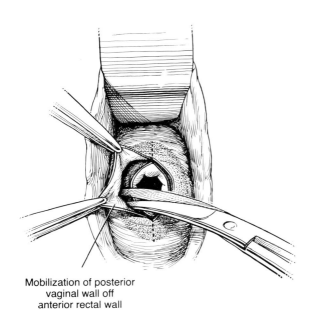

Mobilization of posterior vaginal wall off anterior rectal wall

Figure 459

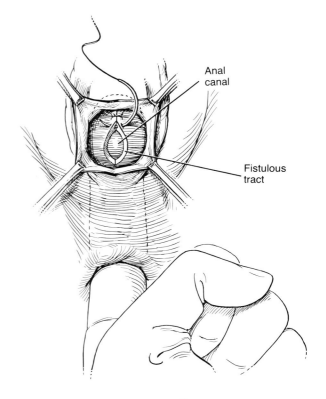

Anal canal

Fistulous tract

Figure 461

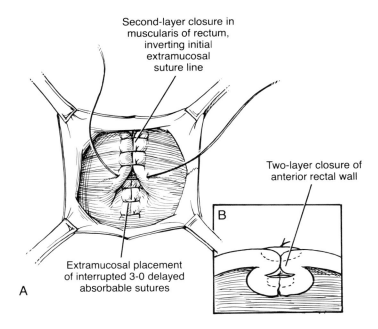

Second-layer closure in muscularis of rectum, inverting initial extramucosal suture line

Two-layer closure of anterior rectal wall

B

Extramucosal placement of interrupted 3-0 delayed absorbable sutures

A

Figure 462

A second layer of inverting sutures, again begun 5 mm above the previously closed suture line and extended 5 mm distal to the fistulous closure, inverts the initial suture line into the rectum (Fig. 462*A*), and no sutures are located within the rectal lumen (Fig. 462*B*). The second layer of the second suture line inverts the initial closure.

Once the wall of the rectum is reconstituted, the lower portion of the puborectalis muscle and the external anal sphincter are approximated to add a

third layer in the closure and help reconstitute the anterior rectal wall (Fig. 463*A*). Care should be taken that this approximation is not carried so far superiorly that it results in a transverse bar across the posterior vaginal wall, which leads to dyspareunia. Once the muscular walls are approximated, the vaginal wall is approximated with fine (4-0) delayed absorbable suture accurately placed so as to promote primary apposition of the fresh edges of the mucosal wall (Fig. 463*B*).

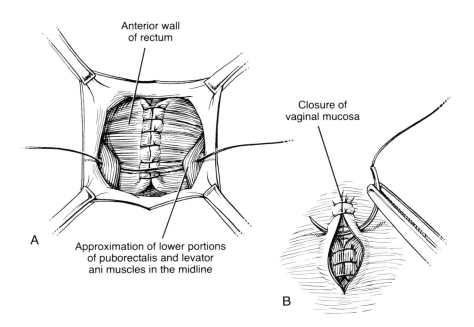

Anterior wall of rectum

Closure of vaginal mucosa

A

Approximation of lower portions of puborectalis and levator ani muscles in the midline

B

Figure 463

Repair of Radiation-Induced Fistula

The usual rectovaginal fistula is located in the lower third of the vagina or just inside the hymenal ring. Less commonly, a sizable rectovaginal fistula is located high in the posterior vaginal wall, frequently associated with a degree of stricture of the rectum and significant perirectal fibrosis and scarring. When this does occur, it is almost always after radiation therapy. Successful closure of the fistula requires aggressive excision of the surrounding tissue damaged by radiation. In selected patients, the fistula is best managed with primary resection and anastomosis of the rectosigmoid through a lower midline incision. In some patients, successful closure can be accomplished by means of a pedicled bulbocavernous muscle with an overlying labial fat pad (Martius procedure); this is performed vaginally.

Figure 464 is a lateral view depicting the usual location of the fistula high in the posterior vaginal wall.

Figure 465 outlines the potential sites from which the pedicled bulbocavernous Martius-type flap is obtained. Initially, an incision is made in the vagina to separate the scarred vagina from the underlying anterior wall of the rectum circumferentially. The edge of the scarred vaginal epithelium adjacent to the edge of the rectal mucosa is excised in anticipation of this being the site of the initial suture line approximating the squamous epithelium from the vulvar flap to the rectum in order to fill the defect in the rectum. With a Mayo scissors, a subcutaneous tunnel is made from the labium majus to the fistula under the labium and vaginal mucosa (Fig. 466). The free end of the muscle is guided through the subcutaneous tunnel with a single absorbable suture placed along its edge to assist in passage through the tunnel. The rectal defect is such that it cannot be closed primarily. Thus, the edge of the squamous epithelium from the vulvar graft is sutured to the edge of the rectal mucosa with 4-0 delayed absorbable sutures. Occasionally, a Schuchardt incision is required in the vagina to obtain adequate exposure for the dissection.

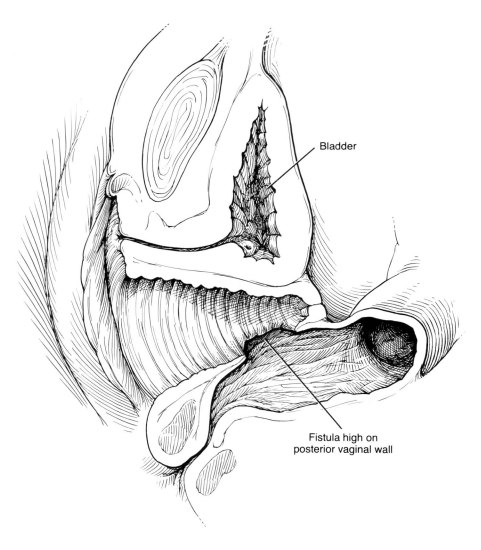

Bladder

Fistula high on posterior vaginal wall

Figure 464

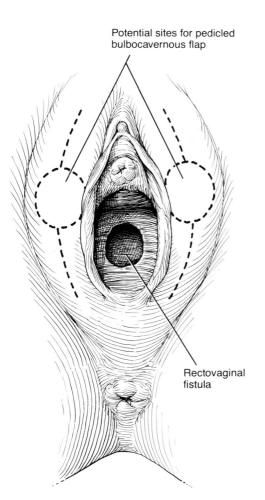

Potential sites for pedicled
bulbocavernous flap

Rectovaginal
fistula

Figure 465

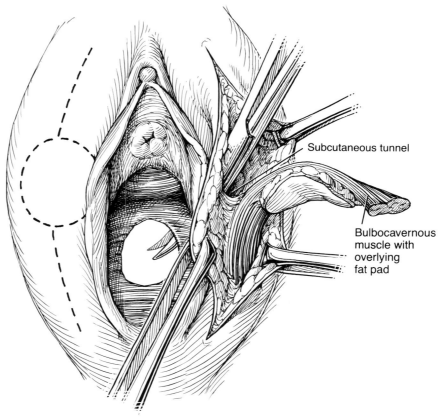

Subcutaneous tunnel

Bulbocavernous
muscle with
overlying
fat pad

Figure 466

The pedicled graft initially is closed, beginning at the 3-o'clock position, in a synchronous fashion such that the entire edge of the fistulous tract is in immediate proximity to the edge of the skin from the vulva (Fig. 467). Once in place, the muscle and subcutaneous tissue of the graft are sutured to the surrounding connective tissue.

To provide coverage for the exposed Martius flap, which has been inserted as a plug into the rectum, a similar pedicled graft is developed from the patient's right side, and this is placed such that the skin of the vulva is approximated to the skin of the vagina (Fig. 468). The edges are placed such that there is no exposed source for granulation tissue (Fig. 469).

A small suction catheter is placed between the two pedicled grafts and brought out through a stab wound lateral to the perineal incision. The vulvar incision is closed in layers with skin approximated with fine interrupted delayed absorbable suture. In patients requiring a pedicled graft, the repair may result in a compromise of the vagina and a degree of colpo-cleisis. This results not only from the encroachment on the vaginal lumen with the pedicled grafts but also from the associated contracture secondary to the underlying cause of the fistula—pelvic radiation. There is a tendency to further contracture and stenosis of the vagina, which may result in significant dyspareunia or apareunia.

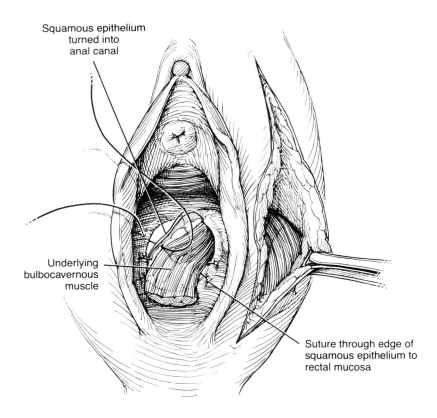

Squamous epithelium turned into anal canal

Underlying bulbocavernous muscle

Suture through edge of squamous epithelium to rectal mucosa

Figure 467

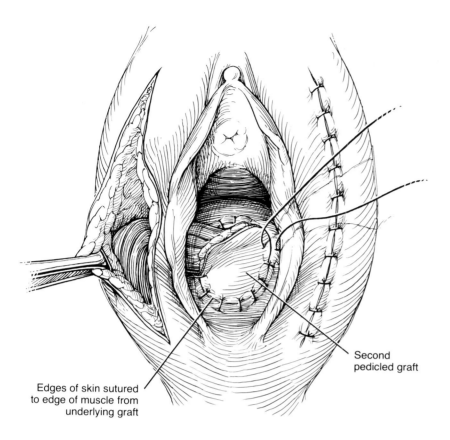

Edges of skin sutured
to edge of muscle from
underlying graft

Second
pedicled graft

Figure 468

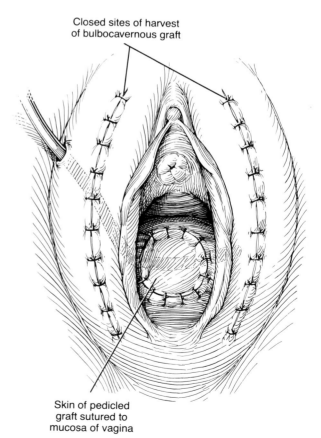

Closed sites of harvest
of bulbocavernous graft

Skin of pedicled
graft sutured to
mucosa of vagina

Figure 469

Presacral Tumor

Perineal Approach

A relatively infrequent heterogeneous group of tumors with a similar clinical presentation may arise in the presacral space. Depending on their origin, size, and degree of invasion, they may be asymptomatic and found only on routine pelvic examination. Diagnostic studies such as sigmoidoscopy, barium enema, and intravenous pyelography generally demonstrate extrinsic compression or distortion of adjacent organs. Computed tomography, although unable to differentiate specific lesions, has improved the ability to determine the extent of the tumor more specifically. It also delineates the extent of bony and soft tissue involvement with invasion of the adjacent structures and thus aids in determination of the proper surgical approach. Depending on the location of the tumor, its size, and its mobility, various surgical approaches can be selected. For tumors as large as 8 cm in diameter that are located low on the sacrum, we prefer a transsacral approach, removing the coccyx when necessary.

The patient is placed in a prone position with the buttocks elevated and the trunk and thighs flexed (Kraske position) (Fig. 470A). A midline incision is made over the sacrum, extending down to the anal ring (Fig. 470B). The coccyx is excised, and the rectum is freed from the hollow of the sacrum. Tumors that are fixed to the sacrum require sharp dissection with an osteotome, and scissors are used to dissect the ligaments, muscles, or portions of the sacrum lateral to the tumor margins. The nerves, especially the pudendal nerve, are protected.

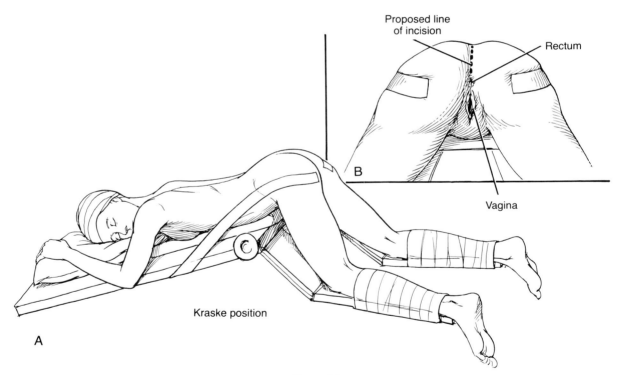

Figure 470

Tumors that are located low on the sacrum can also be approached with the patient in the lithotomy position. The initial perineal incision is much like that of a Schuchardt incision extended around the rectum and entering the presacral space (Fig. 471*A*). With sharp dissection, the rectum and vagina are elevated and displaced to either the patient's right or left, depending on the location of the tumor (Fig. 471*B*). This approach exposes the tumor, now freed on its anterior surface, and permits the use of sharp

dissection to free it from the anterior surface of the sacrum under direct vision.

Careful hemostasis is obtained. A suction catheter is placed in the bed of the hollow of the sacrum and brought out through a separate stab wound; the rectum and vagina are returned to place; and the incision is closed with fine delayed absorbable suture placed in several layers.

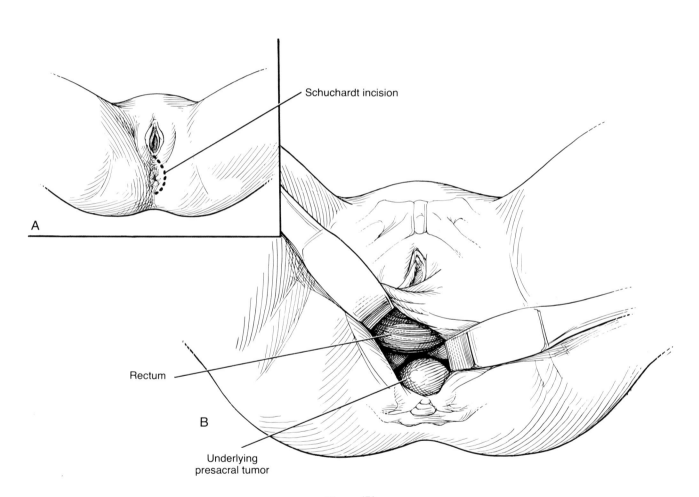

Schuchardt incision

A

Rectum

B

Underlying
presacral tumor

Figure 471

Abdominal Approach

For tumors high on the sacrum or of significant size or fixation, an abdominal approach permits a thorough evaluation of the abdomen and upper pelvis and allows safe and accurate mobilization of the rectum and ureters from the upper and anterior surfaces of the tumor. Frequently, the anterior division of the internal iliac artery is ligated as the perirectal and perivesical spaces are developed and the tumor is set up for excision. In Figure 472, a neurofibroma is located on the right posterior surface of the pelvic side wall and sacrum, and the ureter is stretched over its superior surface. The sigmoid colon is mobilized to the patient's left. With sharp and blunt dissection, the left lateral and anterior surfaces of the tumor are freed from the sigmoid colon and the hollow of the sacrum.

On the right side of the tumor, the peritoneum is incised, and a short remnant is left adjacent to the ureter to ensure maintenance of an adequate blood supply (Fig. 473). With sharp dissection, this incision is continued distally; this approach permits the ureter to be lifted off the lateral surface of the tumor at the appropriate time and prevents potential damage to the ureter. The anterior division of the interior iliac artery is clamped, cut, and ligated (Fig. 474).

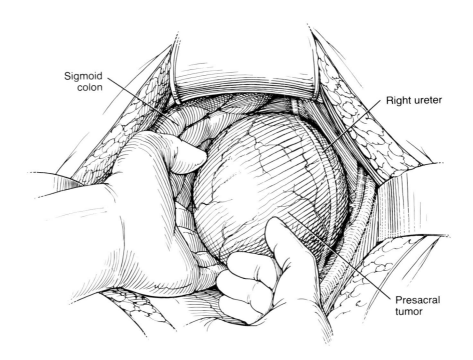

Figure 472

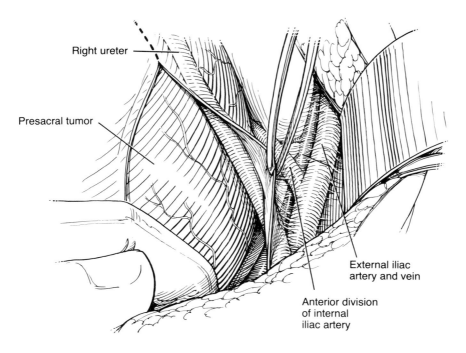

Right ureter

Presacral tumor

External iliac
artery and vein

Anterior division
of internal
iliac artery

Figure 473

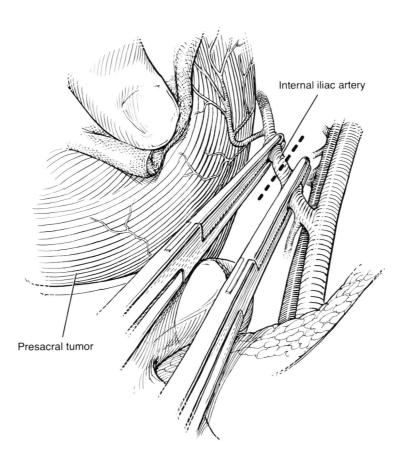

Internal iliac artery

Presacral tumor

Figure 474

Once the sigmoid colon is mobilized laterally (Fig. 475), the location of the left iliac vessels and left ureter must be defined to ensure that they are freed from the site of potential injury (Fig. 476).

Troublesome bleeding deep in the pelvis can complicate the safe and accurate resection of presacral tumors. If significant venous bleeding does occur, we prefer to place a small sponge over the site of the bleeding and compress it under a retractor. This method permits complete excision of the tumor, after which accurate and complete hemostasis can be obtained at the bleeding site. Frequently, this requires a combination of techniques, including a suture ligature, placement of fine silver clips, and cautery on the appropriate-sized vessel (Fig. 477).

Combined Approach

Occasionally, a combined abdominal-perineal approach is required for safe and complete en bloc removal. The abdominal operation just described is done first. When the tumor is freed as completely as possible through this approach, the incision is closed and the patient is turned. A transsacral or transperi-

neal dissection is done for perineal removal of the tumor mass. Occasionally, during the primary transsacral or transperineal approach, it becomes apparent that a concomitant abdominal incision is required for a complete resection of the tumor; if the patient is in the lithotomy position, a supplemental abdominal incision can easily be accomplished. Some surgeons prefer a synchronous approach, noting that it provides maximal flexibility for tumors in this rather inaccessible area and allows protection of the rectum, ureters, and major blood vessels. Lesions in the upper presacral area and those extending up to the pelvic brim or above initially require an abdominal approach for safe dissection of the upper reaches of the tumor. When this is done, the entire tumor can often be readily excised from above. Complete and preferably en bloc excision should be performed to eliminate the possibility of recurrent or persistent tumors. Tumors that act as "pushers"—benign tumors that displace contiguous structures—can safely and expeditiously be removed with minimal risk of bleeding and postoperative complications. Treatment of malignant tumors or "invaders," with their associated fixation, complications, and frequent recurrence, leads to disappointing results.

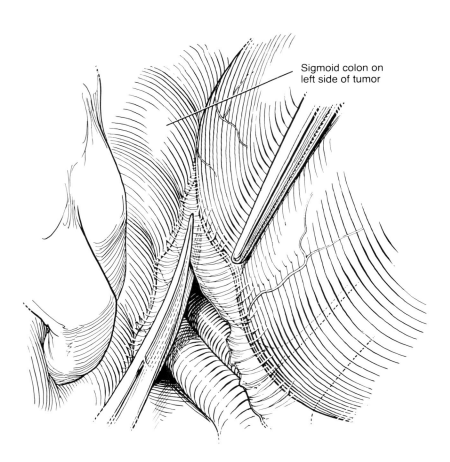

Sigmoid colon on left side of tumor

Figure 475

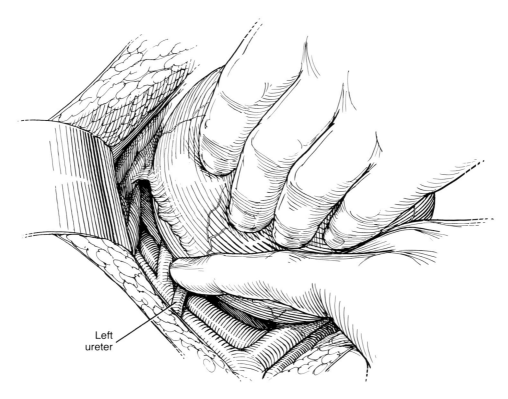

Left
ureter

Figure 476

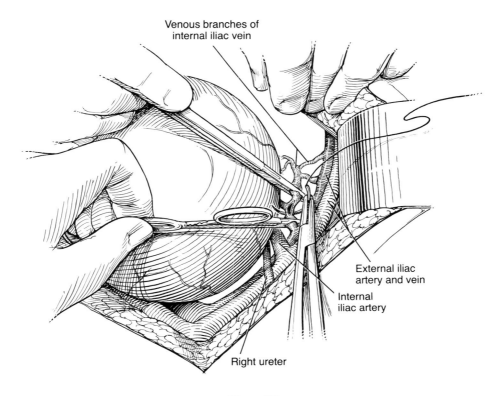

Venous branches of
internal iliac vein

External iliac
artery and vein

Internal
iliac artery

Right ureter

Figure 477

Appendectomy

The gynecologic pelvic surgeon performs appendectomy in most instances as a prophylactic procedure. Gentle traction is placed on the cecum with gauze held by the first assistant; this delivers the appendix and cecum into the incision. A Babcock clamp placed on the distal end of the appendix aids in further exposure and fans out the mesentery of the appendix (Fig. 478). We prefer to ligate the appendiceal artery at the beginning of the procedure; this ligation is accomplished with placement of a single clamp across the mesentery, which is cut. The mesoappendix is ligated with a single 2-0 delayed absorbable suture. Occasionally, the long appendix and mesoappendix are taken in several bites. A pursestring suture is

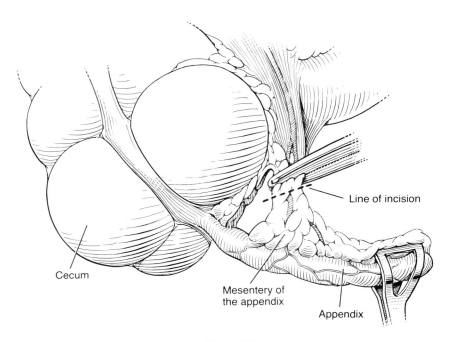

Line of incision

Cecum

Mesentery of
the appendix

Appendix

Figure 478

placed around the base of the appendix. A straight Kocher clamp is used to crush the appendix at its junction with the cecum. The clamp is moved a few millimeters distal, and the stump is tied with a single 2-0 delayed absorbable suture flush with the wall of the cecum (Fig. 479A). A pointed clamp is placed on the ligature at the base of the appendix, and a second Kocher clamp is placed across the appendix. The

wound edges are protected as the appendix is amputated. Contaminated instruments and the specimen are removed from the table; at the same time, traction is maintained on the cecum to facilitate treating the stump of the appendix with two separate iodine applications. The stump of the appendix is then inverted into the pursestring suture, which is pulled tightly and tied, and the suture is cut (Fig. 479B).

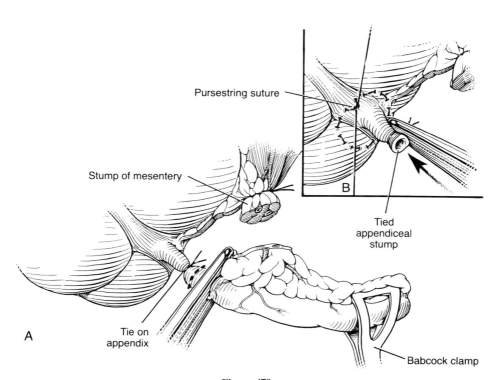

Figure 479

Small Intestine

Injury

Minor trauma to the small bowel is not infrequent in gynecologic surgery, especially in adhesive conditions such as pelvic inflammatory disease or endometriosis. It is especially common in patients who have had irradiation or patients undergoing operation for ovarian carcinoma. If the lumen of the intestine is entered, the site of injury is isolated to reduce contamination of the peritoneal cavity (Fig. 480*A*). The injury to the small intestine should be closed in a transverse manner with an inner row of 3-0 delayed absorbable suture and an outer inverting row of 3-0 silk suture (Fig. 480*B*). No drains would normally be used at the operative site.

Obstruction

In the procedure depicted, a stricture of the small bowel occurred after prior hysterectomy and radiation therapy. A wedge of mesentery is outlined well beyond the strictured area (Fig. 481).

Resection with End-to-End Anastomosis

The peritoneum is incised, and the vessels coursing through the mesentery are easily identified by lifting the mesentery and projecting a light from its posterior surface. The individual vessels are clamped, cut, and ligated with a single interrupted 2-0 delayed absorbable suture. Straight Kocher clamps with an angled rubber-shod clamp are placed across the bowel, which is divided between the clamps (Fig. 482); an appropriate cuff is left to enable the anastomosis to be accomplished. The everted edges of the bowel mucosa are wiped with iodoform solution before the end-to-end anastomosis is performed.

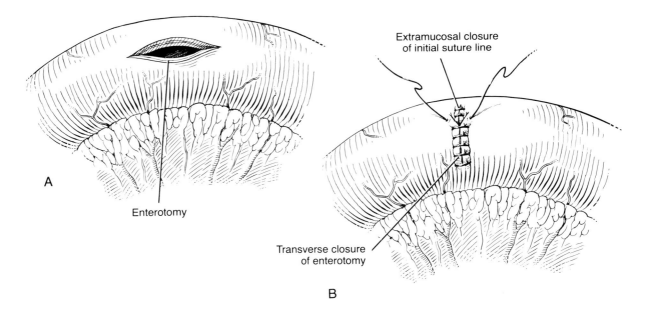

A — Enterotomy

B — Extramucosal closure of initial suture line — Transverse closure of enterotomy

Figure 480

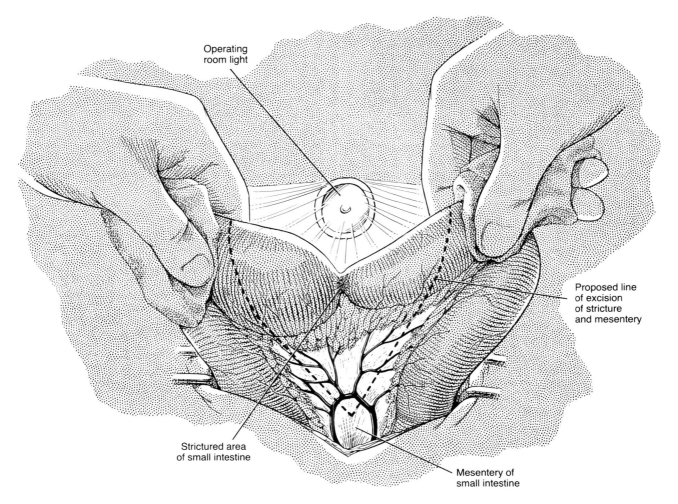

Operating
room light

Proposed line
of excision
of stricture
and mesentery

Strictured area
of small intestine

Mesentery of
small intestine

Figure 481

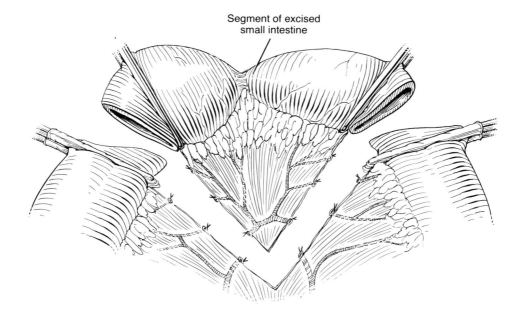

Segment of excised
small intestine

Figure 482

Silk sutures (3-0) are placed in the mesenteric and the antemesenteric ends of the bowel and represent the corners of the anastomosis. As the bowel is held together by the clamps, the edges are everted to expose the serosal surface, in which interrupted seromuscular sutures (3-0 silk) are placed; this area will be the posterior wall (Fig. 483A). The inner layer of 3-0 delayed absorbable sutures is placed as described for small bowel anastomosis (Fig. 483B and C), after which the outer row of interrupted silk sutures is placed (Fig. 483D). The mesentery is closed with a running 3-0 delayed absorbable suture (Fig. 483E), and care is taken not to injure any of the vessels within the mesentery. The adequacy of the lumen of the bowel at the point of the anastomosis can be tested with the thumb and index finger. The bowel is replaced into the abdomen in its usual position, the abdomen is irrigated, and the incision is closed in the customary fashion.

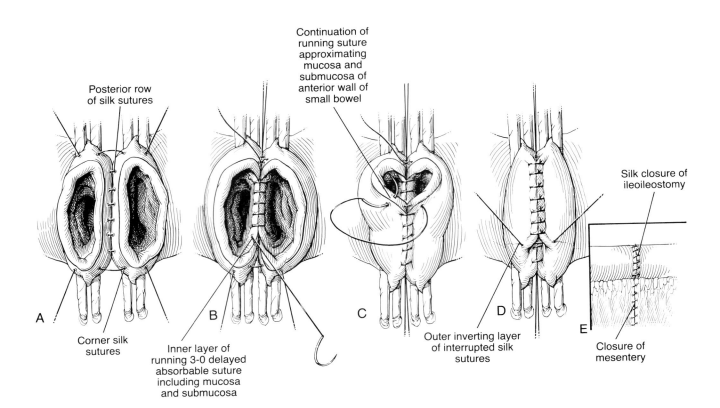

Figure 483

Bypass Procedure with Side-to-Side Anastomosis

Occasionally, the adhesive mass of obstructed small intestine is such that it is appropriate to leave it undisturbed and bypass the area with a side-to-side anastomosis. In Figure 484A, the midileum is anas-

tomosed to the ascending colon with this type of anastomosis. It is constructed in the same fashion as previously described; an inner suture line approximates the mucosa and submucosa with a running 3-0 delayed absorbable suture (Fig. 484A) and an outer seromuscular layer of interrupted 3-0 silk sutures (Fig. 484B).

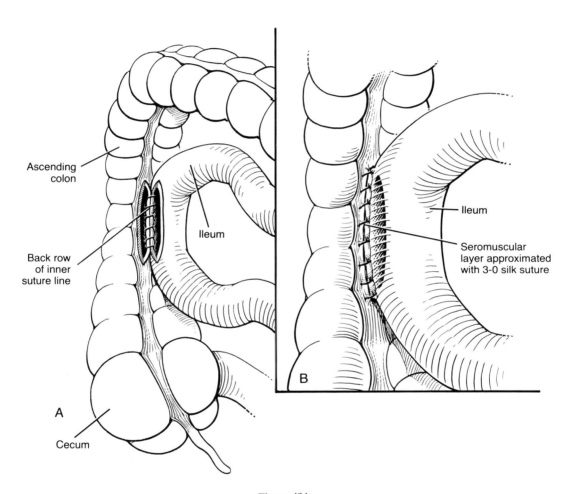

Figure 484

Large Intestine

Injury

During a difficult dissection or if recurrent tumor is suspected, a lesion may be excised and the colon purposely or accidentally opened (Fig. 485A). The colotomy may be simply closed with a running 3-0 delayed absorbable suture approximating the mucosa and submucosa; this suture line is inverted with a second layer of interrupted 3-0 silk sutures, with each lateral suture placed distal to the lateral margins of the original suture line (Fig. 485B). The pelvis should be appropriately irrigated, and the operative site is drained depending on the individual circumstance.

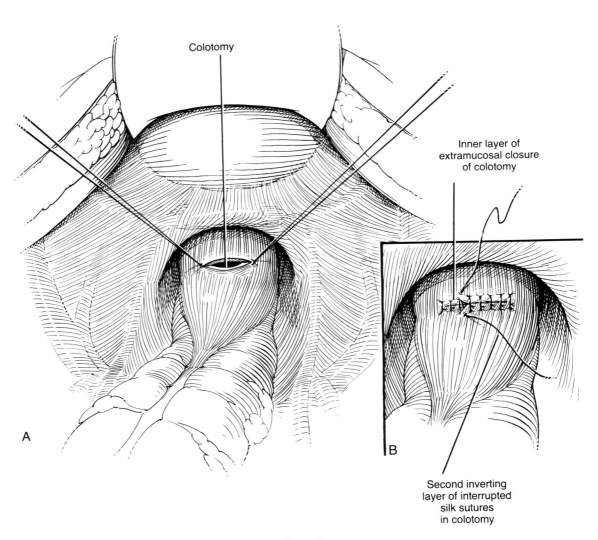

Colotomy

Inner layer of extramucosal closure of colotomy

Second inverting layer of interrupted silk sutures in colotomy

A

B

Figure 485

Right Hemicolectomy for Volvulus of Cecum

Conditions requiring resection of the right colon are usually treated by removal of the terminal ileum, cecum and ascending colon, hepatic flexure, and proximal portion of the transverse colon. Intestinal continuity is reestablished by performing an ileotransverse colostomy. The advantages of complete resection are that (1) the excellent blood supply to the terminal ileum ensures integrity of the anastomotic

suture line, (2) the ascending colon is incompletely covered with peritoneum and therefore is less suitable for anastomosis, and (3) an ileotransverse colostomy may be technically easier to perform than an ileoascending colostomy.

The right hemicolectomy depicted is for volvulus of the cecum that developed after a gynecologic operation. After preparation and draping, a midline incision is made with the patient in the Trendelenburg position (Fig. 486A). After appropriate abdominal

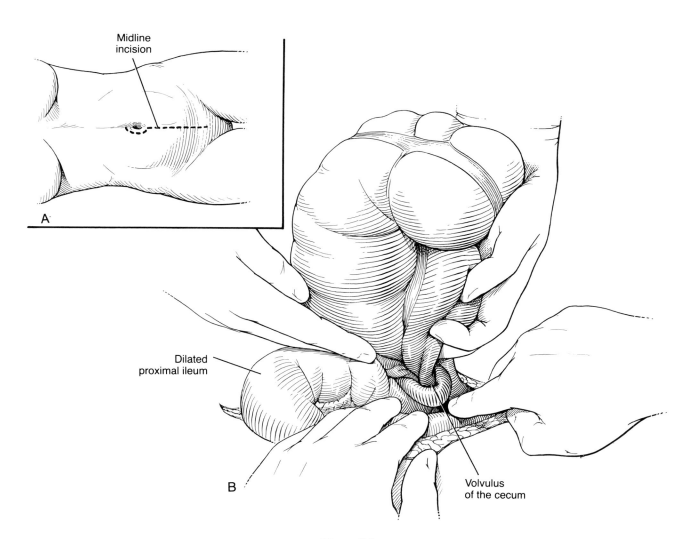

Figure 486

exploration, traction is applied on the right colon toward the midline (Fig. 486*B*); an incision is made through the lateral peritoneal attachment along the right lateral margin of the cecum and ascending colon (Fig. 487). The cecum and ascending colon are then further rotated medially, and with blunt dissection the retroperitoneal fat and lymphatics are freed from the bowel. Care should be taken to avoid injury to the right kidney and ureter and underlying ovarian vessels. The lateral peritoneal attachments of the hepatic flexure are incised to mobilize the flexure inferiorly and medially. Again, care must be taken that the underlying duodenum and kidney are avoided during this portion of the dissection. After full mo-

bilization of the cecum and ascending colon and hepatic flexure, the terminal ileum is located, and traction is applied so that the vessels in the mesentery can be identified. The mesentery and its vessels are divided and ligated with 3-0 delayed absorbable suture (Fig. 488*A*). The ileum is transected between a rubber-shod clamp and a crushing clamp (Fig. 488*B*). The transverse colon is divided between a crushing clamp on the proximal portion and a rubber-shod clamp on the distal portion (Fig. 488*C*). The point of transection is carefully selected to ensure that the blood supply is adequate to the cut end that is to remain. The cut ends of intestine are cleaned with iodine applications. A primary end-to-end anasto-

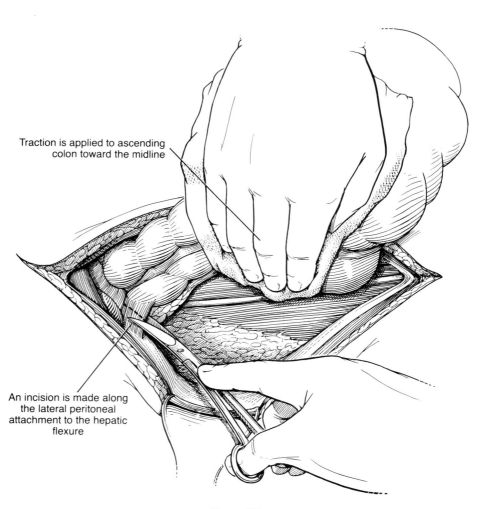

Traction is applied to ascending colon toward the midline

An incision is made along the lateral peritoneal attachment to the hepatic flexure

Figure 487

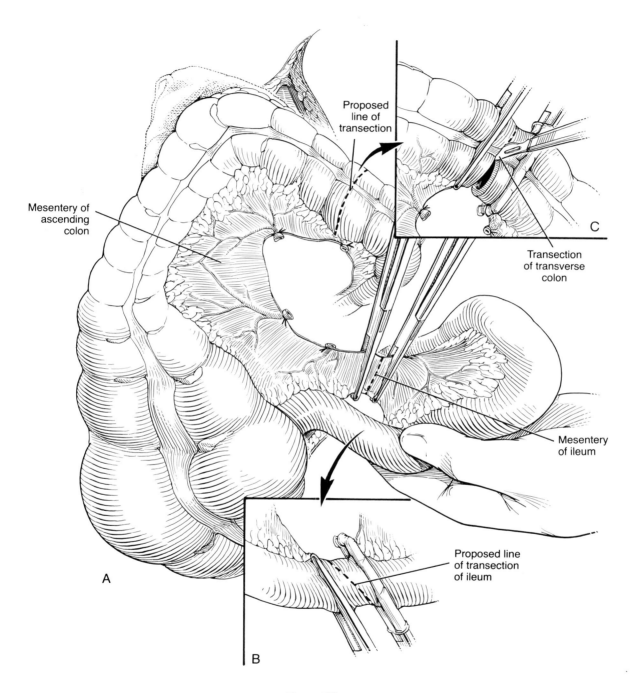

Mesentery of
ascending
colon

Proposed
line of
transection

Transection
of transverse
colon

Mesentery
of ileum

A

B

Proposed line
of transection
of ileum

C

Figure 488

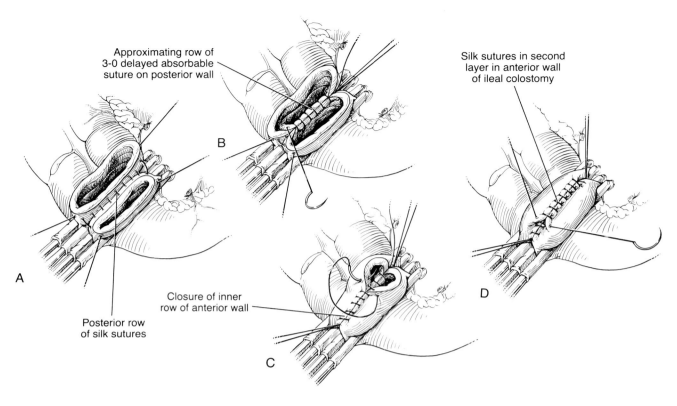

Approximating row of
3-0 delayed absorbable
suture on posterior wall

Silk sutures in second
layer in anterior wall
of ileal colostomy

Posterior row
of silk sutures

Closure of inner
row of anterior wall

Figure 489

mosis is done with an inner layer of 3-0 delayed absorbable sutures and an outer layer of interrupted 3-0 silk sutures; the mesentery is closed with a running 3-0 delayed absorbable suture (Fig. 489).

Loop Transverse Colostomy

A loop transverse colostomy is indicated if the colonic contents are to be diverted. Appropriate in various circumstances, its placement is determined primarily by the site of obstruction, perforation, or the area to be protected.

Through an appropriate incision placed directly over the transverse colon (Fig. 490A), a portion of the colon is identified and pulled anteriorly through the abdominal wall (Fig. 490B). A scissors is introduced through an avascular space in the mesocolon immediately adjacent to the bowel to permit the passage of a bridge, which is sutured into position on the skin. The fascial edges of the incision are closed with 2-0 delayed absorbable suture until they approximate the serosa of the bowel. The colostomy can be opened promptly or in the next 24 hours by a cautery incision along the taenia (Fig. 491).

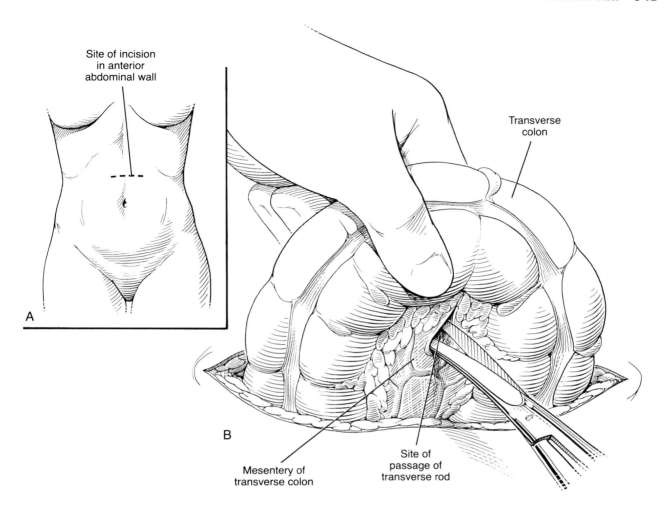

Site of incision
in anterior
abdominal wall

Transverse
colon

A

B

Mesentery of
transverse colon

Site of
passage of
transverse rod

Figure 490

Taenia
of colon

Cautery
opening taenia

Distal
colotomy

Proximal
colotomy

Rod fixed
to skin

A

B

Figure 491

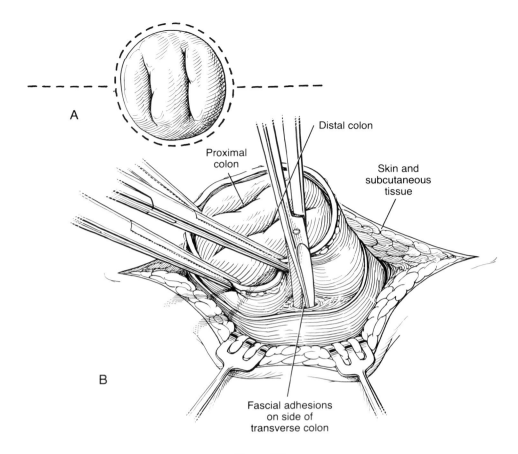

Figure 492

Closure of the colostomy is usually done in a transverse fashion such that the colon is not narrowed. An elliptic incision is made around the colostomy (Fig. 492*A*). Straight Kocher clamps are placed along the incised peristomal skin edges bilaterally and held on traction by the surgeon as small rakes are positioned along the outside wound edges to provide countertraction and exposure (Fig. 492*B*). The skin and subcutaneous tissues are dissected down and freed from the fascia circumferentially. The fascia and peritoneum are separated from the serosa, and any fibrous adhesions surrounding the extruded colon are excised. Once the colon is completely mobilized, the thin collar of skin and subcutaneous tissue about the stoma are sharply excised with scissors. The anterior half of the colon is then closed with a running 3-0 delayed absorbable mucosal and submucosal suture; this is inverted with a second layer of interrupted 3-0 silk sutures, approximating the adjacent seromuscular layers (Fig. 493).

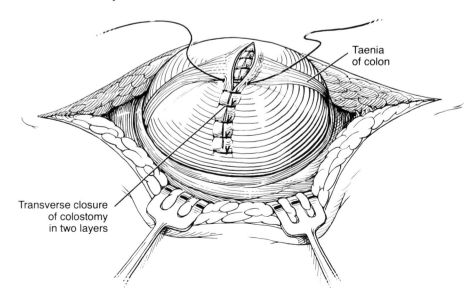

Figure 493

The colostomy is replaced in the abdominal cavity, and the abdominal wound is closed in the customary fashion. A small suction catheter can be placed on the fascia and brought out through a stab wound inferior to the incision, and the skin is closed with running subcuticular suture.

Sigmoidovaginal Fistula: Sigmoid Resection with Sigmoidorectostomy

Fistulas between the sigmoid colon and the vagina occur infrequently, but the overwhelming majority result from diverticulitis of the sigmoid colon in a patient who has previously had a hysterectomy. Generally, the sequence of events consists of the patient experiencing repeated bouts of acute diverticulitis that finally result in perforation of a diverticulum and abscess formation with a fistulous tract communicating to the vagina. Passage of fecal material or gas through the vagina in the absence of a rectal communication should lead one to suspect a fistula arising from the sigmoid colon or small intestine. A proctoscopic examination should be done, although it is often impossible to visualize the fistulous orifice because of narrowing or fixation resulting from the inflammatory condition. Surgical intervention is indicated for a sigmoidovaginal fistula that is large enough to permit the passage of fecal material. In a few selected patients, a colostomy may be the only treatment, or the fistula may be divided and the sigmoidal defect closed with or without a temporary colostomy. In the overwhelming majority of patients, we prefer a sigmoid resection with primary anastomosis and closure of the opening into the vagina. The need for a temporary protective colostomy is determined on an individual basis.

Primary Anastomosis

Through a lower midline incision with the patient in a steep Trendelenburg position, the small bowel is packed out of the pelvis to provide excellent exposure. The surgeon can identify the multiple diverticula of the sigmoid colon with a fixed, inflammatory mass involving the back of the bladder and the top of the vagina (Fig. 494). With strong traction on the sigmoid colon in a cephalad and anterior direction, the peritoneum along the base of the mesosigmoid is incised.

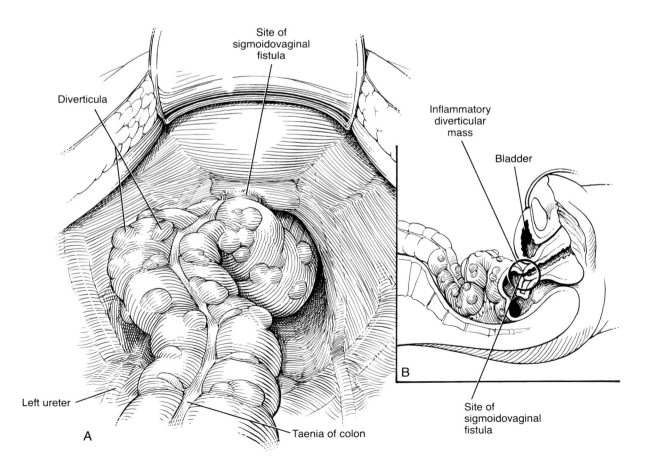

Figure 494

With appropriate traction and lifting of the rectosigmoid with a scissors, the surgeon assists the air dissection to develop the natural plane posterior to the sigmoid colon and rectum and yet anterior to the presacral venous plexus (Fig. 495A). With similar traction, the surgeon pulls the rectosigmoid to the patient's right side in a cephalad direction and incises along the white line (Toldt's white line), sweeping the lateral peritoneal attachments off the left side of the sigmoid colon and rectum as the ipsilateral ureter is visualized. This approach effectively frees the sigmoid colon and upper rectum laterally and posteriorly and provides additional mobility. With a wide Deaver retractor applying traction to the back of the bladder, the surgeon, with a gauze-lined left hand, applies countertraction (toward the patient's head) on the sigmoid colon to facilitate sharp dissection of the anterior wall of the sigmoid colon from the back of the bladder and the top of the vagina, transecting the sigmoidovaginal fistula (Fig. 495B). Traction is placed on the top of the vagina, and the vagina is pulled toward the patient's feet; the surgeon applies countertraction on the sigmoid colon toward the patient's head, and the sigmoid colon can be freed further from the top and back of the vagina. Thus, mobility of the rectum is gained and anastomosis is facilitated. Once the rectosigmoid is freed from the back of the vagina, the surgeon may want to slide the right hand down behind the rectum over the presacral veins, using finger dissection bilaterally to lift the rectum further out of the hollow of the sacrum and gain additional mobility.

With the rectum mobilized circumferentially, maximal mobility is obtained. The appropriate blood supply within the sigmoid colon is clamped, cut, and tied with 0 delayed absorbable sutures. At this point, both the distal and the proximal bowel have been carefully cleaned and prepared for subsequent anastomosis. A curved rubber-shod clamp is placed across the rectum 2 cm below the site of the proposed resection; a Pemberton right-angled clamp is placed proximal to the rubber-shod clamp (Fig. 496A). The transection is done with a right-angled scalpel flush with the Pemberton clamp. The Pemberton clamp is then rotated in a cephalad direction. The surgeon then places a second rubber-shod clamp and then a right-angled Pemberton clamp distal to the rubber-shod clamp at the previously cleaned proximal sigmoid colon. The surgeon uses a scalpel to transect the colon between the right-angled Pemberton clamp and the rubber-shod clamp as the second assistant hands the specimen off the table.

The lumina of the bowel are cleaned with an iodoform solution (Fig. 496B). The anastomosis is done as already described, with initial placement of the posterior row of interrupted 3-0 silk sutures. The mucosa and submucosa are closed with a continuous running 3-0 delayed absorbable suture placed such that it provides perfect mucosal approximation. The outer anterior row of interrupted 3-0 silk sutures is then placed. Generally, after the anastomosis has been completed (in this case it was closed before), the previous fistula site in the vagina is carefully resected,

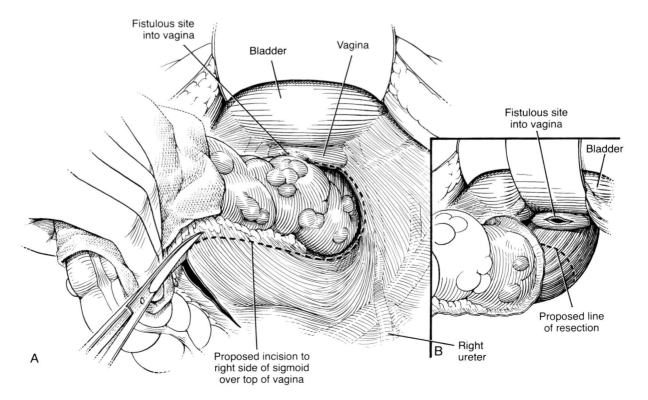

Figure 495

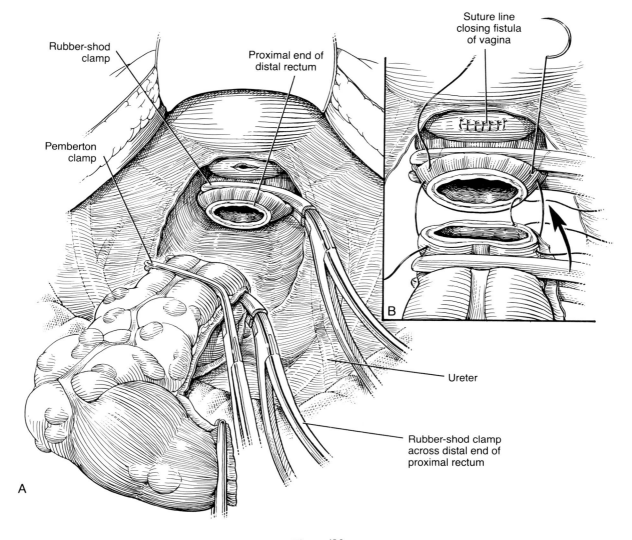

Figure 496

and the vagina is closed with two rows of 3-0 delayed absorbable suture (Fig. 497). The peritoneum from the back of the bladder may be pulled over the suture in the vagina and fixed with 2-0 delayed absorbable sutures. The pelvis is irrigated and drained with two large Jackson-Pratt drains (close to but not touching the anastomosis) brought out through stab wounds lateral to the midline incision. The need for a temporary protective loop colostomy (to protect the anastomosis) is determined on an individual basis.

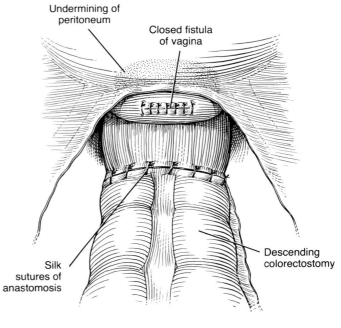

Figure 497

Hartmann Procedure

Under some circumstances, the infected, inflammatory process is such that the sigmoid mass may be excised, but a primary anastomosis is ill advised. It may be more appropriate to excise the diseased colon, close the fistula in the vagina, and oversew the proximal end of the distal rectal stump. This procedure is accomplished with an inner layer of running 3-0 delayed absorbable suture inverted with a second layer of interrupted 3-0 silk sutures. The tails on the tied silk sutures are left long to facilitate later identification of the rectal stump during reoperation (Fig. 498). The distal end of the descending colon is brought out as a colostomy, which is matured at that time. Later, usually after 2 to 3 months, reoperation can be done through the previous incision. The long ends of the silk ties facilitate identification of the proximal end of the distal rectal stump, which may be difficult to identify otherwise. Placement of a gauze pack in the vagina with a large rectal tube in the anal stump may also help to identify these structures. Once identified, the descending colon is freed from the splenic flexure in a sufficient fashion to permit the primary descending colorectostomy in a noninfected field as a closing step in this two-stage procedure.

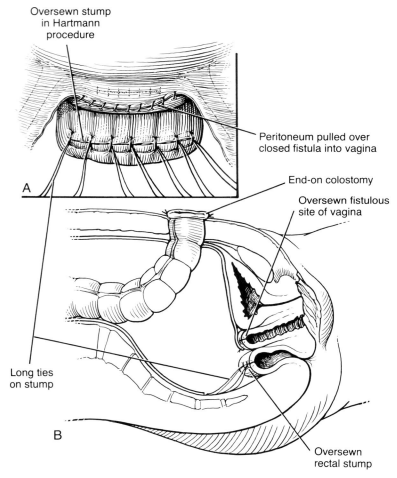

Figure 498

Index

Note: Numbers in *italic* refer to illustrations.